To Bill Sirons,

with very best wishes

from

Fred M

Mick Wright.

September 1997

The Gut as a Model in Cell and Molecular Biology

FALK SYMPOSIUM 94

The Gut as a Model in Cell and Molecular Biology

EDITED BY

F. Halter
Abteilung für Gastroenterologie
Department Innere Medizin
Universitat Bern
Inselspital
Bern
Switzerland

D. Winton
CRC Human Cancer
Genetics Research Group
Addenbrooke's Hospital
Cambridge UK

N.A. Wright
Department of Histopathology
Royal Postgraduate Medical School
London
UK

Proceedings of the Falk Symposium No. 94 (Part III of the Gastroenterology Symposia 1996) held in Freiburg-im-Breisgau, Germany, October 25–26, 1996

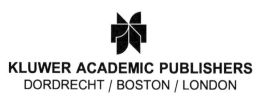

KLUWER ACADEMIC PUBLISHERS
DORDRECHT / BOSTON / LONDON

Distributors

for the United States and Canada: Kluwer Academic Publishers, PO Box 358, Accord Station, Hingham, MA 02018-0358, USA

for all other countries: Kluwer Academic Publishers Group, Distribution Center, PO Box 322, 3300 AH Dordrecht, The Netherlands

A catalogue record for this book is available from the British Library

ISBN 0-7923-8726-0

Published in the United Kingdom by Kluwer Academic Publishers, PO Box 55, Lancaster, UK.

Kluwer Academic Publishers BV incorporates the publishing programmes of D. Reidel, Martinus Nijhoff, Dr W. Junk and MTP Press.

Typeset by Speedlith Photo Litho Ltd., Stretford, Manchester, UK
Printed and bound in Great Britain by Hartnolls Ltd., Bodmin, Cornwall.

Contents

SECTION III: EPITHELIAL MESEMCHYMAL INTERACTIONS

CONTENTS

List of Principal Contributors

J.-F. Beaulieu
Departmente d'anatomie et de biologie
  cellulaire
Faculté de médicine
Université de Sherbrooke
Sherbrooke, QUE J1H 5N4
Canada

M. Bjerknes
Department of Anatomy and Cell Biology
Medical Sciences Building
University of Toronto
Toronto, ONT M5S 1A8
Canada

R.J. Coffey
Gastrointestinal Division
Department of Medicine
Vanderbilt University
C2104 Medical Center North
Nashville, TN 37232-2279
USA

J.R. Dorin
MRC Human Genetics Unit
Western General Hospital
Crewe Road
Edinburgh EH4 2XU
UK

J.G. Forte
Department of Molecular and Cell Biology
241 LSA University of California
Berkeley, CA 94720-3200
USA

J. Gum, Jr
Gastrointestinal Research Laboratory
University of California VA Medical Center
4150 Clement Street (151M2)
San Francisco, CA 91421-1598
USA

F. Halter
Abteilung für Gastroenterologie
Department Innere Medizin
Universität Bern
Inselspital
CH-3010 Bern
Switzerland

S.J. Henning
Department of Pediatrics
Baylor College of Medicine
One Baylor Plaza
Houston, TX 77030-3498
USA

M. Kedinger
Unité de Recherche de Physiopathologie
  Digestive
INSERM - U 381
3, Ave. Molière
F-67200 Strasbourg
France

I.M. Modlin
Department of Surgery
Yale University School of Medicine
New Haven, CT 06520-8062
USA

A.J. Ouellette
Department of Medicine
Harvard Medical School and
  Gastrointestinal Unit
Medical Services
Massachusetts General Hospital
Fruit Street
Boston, MA 02114
USA

C. Paraskeva
CRC Colorectal Tumour Biology
   Research Group
Department of Pathology and Microbiology
University of Bristol
University Walk
Bristol BS8 1TD
UK

G. Perozzi
Istituto Nazionale della Nutrizione
Via Ardeatina 564
I-00178 Roma
Italy

M. Pignatelli
Cell Adhesion Laboratory
Department of Pathology
Royal Postgraduate Medical School
Du Cane Road
London W12 0NN
UK

P. Poulsom
Histopathology Unit
Imperial Cancer Research Fund
   Laboratories
44 Lincoln's Inn Fields
London WC2A 3PX
UK

J-C Reubi
Institute of Pathology
Department of Cell Biology and
   Experimental Cancer Research
University of Berne
CH-3010 Berne
Switzerland

D.C. Rubin
Washington University
School of Medicine
PO Box 8124
660 S Euclid Avenue
St. Louis, MO 63110
USA

T.C. Savidge
Department of Cellular Physiology
The Babraham Institute
Babraham Hall
Cambridge CB2 4AT
UK

E. Sterchi
Institut für Biochemie und
   Molekularbiologie
Bühlstr. 28
C H-3012 Bern
Switzerland

P.G. Traber
Department of Internal Medicine
Division of Gastroenterology
University of Pennsylvania
600 Clinical Research Building
415 Curie Boulevard
Philadelphia, PA 19104-6144
USA

J.T. Troelsen
Department of Medicine, Biochemistry
   and Genetics
Panum Institute
University of Copenhagen
Blegdamsveg 3
DK-2200 Copenhagen N
Denmark

M.M. Weiser
Gastroenterology Section
Department of Medicine
Buffalo General Hospital
Bldg E3, 10 High Street
Buffalo, NY 14203-1154
USA

R.H. Whitehead
Ludwig Institute for Cancer Research
Tumor Biology Branch
PO Royal Melbourne Hospital
Victoria 3050
Australia

E.D. Williams
Department of Pathology
University of Cambridge
Addenbrooke's Hospital
Box 235, Hills Road
Cambridge CB2 2QQ
UK

D.J. Winton
CRC Human Cancer Genetics Research
   Group
Level 3 Lab. Block
Addenbrooke's Hospital
Box 238, Hills Road
Cambridge CB2 2QQ
UK

LIST OF PRINCIPAL CONTRIBUTORS

N.A. Wright
Department of Histopathology
Royal Postgraduate Medical School
Du Cane Road
London W12 0NN
UK

Preface

It was the concept of the organisers of Falk Symposium No. 94 to propose the gut as an appropriate model for investigating general problems in differentiation, growth control, stem cell biology, epithelial regeneration and adaptive responses. We attempted to define the objectives of the next five to ten years by bringing together both basic scientists and clinicians whose research is focused on gut biology, with a view to identifying areas which are currently being utilized and need to be further exploited, such as transgenic and knockout approaches, retrovirus delivery systems and model cell/tissue systems.

The main themes of the meeting were gastrointestinal development and differentiation, gut stem cell biology and the control of gut growth in normal and abnormal situations. Throughout the meeting much emphasis was placed on relating the more basic studies to the clinic. A session with excellent posters clearly demonstrated the great interest this symposium found amongst young cell and molecular biologists interested in the gut and gastroenterologists with their more clinical outlook. It is hoped that this symposium on gut biology will be the first of similar future and successful meetings.

The Editors

Section I
Stem cells

1
Intestinal stem cells and clonality

D. J. WINTON

INTRODUCTION

In the bottom part of each small intestinal crypt there appears to be a region of stability where cells are not obliged to undergo upward migration. It is clear that proliferating cells within this region will supply cells to undergo amplification and differentiation to fulfil the future needs of the epithelium in terms of cellularity and integrated function[1-3]. The property of maintaining future needs is a function of stem cells. We know little about the properties of the putative stem cells, including the extent to which there is heterogeneity between individual proliferative stem cells in their degree of commitment to particular lineages, the size of the territories which their progeny occupy and how these territories relate to the anatomy of the epithelium.

One problem in investigating stem cell biology is that their presence can only be inferred retrospectively by virtue of their ability to produce a number of cells over time. Consequently, it would seem that a useful tool in determining their properties would be to induce expression of a cell autonomous marker in an individual stem cell which is inherited by its daughters on division. In this way, all the surviving progeny of a single cell would be identified as a coherent cellular clone, the fate of which should reflect the fate of the original marked stem cell.

The methods used to mark clones of cells in this way have been described previously[4,5] and depend on mutation of polymorphic genetic loci which cause loss of a visually detectable gene product. In mouse intestinal studies only two genetic loci have been used in marking studies i.e. G6PD and *Dlb-1*. (Studies arising from the former are described in Chapter 2). *Dlb-1* determines a lectin binding polymorphism (for *Dolichos biflorus* agglutinin (DBA)) which has been described extensively elsewhere[6,7]. In essence, the marking assay depends on detecting clonal loss of lectin binding (using a peroxidase conjugate of DBA) by mutation affecting a single allele determining expression of the lectin binding site in intestinal epithelium. This chapter will summarize the important findings made in these studies and discuss the limitations of the approach.

3

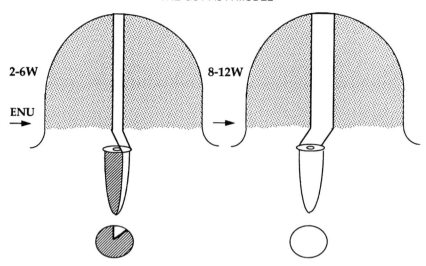

Figure 1 Schematic demonstrating clonal marking in small intestine. Mutation of a single allele determining a visualizable gene product results in the formation of mutant clones which are recognized by the appropriate histochemical method. Clones can be analysed in tissue sections or in wholemount preparations either on the villus epithelium or within intestinal crypts. Clones can be analysed with time following a mutagenic stimulus during which the territory occupied by the clone may change. Alternatively, spontaneously occurring clones can be analysed during life

MONOCLONALITY OF CRYPTS

The concept of marking a proliferative cell and inferring its fate from the resultant clone seems simple (Figure 1). However, the problem is when, following muta-genesis, to begin a clonal analysis and when to finish it. From the initial per-spective, the manner in which the clonal pattern corresponds to the anatomy of the intestine, and in particular to the crypt, is important. This is because the population of an anatomically defined structure like the crypt appears to represent a likely maximum limit on a cell's clonal expansion. Further, reaching this maxi-mum limit implies heterogeneity in the fate of the population of 4–16 stem cells postulated from kinetic studies[8]. This would then be consistent with the picture of stem cell organization in the haemopoietic system of long-lived stem cells and shorter-lived committed progenitor cells which serves as the stem cell paradigm.

Two categories of experiment indicate that crypts are clonal in origin. First is the spontaneous accumulation of wholly mutant crypts (in which the entire crypt epithelium is populated by the mutant epithelium) in untreated mice with time, and the second their induction following mutagen treatment (Figure 2). Mutant

Figure 2 (Opposite) Quantitation of clones mutated at *Dlb-1* in intestinal wholemounts of *Dlb-1*[h]/*Dlb-1*[a] heterozygous mice. Clones are recognized by their inability to bind a lectin-peroxidase conjugate which is determined by a *Dlb-1*[h] allele in these mice. (a) In untreated mice there is an accumulation of crypts entirely populated by the mutant epithelium (solid line) while partially populated crypts remain at a constant frequency (dashed line). (b) Following mutation with *N*-nitroso-*N*-ethylurea (50 mg/kg) both types are induced but partially populated crypts return to background levels while wholly populated ones persist. Note the long time periods over which mutant clones appear following mutagenesis

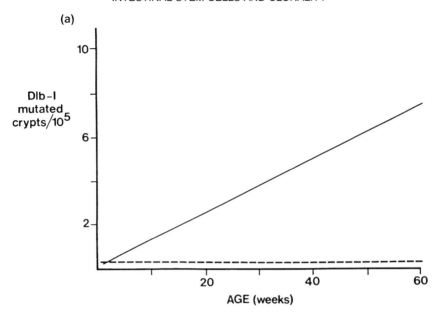

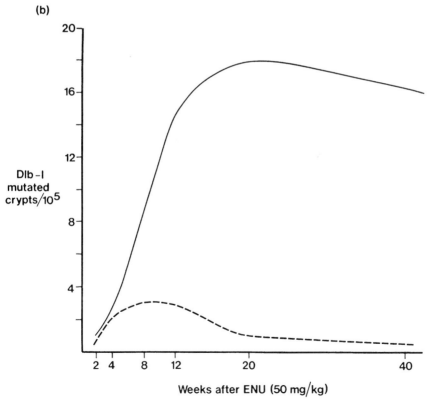

crypts can be identified either in tissue sections or in appropriately pre-pared wholemount preparations. A striking feature of the mutation experiments is the long time period over which their numbers increase in frequency (around 12 weeks). The immediate implication of these observations is that the crypt is derived from the progeny of a single pluripotential stem cell. Subsequent work on both small and large intestine has concentrated on trying to determine the mechanism in terms of the sequence of cellular replacement by which crypts become mono-clonal. However, the nature of these experiments requires that one variable is the choice and dose of the genotoxic chemical administered and another the latent period prior to analysis. Both of these variables can influence the observations made and their interpretation.

TIME AND TOXICITY

The identification of small intestinal crypts as a 'clonal unit' is made many weeks after mutagenesis. It is self-evident that the population of the crypt by the progeny of a single cell cannot proceed to completion instantly. The question then arises of whether, prior to the appearance of monoclonal crypts, a smaller 'clonal unit' can be identified (Figure 1). In intestinal wholemounts stained for *Dlb-1* mutants, intermediate forms containing both mutant and non-mutant epithelium can be identified. The frequency of these remains low relative to the number of mono-clonal crypts (Figure 2b). There are different interpretations of this, including a rapid resolving time for intermediates[9] or that there is a high detection threshold in identifying partially mutant crypts in wholemounts which would underestimate their numbers[10].

An alternative method of analysis involves measuring the width of mutant clones on intestinal villi after they have been exported from the crypt (Figure 3). The width of mutant clones some 12 weeks after mutagenesis correlates to the average crypt output (85% of crypts are monoclonal at this time). Consequently, at earlier times the width of mutant clones can be compared with this end-point or indeed with the estimated width as determined by calculations of crypt cell output (Table 1). At 12 weeks after administration of mutagen *N*-nitroso-*N*-ethylurea (NEU; 50 mg/kg) the average clone width is 7 cells across, while at 10 days (selected arbitrarily) it is two cells across (29% in output compared with that seen at 12 weeks). Comparison with published estimates of the number of cells produced per crypt indicates that the number of mutant cells present in an intestinal villus is equal to roughly 20–25% of crypt output[11]. Both of these results suggest that crypt output is maintained by around 3–5 stem cells surviving from the time of mutagenesis. Clearly this implies a clonal unit smaller than an entire crypt. Measurements at earlier times may detect small clones and thereby a larger number of stem cells per crypt. The 10 day time is selected as representing twice the transit time of cells to migrate from the lower crypt to the villus tip.

Apoptotic cell death following treatment with the same doses and chemicals as used in cell marking studies has been demonstrated[12,13]. Further, it is apparent that the toxicity associated with increasing doses of mutagen can affect clone measurement, as shown in Table 2 for *Dlb-1* mutant clone widths following i.p. administration of the direct acting genotoxin, methyl-*N*-nitro-*N*-nitrosoguanidine

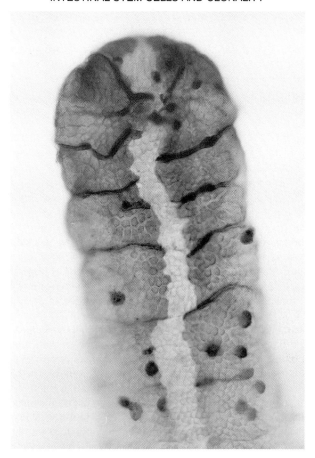

Figure 3 Photomicrograph of a jejunal villus containing a *Dlb-1* mutant clone. The villus has been dissected from an intestinal wholemount stained with a peroxidase conjugate of *Dolichos biflorus* agglutinin to allow recognition of the mutant clones. Measurements of the width at different times following NEU treatment allow estimates of the number of 'clonal units' (or number of stem cells surviving from the time of mutagenesis) per crypt to be estimated

Table 1 Calculation of the percentage of crypt output contributed by *Dlb-1* mutant stem cells at 10 days after NEU mutagenesis

	Position in small intestine	
Small intestinal parameters[a]	25%	50%
Villus row count	75	55
Total cells/clone[b]	150	110
Villus 'transit' time (h)	37	45
Cells/clones/24 h	97	59
Crypt cell production rate/24 h	394	278
% crypt output	25%	21%

[a]From Ref. 11.
[b]The average clone is two cells across at 10 days post-NEU treatment (50 mg/kg)

7

Table 2 Effect of dose of *N*-methyl-*N*-nitro-*N*-nitrosoguanidine on clone width

Dose (mg/kg)	No. observed	Clone width	
		Median range	*Mean (SE)*
10	45	4–4.9	5.4 (0.5)
25	72	5–5.9	5.4 (0.3)
50	50	5–5.9	5.9 (0.3)
100	50	6–6.9	7.5 (0.4)

*Arbitrary units

(MNNG). Clearly this suggests that some of the cells acting as targets in the assay are ablated and, therefore, calculations of the kinetics of clonal growth are affected. One implication, based on evidence of recruitment of non-stem cells back into the stem cell compartment after extensive cell death[14], is that a proportion of clones measured may arise from cells that were not stem cells at the time of mutagenesis. The more obvious consequence is, however, that replacement of ablated stem cells probably requires recruitment of both daughters of a proportion of dividing stem cells to the stem cell population, resulting in clone width measurements which overestimate the contribution of an individual stem cell.

The implications of the above for the design of clonal marking studies are far-reaching. In order to minimize toxicity effects a series of compromises need to be accommodated. First, the dose and agent administered must give a reasonable increment above background frequencies of mutant clones at both the start and the end of time courses. If the spontaneous mutation rate is relatively high, as for *Dlb-1* (one new mutant clone/10^5 crypts/month) and the time course is long (~12 months), then around 120 induced mutant clones would give a 10-fold increase for analysis. This requires a substantial mutational stimulus. On the other hand, a lower background may also reflect a lower event rate on chemical mutagenesis. Ideally, the consequences of dose should be determined in advance to establish whether there is an area of the dose–response curve in which a reasonable increment is achievable without a concomitant increase in clone size.

Finally, with regard to toxicity, the net effect may be to speed up the normal rates of clonal expansion in the early part of a time course. In this case later kinetic measurements, after a steady state has been re-established, reflect normal physiological events.

MECHANISM

In essence, three mechanisms of stem cell replacement have been proposed to explain the above observations or their counterpart in the colon[9,15,16]: (1) population of the crypt by an individual stem cell predestined to do so; (2) population by a single stem cell successful in stochastic competition with its neighbours, possibly with the imposition of a degree of ordering directed by a stem cell niche (see Chapter 2); (3) segregation of clones via crypt fission. Inevitably a combination of any of the three mechanisms could be proposed. The models can accommodate very different modes and rates of division: for example, a lower limit of once every 12 weeks (model 1) and an upper limit of once every 24 h (model 2).

It is not possible currently to distinguish unequivocably between these alternatives. One particular difficulty in distinguishing between models (1) and (2) above is that their quantitative predictions for stem cell replacements are probably the same[17]. Another problem is that the behaviour of the stem cell population may change due to toxic effects, e.g. by creating or increasing the degree of competitiveness. Some discrimination may be possible with a more idealized system in which a minimally cytotoxic but potent mutagen and/or a reporter gene with low background reversion rates but high susceptibility to induction of mutation should allow analysis with minimal perturbation. This may be best achieved where the genetic basis of the molecular event is known, allowing selection of a mutagen known to induce the appropriate lesion.

PROPERTIES OF INTESTINAL STEM CELLS

There is considerable speculation about the extent to which stem cells have unique properties which affect their susceptibility to mutation. This exists because of the difficulty in isolating epithelial stem cells and determining their properties directly. Dose-sparing effects in early irradiation mutagenesis experiments using the *Dlb-1* assay demonstrated that the stem cell targets are capable of repairing some damage when irradiation is administered at low dose rates[18]. Consequently, we became interested in the extent to which in vivo mutation assays can identify intrinsic properties of stem cells which predispose them to mutation and simultaneously discover the extent to which they are the same as or different to their proliferative descendants.

In respect of carcinogens requiring metabolic activation, we attempted to elucidate whether stem cells participated in localized activation and thereby effectively conspired in their own mutation. Pathways of activation are complex and we concentrated on the initial steps which are mediated by the cytochrome P450 family. Two heterocyclic aromatic hydrocarbons, 2-amino-3,8-dimethyl-imidazo[4,5f]quinoxaline (MeIQx) and 2-amino-1-methyl-6-phenylimidazo-[4,5b]pyrimidine (PhIP) are genotoxic and found in cooked food. The initial activation step is mediated by CYP1A2. Interestingly, MeIQx induces liver cancers in rodents and PhIP induces mainly extrahepatic tumours. MeIQx is not mutagenic in the *Dlb-1* assay and PhIP is (Table 3). Correlation with the pattern of CYP1A2 detected by immunocytochemistry using anti-peptide antibodies indicated that CYP1A2 is constitutively expressed in the liver and in a few sporadically distributed cells in villus epithelium in the proximal small intestine and is not induced by mutagen treatment. Proximal and distal small intestine show equal susceptibility to PhIP mutagenesis, so there is no correlation with the small number of CYP1A2-expressing cells in proximal intestine. This implies that the proximate metabolite of PhIP is systemically delivered, probably from the liver via the circulatory system, to the gut[19]. (Reactive metabolites of MeIQx are too unstable to be delivered in the same way.)

For another chemical, benzo[a]pyrene (B[a]P), the possible routes of activation are more complicated, but CYP1A1 is primarily implicated and is not consti-

Table 3 *Dlb-1* mutations after exposure to 2-amino-1-methyl-6-phenylimidazo[4,5-b]pyridine (PhIP) or benzo[a]pyrene (B[a]P)

Treatment	No. of doses[a]	No. of mice	total clones	Dlb-1 *mutation/* 10^5 *crypts*	SE
PhIP	2	4	49	12.9	2.0
	4	4	70	23.4	5.6
	6	5	202	48.4	8.7
	10	5	284	69.1	13.8
B[a]P	2	4	318	92.5	10.2
	4	5	812	206.4	33.5
	6	5	1564	358.3	41.5
Control	–	5	12	3.3	0.5

[a]Each dose of PhIP was 20 mg/kg and of B[a]P 40 mg/kg administered by i.p. injection

tutively expressed. B[a]P is a highly potent intestinal mutagen (Table 3) and after i.p. administration strongly induces CYP1A1 expression in the bottom of the crypt. Although other routes of activation including systemic delivery are equally possible, the results are consistent with localized mediation of the first step of B[a]P activation by the stem cells themselves. Identifying the contribution of other metabolizing systems and of Phase II detoxification mechanisms within the stem cell population remains a challenge for the future.

Another way of elucidating properties of intestinal stem cells comes from comparing the responsiveness of a genotoxic agent in normal animals and animals deficient in respect of DNA repair pathway or tumour suppressor gene function due to gene targeting. For example, *p53* deficient animals appear more susceptible to *Dlb-1* mutagenesis only at high doses of irradiation. This may imply that the role of *p53* in intestinal stem cells is only protective at high levels of damage.

SPATIAL ASPECTS OF DAMAGE AND REPAIR

A useful feature of the organization of the cells in the crypt is that their position defines the extent of progression along a differentiative/proliferative gradient. Another way of determining the properties of the cells occupying the stem cell region of the crypt (if not the actual stem cells themselves) would be to compare the properties of cells in a quantitative way along this gradient.

In order to assay DNA damage and repair along the vertical axis of the crypt we have devised an assay which detects DNA strand breaks in intact isolated crypts. The assay is a modified form of the single-cell gel electrophoresis or 'comet' assay[20,21]. The value of the assay is (1) that it measures a ubiquitous element of DNA repair allowing a diverse range of genetic lesions and agents to be detected; (2) the endpoint is quantitative and allows differences in the degree of responsiveness to be determined; (3) it retains the spatial relationship between cells. In the assay strand breaks can be generated directly or by manipulating DNA repair pathways, e.g. by inhibiting DNA polymerase[22].

In initial experiments we have determined that isolated crypts remain repair competent in respect of both UV and gamma irradiation. Clear spatial differences in responsiveness are found with low doses of hydrogen peroxide and with a

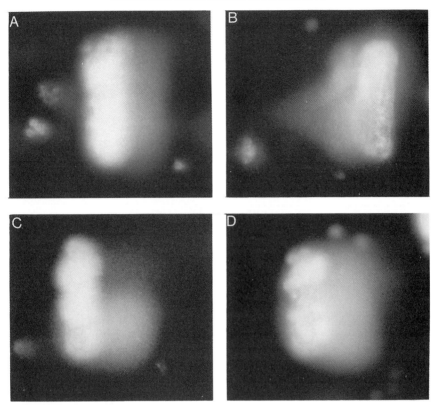

Figure 4 Crypt comet. Examples of the different spatial pattern of damage induced by different agents. (A) UV-C irradiation, (B) etoposide, (C) hydrogen peroxide, (D) gamma irradiation

topoisomerase II inhibitor, etoposide (Figure 4)[23]. The assay has the ability to detect differences between cells and in their subsequent repair response, which in the crypt may vary by position with their proliferative or differentiative status (Figure 5)[23]. In the future increased discrimination of the cells which are responding in the assay could be achieved using bromodeoxyuridine incorporation to detect migration only of labelled DNA.

Acknowledgements

DJW is supported by a programme grant from the Cancer Research Campaign [CRC].

References

1. Cheng H, Leblond CP. Origin, differentiation and renewal of the four main epithelial cell types in the mouse small intestine. I. Columnar cell. Am J Anat. 1974;141:461–80.

11

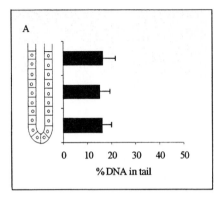
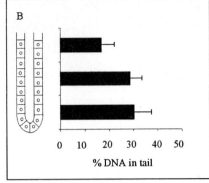
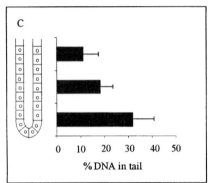
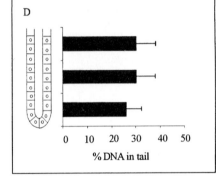

Figure 5 Schematic representation quantitatively showing responsiveness of stem cell, proliferative and maturation zones of the crypt to (A) UV-C irradiation, (B) etoposide, (C) hydrogen peroxide, (D) gamma irradiation

2. Cheng H, Leblond CP. Origin, differentiation and renewal of the four main epithelial cell types in the mouse small intestine. V. Unitarian theory of the origin of the four epithelial cell types. Am J Anat. 1974;141:537–62.
3. Bjerknes M, Cheng H. The stem cell zone of the small intestinal epithelium. III. Evidence from columnar, enteroendocrine and mucosa cells in the adult mouse. Am J Anat. 1981;160:77–91.
4. Winton DJ, Blount MA, Ponder BAJ. A clonal marker induced by mutation in mouse intestinal epithelium. Nature. 1988;333:463–6.
5. Griffiths DFR, Davis SJ, Williams D, Williams GT, Williams ED. Demonstration of somatic mutation and colonic crypt clonality by X-linked enzyme histochemistry. Nature. 1988;333:461–3.
6. Ponder BAJ, Festing MFW, Wilkinson MM. An allelic difference determines reciprocal patterns of expression of binding sites for *Dolichos biflorus* lectin in inbred strains of mice. J Embryol Exp Morphol. 1985;87:229–39.
7. Uiterdijk HG, Ponder BAJ, Festing MFW, Hilgers J, Skow L, Van Nie R. The gene controlling the binding site of *Dolichos biflorus* agglutinin, *Dlb-1*, is on chromosome 11 of the mouse. Genet Res Camb. 1986;47:125–9.
8. Potten CS, Loeffler M. A comprehensive model of the crypts of the small intestine of the mouse provides insight into the mechanisms of cell migration and the proliferation hierarchy. J Theor Biol. 1987;127:381–91.
9. Winton DJ, Ponder BAJ. Stem-cell organization in mouse small intestine. Proc R Soc Lond B. 1990;241:13–18.

10. Loeffler M, Birke A, Winton D, Potten C. Somatic mutation, monoclonality and stochastic models of stem cell organization in the intestinal crypt. J Theor Biol. 1993;160:471–91.

11. Wright NA, Irwin M. The kinetics of villus cell populations in the mouse small intestine. Cell Tissue Kinet. 1982;15:595–609.

12. Li YQ, Fan CY, O'Connor PJ, Winton DJ, Potten CS. Target cells for the cytotoxic effects of carcinogens in murine small bowel. Carcinogenesis. 1992;13:361–8.

13. Potten CS, Li YQ, O'Connor PJ, Winton DJ. A possible explanation for the differential cancer incidence in the intestine, based on distribution of the cytotoxic effects of carcinogens in the murine large bowel. Carcinogenesis. 1992;13:2305–12.

14. Potten CS, Loeffler M. Stem cells: attributes, cycles, spirals, pitfalls and uncertainties. Lessons for and from the crypt. Development. 1990;110:1001–20.

15. Williams ED, Lowes AP, Williams D, Williams GT. A stem cell niche theory of intestinal crypt maintenance based on a study of somatic mutation in colonic mucosa. Am J Pathol. 1992;141: 773–6.

16. Park HS, Goodlad RA, Wright NA. Crypt fission in the small intestine and colon – a mechanism for the emergence of G6PD locus mutated crypts after treatment with mutagens. Am J Pathol. 1995;147:1416–27.

17. Winton DJ. Mutation induced clonal markers from polymorphic loci: application to stem cell organisation in the mouse intestine. Semin Dev Biol. 1993;4:293–302.

18. Winton DJ, Peacock J, Ponder BAJ. Effect of gamma-radiation at high and low dose rate on a novel in vivo mutation assay in mouse intestine. Mutagenesis. 1989;4:404–6.

19. Brooks RA, Gooderham NJ, Zhao K et al. 2-Amino-1methyl-6-phenylimidazo[4,5-b]pyridine is a potent mutagen in mouse small intestine. Cancer Res. 1994;54:1665–71.

20. Ostling O, Johanson KJ. Microelectrophoretic study of radiation-induced DNA damages in individual mammalian cells. Biochem Biophys Res Commun. 1984;123:291–8.

21. Singh NP, McCoy MT, Tice RR, Schneider EL. A simple technique for the quantitation of low levels of DNA damage in individual cells. Exp Cell Res. 1988;175:184–91.

22. Gedik CM, Ewen SWB, Collins AR. Single-cell gel electrophoresis applied to the analysis of UV-C damage and its repair in human cells. Int J Radiat Biol. 1992;62:313–20.

23. Brooks RA, Winton DJ. Determination of spatial patterns of DNA damage and repair in intestinal crypts by multi-gel electrophoresis. J Cell Sci. 1996;109:2061–8.

2
The stem cell niche hypothesis, mutation and neoplasia

E. D. WILLIAMS

The mechanisms that maintain the structure of the intestinal mucosa are of considerable importance not only to our knowledge of the biology of stem cell tissues, but also to our understanding of the mechanisms leading to the development of malignancy. The structural unit in both small and large intestines, the crypt, is anatomically clearly defined, and known to form an escalator for cells passing from the base to the mucosal surface. Early observations using tritiated thymidine as a label demonstrated this cell movement, providing evidence that the stem cells were situated at or near the base of the crypt. Detailed kinetic and modelling studies suggested that there were multiple stem cells in each crypt – up to 16 in the small intestine, and up to three in the large intestine[1]. The existence of multiple stem cells was questioned when two separate studies, one in the small intestine and one in the large intestine, showed that all the cells in a crypt were derived from the same cell[2,3]. Both groups had recognized that a phenotypic change induced by a mutagen could be used to trace cell lineage; the small intestinal study used loss of lectin binding in heterozygous mice, the large intestinal study used loss of activity of the X linked enzyme glucose-6-phosphate dehydrogenase (G6PD). Further studies demonstrated a human polymorphism for O-acetylation of sialic acid, and showed that mutation in heterozygotes induced a phenotypic change due to loss of O-acetylation activity that affected all the cells in a colonic crypt, demonstrating that all the cells in a human crypt were also derived from one cell[4].

It was later realized that the concept of crypts maintained by multiple stem cells and yet maintained by the daughters of single stem cells could be combined in a concept of a crypt niche. In this proposal the crypt is maintained by a group of stem cells, the control of stem cell asymmetry of division is extrinsic rather than intrinsic, and the loss of a cell from the stem cell niche is random, or at least partly random[5]. It can easily be shown that this will fit the observed facts. In this proposal the crypt is maintained by multiple stem cells, defined by their ability to continue to divide indefinitely, but retaining this property only while situated within the site of the niche. The descendant of one stem will come to occupy the whole niche on a purely chance basis because of an element of randomicity in the loss of cells from the niche. After mutagen administration it is likely that only one stem cell in a niche will be mutated: this will give rise to crypts with a mixed phenotype, but with successive stem cell division the mixed phenotype crypts will reduce in number, giving rise to monophenotypic crypts, either normal or mutated. The evidence presented to support the crypt niche concept was based on the observation of mixed phenotype crypts after mutagen administration: as they declined in frequency the number of crypts showing only the mutated phenotype increased in frequency, stabilizing when the mixed phenotype crypts had effectively disappeared[5]. The finding that the time to this plateau was considerably longer in the small than the large intestine[5,6] would fit with the earlier observations that there are many more stem cells in the small intestinal crypt than the large. The crypt stabilization time was found to be 1 year or more in the human colon. This was deduced from studies of colons from patients who had received radiation 4 weeks to many years before colectomy, and quantifying whole and partially involved crypts with the mPAS technique[7].

A stem cell niche is, therefore, a pattern of organization that is compatible with the observed features of crypt replacement by a mutated phenotype. A crypt maintained by a single stem cell would be expected to show peaks of involvement of mutated phenotype crypts at different times after mutagen administration. The first would be at about the end of one stem cell cycle time, when cells with a mutated phenotype derived from a mutation in the immediate substem cell, or passed from the stem cell to its differentiating daughter cells, were beginning to be replaced by normal phenotype cells. A second would be expected at about the end of a second stem cell cycle, when cells derived from a stem cell daughter that had retained the mutation were completing the occupation of the whole of the crypt on a permanent basis.

None of the studies of the time course of the replacement of crypts by cells with mutated phenotype have shown this biphasic course; in particular the synchronous appearance of wholly mutated crypts which would be expected when a short acting mutagen is given on a single occasion to crypts maintained by a single stem cell is not seen. A stem cell niche hypothesis, with random or partially random loss of cells from the niche, in contrast, would be expected to show a smooth drop with time in the number of partially involved crypts, and a progressive increase in the number of crypts entirely replaced by a mutated phenotype. This is what has been found in mouse and in man, and we can therefore conclude that a stem cell niche with an element of randomicity in the loss of stem cells from the niche is likely to be the mechanism maintaining the small and large mammalian intestinal crypt.

We have therefore set out to investigate possible ways in which the crypt niche hypothesis could influence thinking about the way in which neoplasia can develop in the intestinal crypt. One of the paradoxes in medicine is the lack of correlation between the division rate of different tissues, and the frequency with which malignancy develops. The sequential acquisition of somatic mutations, with clonal progression, is accepted as the model for carcinogenesis; most somatic mutations occur in cycling cells during S phase. The frequency of malignancy in the small intestine in man is surprisingly low, given the very high rate of cell division, the presence of stem cells which divide and whose progeny persist throughout the lifetime of the individual, giving rise to many millions of daughter cells, and the exposure of food containing mutagenic substances. In the colon, carcinoma is relatively common in the western world. This relative frequency could be related to a greater exposure to carcinogens, a greater exposure to mucosal damage, a difference in inherent mutability or in mucosal organization or to other factors. A defect in a DNA repair gene is associated with one form of an inherited liability to colon cancer, and a defect in a tumour suppressor gene is associated with another. Colon cancer is also more common in patients with ulcerative colitis, where mucosal damage is associated with repeated growth, and formation of new crypt units.

One possible way in which the crypt niche could modify response to mutagenesis would be if stem cells carrying a potentially carcinogenic mutation were preferentially lost from the niche. One of the characteristics of neoplasia is a loss of cell contact adhesiveness, and the 'preferential loss of oncogenic mutations' (PLOOM) is a plausible mechanism to reduce the chance of neoplasia developing in stem cell systems. This mechanism would be subverted if only one stem cell was available to populate a crypt, as would be expected in regenerative growth, or growth following extensive stem cell death, when some crypts would have only one surviving stem cell. Any advantage accruing from PLOOM would then be lost. To investigate this possibility we have carried out two studies, one on the effect of regenerative growth on the retention of a growth neutral mutation, and one on the effect of regenerative growth on the retention of oncogenic mutations, as shown by the development of atypical crypt foci.

The growth neutral mutations were studied by quantifying the number of crypts showing loss of G6PD activity. G6PD is normally uniformly expressed in colonic mucosal cells, and we have shown that following mutagen administration to mice there is a dose dependent development of individual scattered crypts which lack histochemically demonstrable enzyme activity[5]. This loss of enzyme activity is present in all the cells of the affected crypt, showing that the change is heritable at a cellular level, and is confined to the cells of one tissue unit. The findings show that this must be a stem cell mutation. We have recently confirmed that the G6PD gene in these crypts shows a somatic mutation[8]. The lack of enzyme activity does not alter the crypt morphology, and in a heterozygous G6PD-deficient mouse the enzyme positive and negative crypts are approximately equal in number, suggesting that G6PD lack is not deleterious to crypt survival[9].

Groups of 12 6-week-old male C57Bl mice were given a single injection of dimethyl hydrazine (DMH), a known mutagen which also causes crypt loss and crypt fission in the colon. Mice were also treated with a single injection of ethylnitrosourea (ENU), a known mutagen which does not cause crypt neogenesis. ENU was given at different times to different groups of rats, bridging the time of regenerative growth. One group received ENU 2 days before the DMH injection, others 1, 2, 3, 4, 6 or 10 days after DMH. One group received DMH only, and a further group received ENU only. The animals were sacrificed 40 days after DMH, the colon was removed, opened and frozen sections cut of a 'series roll' of the whole colon. Loss of function mutations in a stem cell G6PD gene result in scattered individual crypts showing loss of G6PD function in all epithelial cells: these were identified by histochemistry using a standard technique[9]. Crypts showing loss of G6PD function were counted in 10 frozen sections, cut at levels of $100\,\mu$m intervals through the whole colon using a $\times 100$ magnification.

The total number of crypts present was calculated by counting the number of crypts present in the central section and multiplying by the number of sections. The results were expressed as the number of mutated crypts $\times 10^{-4}$.

A second study used the same strain of mice and the same timing of injections of ENU in relation to DMH, but the groups of mice were killed after 6 months, the colons removed and fixed, and serial sections cut at the same intervals as before. The sections were stained with haematoxylin and eosin and atypical crypt foci were identified and counted. These were identified as one or more crypts clearly distinguished from their neighbours by crowded nuclei and loss of differentiation. They were counted at a magnification of $\times 100$, and expressed as numbers of foci per animal.

The third study was similar to the second, but the cycle of injections was repeated three times on alternate weeks only for animals given ENU 2 days before, 2 days after or 4 days after DMH. The mice were killed 6 months after the first DMH injection and ACF quantified as for the second study. All counts were made without knowledge of the treatment received.

The results we have obtained show that regenerative growth is associated with an increased susceptibility to stem cell mutations. The increase seen with a growth neutral mutation is localized to a short period after the regenerative stimulus, which is just before the time when crypt fission is seen. This is likely to correspond to the time of maximum stem cell growth with loss of probability of self maintenance, so that stem cells divide to replace lost stem cells within a niche, and divide to increase niche size preparatory to crypt fission. The risk increase is of the order of 40% above that seen when the same dose of the two mutagens was given, but the pure mutagen ENU preceded administration of the regeneration inducing agent, DMH. When ENU was given at this time, in the absence of regenerative growth, the mutation frequency in the animals given both ENU and DMH was very close to that predicted by summing the frequency seen when ENU and DMH were given to separate groups of animals. This study shows the importance of the time of administration of a mutagenic agent in relation to regeneration. The increased retention of mutations seen could in theory occur whether there was one or more stem cells to each crypt.

When a similar study was carried out using the frequency of atypical crypt foci (ACF) as the end-point, a similar pattern of sensitivity was seen in relation to time of administration of mutagen. However, preliminary results suggest that the increase in frequency of ACF was relatively very much greater than that seen with a neutral mutation. This increase, of the order of 5–10 times greater than the increase seen with the frequency of a growth neutral gene mutation, provides supporting evidence for the existence of a PLOOM mechanism, which is partially abrogated in regenerative growth, and which could only operate if the control of stem cell asymmetry was extrinsic, as in a stem cell niche, rather than intrinsic. A similar qualitative result was seen in the animals given a single injection of each mutagen and in the animals given three rounds of injections; in the latter there were a number of large lesions, but only in the group given ENU at 2 days after DMH.

When the consequences of a single stem vs. a multiple stem cell are considered, it can be seen that there are many advantages in a multiple stem cell system with extrinsic control of asymmetry. If a toxic agent such as a chemical

17

or radiation kills say 1% of stem cells, then 1% of crypts will die if they are maintained by one stem cell. If they are maintained by three stem cells then only about 0.003% of crypts will lose all three stem cells and die, while approximately 0.09% of crypts will lose two of the three stem cells, and 2.8% of crypts will lose one of the three stem cells. Crypt loss and regeneration would be much greater in the single stem cell model but in the multiple stem cell model a significant number of crypts would be left with a single surviving stem cell. If a mutagen was present while regeneration was taking place the chances that mutated stem cells would persist would be increased.

A stem cell niche hypothesis could also in theory be detrimental to the organism, as in the absence of a PLOOM mechanism a more rapidly dividing stem cell would have a greater chance of coming to occupy the whole niche than a more slowly dividing cell. If there are, for example, two cells in a niche, then 100 crypts with one mutated stem cell would give rise after several rounds of stem cell division to 50 crypts with two mutated cells. If the mutation led to a two-fold increase in the mitotic rate of the mutated stem cell, then about two-thirds of the 100 crypts would be left with two mutated stem cells. If the mutation led to a two-fold increase in the chance of the mutated cell being lost from the crypt then about 30% of the crypts with one mutated stem cell would give rise to crypts with two mutated stem cells. It can be seen that the chance of a mutated stem cell remaining within a niche will depend on the degree to which the mutation influences the rate of cell division and the degree to which it influences the chance of cell loss. Interestingly it has been shown that the *APC* gene, a tumour suppressor gene in the colon which shows a germline mutation in familial polyposis coli, interacts with the cellular adhesion molecule β catenin[10], providing a possible mechanism through which a tumour suppressor gene mutation could influence cell adhesiveness, and therefore influence the chance of a mutation bearing stem cell remaining in the niche.

This chapter has reviewed some of the evidence on which the stem cell niche theory for the maintenance of intestinal crypts is based. Comparison of evidence from studies with tritiated thymidine, in which dividing cells are labelled but the label is diluted at each subsequent cell division and eventually lost, with studies using a mutagen induced phenotypic change which is heritable at the cellular level strongly supports a mechanism for crypt maintenance based on a stem cell niche with at least partially random loss of cells from the niche. The stem cell niche is presumed to be based on interaction between stem cells, basement membrane and pericryptal fibroblasts, with 'stemness' dependent on cells remaining in the niche. Control of the asymmetry of stem cell division is therefore extrinsic, and the cell that leaves the niche is not necessarily the most recently divided cell. The number of stem cells in a niche may in part explain differences in crypt cell replacement time between small and large intestine in mice, and between colon in mouse and man. This mechanism for crypt maintenance is important in the understanding of carcinogenesis, and the ability to quantify induced mutations has allowed a study of the interplay of regenerative growth, the retention of mutations and the development of atypical crypt foci in the mouse colon. The frequency of a growth neutral mutation after administration of a mutagen is raised if the mutagen is given shortly after regenerative growth has been induced, but the frequency of neoplasia is very much enhanced by this timing. It is suggested that this difference is due to a mechanism for the preferential loss of stem cells bearing oncogenic mutations from the niche. The advantage that this gives is partly nullified by regenerative growth leading to crypt neogenesis, or by stem cell death, as either event may lead to the repopulation of the crypt niche from a single mutated stem cell. This mechanism is relevant to the increased frequency of colon carcinomas in ulcerative colitis, as well as the increased frequency seen in chronic regenerative conditions in other stem cell tissues. It is also relevant to the critical importance of the timing of administration of initiator and promoter in experimental carcinogenesis, and may be important in diet-related colon carcinogenesis.

Acknowledgement

Support from the Biotechnology and Biosciences Research Council is acknowledged.

References

1. Potten CS, Loeffler M. A comprehensive model of the crypts of the small intestine of the mouse provides insight into the mechanisms of cell migration and the proliferative hierarchy. J Theor Biol. 1987;127:381–91.
2. Griffiths DFR, Davies SJ, Williams D, Williams GT, Williams ED. Demonstration of somatic mutation and colonic crypt clonality by X-linked enzyme histochemistry. Nature. 1988;333:461–3.
3. Winton DA, Blount MA, Ponder BAJ. A clonal marker induced by mutation in mouse intestinal epithelium. Nature. 1988;333:463–6.
4. Campbell F, Fuller CE, Williams GT, Williams ED. Human colonic stem cell mutation frequency with and without radiation. J Pathol. 1994;174:175–82.
5. Williams ED, Lowes AP, Williams D, Williams GT. A stem cell niche theory of intestinal crypt maintenance based on a study of somatic mutation in colonic mucosa. Am J Pathol. 1992;141: 773–6.
6. Winton DA, Ponder BAJ. Stem cell organisation in mouse small intestine. Proc R Soc Lond B. 1990;241:13–18.
7. Campbell F, Williams GT, Appleton MAC, Dixon MF, Harris M, Williams ED. Post irradiation somatic mutation and clonal stabilisation time in the human colon. Gut. 1996, in press.
8. Kuraguchi M, Thomas GA, Williams ED. Stem cell somatic mutations in the G6PD gene. Mutation Res. 1997, in press.
9. Thomas GA, Williams D, Williams ED. The demonstration of tissue clonality by X-linked enzyme histochemistry. J Pathol. 1988;155:101–8.
10. Rubinfeld B, Albert I, Porfiri E, Fiol C, Munemitsu S, Polakis P. Binding of GSK 3B to the APC-B-Catenin complex and regulation of complex assembly. Science. 1996;272:1023–6.

3
Mutant stem cells

M. BJERKNES and H. CHENG

INTRODUCTION

As discussed in Chapters 1 and 2, there is much to be learned about intestinal epithelial stem cell behaviour from studies of crypts derived from clones of mutant stem cells. These workers have used physiologically neutral mutations which were used as lineage markers. There are, however, several genes whose mutation leads to important physiological changes; for example the *APC* and *K-RAS* genes[1-10]. Appropriate mutations of either of these genes lead to production of morphologically distinctive crypts which have been recognized for some time as potential adenoma precursors[2,9,11-13]. In man, these are referred to as micro-adenomas[11,12] while in animals they have been called aberrant crypt foci (ACF)[13].

In this chapter we will summarize recent work which has attempted to characterize the mode of growth, the rate of growth, and the clonality of these populations of mutant stem cells.

THE CRYPT CYCLE

Normal crypts

It is now widely recognized that the dominant mode of growth of the intestinal epithelium in the mouse involves a process of crypt replication called the crypt cycle. The evidence that crypt replication is a normal event in mice is now compelling. The most direct evidence comes from observations of a population of 328 crypts in three animals over a period of 3 weeks. After one week there were 348 crypts, and by three weeks there were 377 crypts. This corresponds, assuming that all crypts are cycling and that the population is growing exponentially, to an average crypt cycle time of about 107 days. Thus, on average, every 107 days a crypt in a young adult mouse replicates to yield two new crypts[14,15].

Other supporting evidence for a crypt cycle, although less direct, comes from the observation of a small but constant proportion of branching crypts throughout life in both mouse and man[16-18], the observation that crypts with a branching morphology tend to be larger than other crypts[15], and the observation of a distribution of crypt sizes which is consistent in form with the notion of continuous crypt replication[15].

Thus newly formed crypts tend to be rather small. As they progress through the crypt cycle they grow in volume until they are roughly twice their original size. At this point the crypt base begins to bud and then over the course of a few days the crypt splits, usually into two new small crypts and the process begins again (Figure 1). In the young adult mouse, the crypt cycle takes about 107 days (it is probably shorter in younger animals and longer in older animals). It is uncertain whether the crypt cycle is driven by expansion of the stem cell pool contained in the crypt (although this is often assumed to be the case)[14,15,19], however, regardless of the mechanism driving crypt cycle, it is likely that the growth of the crypt population resulting from the crypt cycle is paralleled by growth of the stem cell pool. The net result is that in the adult mouse the stem cell population is continuously expanding.

Mutant crypts

Current evidence indicates that the dominant mode of growth of mutant crypts in microadenomas or ACF is also based on a crypt cycle. For example, studies of the number of crypts contained in each mutant clone found at various times after administration of mutagens have shown an increase[13]. Branching mutant crypts have also been reported[17,18]. Little is known, however, about the rate of expansion of the mutant stem cell population relative to the normal stem cell population.

A MODEL TO ASSESS THE RELATIVE GROWTH RATE OF MUTANT VS. NORMAL STEM CELL POPULATIONS

Assuming that the mutant stem cell population grows as a result of replication of the crypts containing them (mutant crypts) and that the mutant crypt cycle is similar to that of normal crypts, we can apply some simple theory in order to obtain lower bounds on the rate of expansion of clones of mutant crypts relative to the rate of expansion of clones of normal crypts[18-21].

It is likely that the background mutation process which results in the production of mutant stem cells, and hence mutant crypts, occurs at a much lower rate than does the crypt production process. In other words, it is likely that the number of new mutant clones produced per crypt per day is probably much lower than the number of new normal crypts produced through the crypt cycle per crypt per day.

With this additional assumption (which is supported by measurements of the rate of accumulation of mutant crypts)[22], the following heuristic argument may be used to extract the conclusion that on average about ½ of all mutant clones should contain only one crypt (the rest would contain two or more mutant crypts) provided that mutant crypts and normal crypts cycle at the same rate. If the mutant crypts cycle faster, then we would expect significantly fewer than 50% of mutant clones to be unicryptal.

To begin our argument, let N be a number so large that on average in the time required for one normal crypt to grow into a population of N crypts, one new

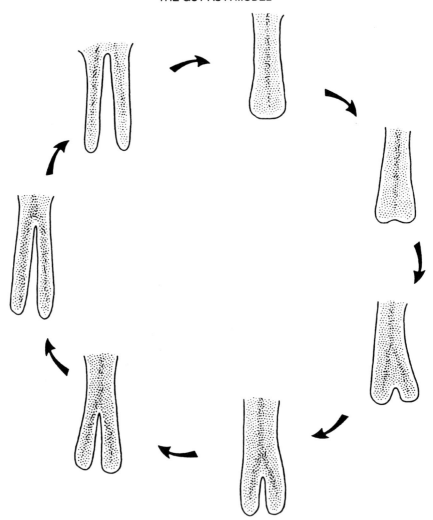

Figure 1 The crypt cycle. Newly formed crypts tend to be small (top left). Over time (months in mice, years in man) crypts increase and eventually contain roughly double the number of stem cells they originally contained (top). At this point, buds begin to form at the base of the crypt (right) and the crypt begins to split (usually in two under normal circumstances) resulting in the formation of two new, smaller crypts. At this point the crypt cycle begins again. This process appears to occur throughout life, although it probably slows with age

mutant clone will arise and develop into a mutant crypt (Figure 2). Within one normal crypt cycle time the population of normal crypts will have doubled to 2N. Furthermore, since in this time we have added N new normal crypts, by our assumption, we will have also, on average, added one new mutant clone. Furthermore, the original mutant crypt will have had time to replicate, producing a poly-

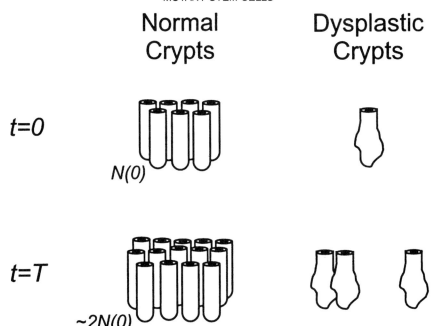

Figure 2 If crypts containing mutant stem cells cycle at the same rate as normal crypts, then with time, ½ of mutant clones should be unicryptal. Thus, if the mutation is in the *APC* gene and results in the formation of dysplastic crypts, with time ½ of clusters of dysplastic crypts (also called aberrant crypt foci, ACF) should be unicryptal. If the mutant crypts cycle faster than normal, fewer than ½ of clones will be unicryptal. The diagram illustrates the process described in the text which acts to maintain the proportion of unicryptal crypts at ½. T is the crypt cycle time.

cryptal clone. In sum, at this point we have one unicryptal and one polycryptal mutant clone in addition to the 2N normal crypts (Figure 2). If we wait another normal crypt cycle time an additional 2N normal crypts will have been produced, so on average we will have also produced an additional two new mutant clones (each of which will be unicryptal). Thus, at this point we have two unicryptal and two polycryptal mutant clones (the unicryptal clone which arose in the previous crypt cycle will have replicated by this time). This process will continue and therefore the fraction of unicryptal mutant clones is stable at ½, provided that the mutant crypts cycle at the same rate as do normal crypts. If the mutant crypts cycle faster than the normal crypt, then the population of polycryptal mutant clones will be larger than that of the unicryptal mutant clones and therefore the fraction of unicryptal mutant clones will be less than ½.

The heuristic argument given can be made rigorous and furthermore detailed dynamics of the changing proportions of differentially sized mutant clones have been derived[18,20,21]. The important point however, is the observation that if the fraction of unicryptal mutant clones is less than ½ then the mutant crypts must be cycling faster than normal crypts and hence the mutant stem cell population is growing faster than normal.

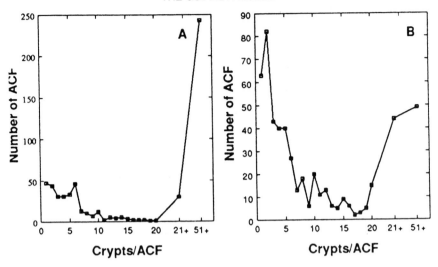

Figure 3 Plots of the number of mutant crypts contained in ACF from FAP patients (A) or nonFAP patients (B). Note that the fraction of unicryptal ACF is much less than ½ of all ACF. The fraction of unicryptal ACF is significantly less in FAP than in nonFAP. From Ref. 18

MEASURING THE RELATIVE GROWTH RATE OF MUTANT VS. NORMAL STEM CELLS

In humans

We have recently applied this theory to both human and mouse colons[18,20]. Two human populations were studied: those with familial adenomatous polyposis (FAP) and non-FAP patients. Most of the ACF (i.e. mutant crypts) found in FAP colons are due to mutation of the *APC* gene[1–4,6,7] while most ACF found in non-FAP patients are due to *K-RAS* and not *APC* mutations[2,9]. This is significant because it is presently thought that most of the *APC* mutant crypts go on to form dysplastic adenomas (cancer precursors) while most *K-RAS* mutant crypts go on to form hyperplastic polyps (benign non-cancerous lesions). Thus by comparing the distributions of ACF crypt content in these two patient populations we may obtain information about the relative growth rates of *APC* vs. *K-RAS* mutant stem cells.

Figure 3 shows the resulting distributions of crypt content in ACF from FAP and non-FAP patients. Note that in both patient populations the fraction of uni-cryptal ACF is much less than ½ of all ACF, leading to the conclusion that both *APC* and *K-RAS* mutant stem cells expand at abnormally rapid rates. More subtle arguments[18] show that the *APC* mutant crypts are expanding at least 11 times faster than normal while *K-RAS* mutant crypts are expanding at least seven times faster than normal. Thus the *APC* mutant stem cells are expanding more rapidly than either normal or *K-RAS* mutant stem cells, which is consistent with their clinical behaviour.

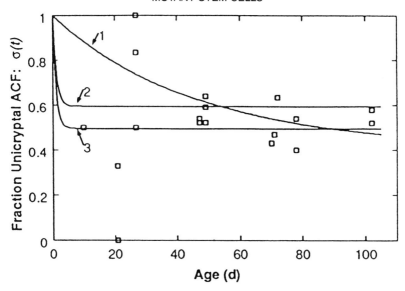

Figure 4 Plot of the dynamics of the fraction of unicryptal ACF in *Apc+/−Msh2−/−* mice. Each open square represents the fraction from one mouse. The three curves represent the range of fits of the model to the data. The value 1/2 falls within the 95% confidence range and therefore this data provides no evidence of any difference in the rate of crypt replication of mutant versus normal crypts in these mice. From Ref. 18

In mouse

There is also a mouse model of FAP[23]. These mice have one defective *Apc* allele and go on to develop multiple intestinal tumours (each of which is due to expansion of a clone derived from a cell in which the second *Apc* allele is lost)[5,10,24]. Mice offer the advantage that animals of different ages can be compared and thus additional dynamic information about the growth of mutant clones is potentially available. Unfortunately, while *Apc* +/− mice developed tumours, their colons contained very few ACF and as a result we were unable to collect enough data to analyse. To increase the ACF frequency, we bred the *Apc* mice with mice in which the DNA mismatch repair enzyme gene *Msh2* was knocked out[18,22]. The resulting *Apc+/−Msh2−/−* offspring showed a 100-fold increase in the rate of ACF production, thus enabling a study[18,22].

Graphs showing the dynamics of the fraction of unicryptal ACF with age as well as fits of a model of those dynamics are presented in Figure 4. The surprising conclusion is that, in contrast to observations in man, this mouse model shows no evidence of an increased mutant crypt replication rate. The mutant crypts contained in ACF appeared to cycle at the same rate as normal crypts as evidenced by the fact that the fraction of unicryptal ACF was stationary at about ½ throughout life.

At face value this finding is somewhat confusing because these mice, like the human FAP patients, developed multiple intestinal tumours. New ACF arose throughout life in these mice (Figure 5), but those produced in the adult do not

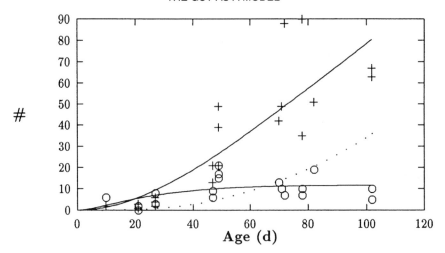

Figure 5 Plot showing the accumulation of ACF (+) and adenomas (O) in *Apc+/–Msh–/–* mice. Each data point represents the total number of ACF or adenomas present in the colon of a single animal. The curves represent fits of models of ACF accumulation and adenoma accumulation, respectively. The models indicate that most ACF arise from postnatal events, but most adenomas arise from perinatal events. From Ref. 22.

appear to be growing sufficiently rapidly to yield macroscopic lesions. This is consistent however, with studies of the dynamics of accumulation of macro-scopic tumours in both *Apc* and *Apc+/– Msh2–/–* mice[22]. The number of adenomas contained in both small and large intestine of animals of various ages and genotypes were scored. The resulting counts were fitted with a simple model of adenoma accumulation. In this model there were two potential sources of new adenomas: (1) postnatally derived nascent tumours (i.e. small clones of mutant cells; Figure 6); (2) perinatally derived nascent tumours. It was assumed that there was an unknown random number of perinatally derived nascent tumours each of which requires a random time to grow into a macroscopic tumour which could be scored (Figure 7). Similarly, postnatally derived tumours were assumed to arise randomly at a constant rate throughout life and to also require a random period of time to grow into macroscopic lesions. We found for all genotypes and for both colon and small intestine that the data was best fitted with a model in which all macroscopic tumours had their origin perinatally (Figure 8)[22].

Thus it would appear that in mouse colon, perinatal *Apc* mutations are able to elaborate into macroscopic tumours, but those mutant clones which arise in the adult have restricted growth rates and do not contribute significantly to the macroscopic tumour population. This is supported by observations in mice that perinatal administration of carcinogens in mice is far more effective than are doses administered in the adult[25].

In contrast, in man it appears that postnatally arising clones grow at abnormally rapid rates and are likely to contribute to the macroscopic adenoma population. The reason for the species difference is not known. It could be genetic. It could be that the normal crypt replication rate in young mice is sufficiently fast that the

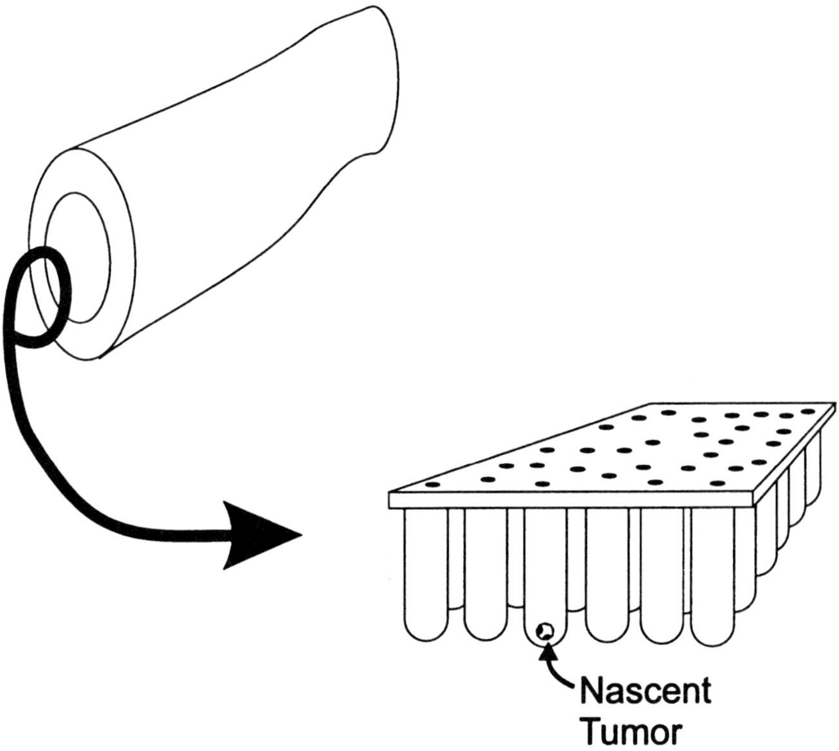

Figure 6 Diagram indicating the idea of nascent tumour, a small clone of mutant cells (initially in a single crypt) which is undetectable with present assays but which can grow into a macroscopic adenoma

loss of *Apc* gene function has no additional impact, or it could be a reflection of the fact that most of these mice die at a very early age (about 100 days) and given more time the ACF in the adult might be able to elaborate macroscopic lesions (especially if subclones acquire mutations in additional genes).

CLONALITY OF DYSPLASTIC CRYPTS IN ADENOMAS

The nature of nascent tumours will serve to lead into our next issue, clonality. It is generally assumed that most tumours arise from a single mutant stem cell. Initially, this mutant cell is found in a crypt dominated by cells with normal genotype (after all, the mutant stem cell originated from a normal cell). With time this mutant stem cell grows into a clone which may dominate the crypt. Little is known about this process, however. In particular, we do not know the degree of clonal homogeneity necessary for the mutant morphology to be recognizable. Work from studies of clonal expansion in normal crypts would lead one to expect that *APC* mutant stem cell clones would quickly dominate the crypt[26-29] (see also Chapters 1 and 2).

27

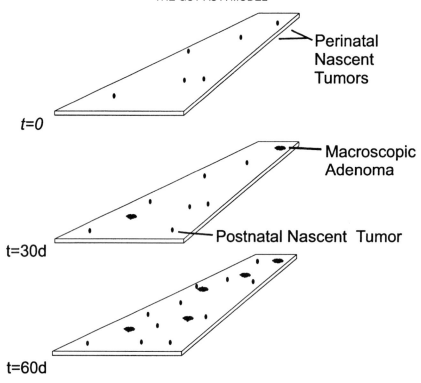

Figure 7 Diagram indicating the ideas behind the adenoma accumulation model. There is a population of nascent tumours present at birth (the perinatal nascent tumour population) which is added to at random points in time in adult life (the postnatal population). Both populations are assumed to be identical in all other respects. In particular, they both require a random time to grow into macroscopic adenomas. By scoring the number of adenomas as animals age, we hope to obtain information about the time of origin of their antecedent nascent tumours.

The initial literature dealing with the clonality of colorectal tumours was confusing. Some claimed evidence of monoclonality while others found evidence of polyclonality. Eventually a consensus emerged that most early tumours were monoclonal and that those studies claiming polyclonality were probably confused by the presence of contaminating stromal tissues (for review see Refs 30, 31). In particular, studies using X-linked mosaic markers found polyclonality if segments of tumours were studied, but monoclonality when workers were careful to isolate dysplastic epithelium[30]. Similarly, *APC* mutations found in different parts of the same tumours were identical[32,33].

Patients with FAP have inherited one defective allele of the *APC* gene[1,3,4,6], which makes them unusually susceptible to development of colorectal adenomas. Most of these adenomas are derived from cells which have incurred either somatic mutation, resulting in protein truncation, or allelic deletion of the remaining wild type allele[34,35]. Thus the carboxyterminus of the normal APC protein product is absent from the mutant cells, and antibodies specific for the carboxyterminus of APC can be used as a marker for mutant cells. In particular, all cells of a normal

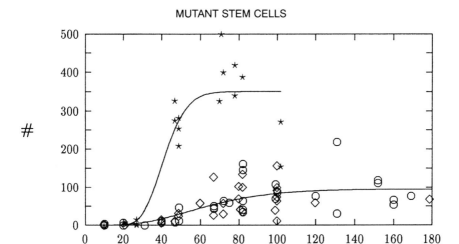

Figure 8 Plot showing the accumulation of macroscopic adenomas in $Apc+/-Msh2-/-$ (stars) and $Apc+/-$ (other points) mice. The curves are fits of the adenoma accumulation model. The best fits are obtained when adenomas arise perinatally. From Ref. 22

phenotype in tissues from FAP patients (that is those cells containing one functional *APC* allele) will stain positively with antibodies specific for the carboxyterminus of APC protein (APC-c), while mutant cells derived from stem cells in which both alleles are dysfunctional will not stain with the antibody. Using this approach we were able to investigate expansion of a mutant clone and study clonal homogenization within dysplastic epithelium[36].

As expected, phenotypically normal crypts in FAP patients stained positively with the anti-APC-c antibody. A careful scan of areas containing no macroscopic lesions will occasionally yield crypts containing both APC-c-positive and -negative cells, presumably representing the early stages in the expansion of a mutant clone (that is, a nascent tumour). Surprisingly, most dysplastic crypts in adenomas of all sizes investigated (up to 1 cm) continued to contain a mixture of APC-c-positive and -negative cells (Figure 9). The majority of cells were APC-c-negative as expected, but a significant number of APC-c-positive cells were present, especially among well differentiated mucous cells. Positively staining mitotic figures were also observed. In combination these observations suggest the presence of a stable normal stem cell compartment within dysplastic epithelium of adenomas from FAP patients. This finding was a surprise since these lesions probably required many months to years to develop and it appears, therefore, that a different mode of clonal expansion/interaction occurs from that found in normal crypts (where studies of X-linked mosaics indicate clonal purification in a matter of weeks in human colon; see Chapter 2).

These results compelled us to seek confirmation using independent methods[36]. To do this we took advantage of the fact that the first half of exon 15 is the most frequent site for mutation in the *APC* gene[37], corresponding to what is called 'segment 3'[35]. We screened adenomas, from FAP patients with germline segment

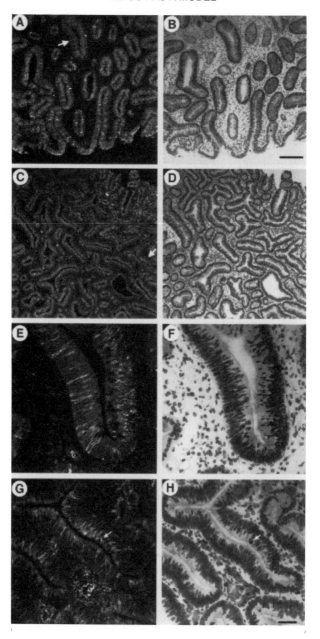

Figure 9 Photomicrographs of fluorescently labelled anti-APC-c staining of adenomas from FAP patients (A, C, E, G) and corresponding haematoxylin-stained images (B, D, F, H). E and G are enlargements of the crypts indicated by arrows in A and C, respectively. Note that while most cells are APC-c-negative and hence are unstained, there is a definite population of APC-c-positive cells in these dysplastic crypts. APC-c-positive mitotic figures are also seen (arrows in G and H). Scale bars: (A–D) $250\,\mu$m; (E–H) $50\,\mu$m. From Ref. 36

3 mutations, for mutations in segment 3 distinct from the germline mutation. Single dysplastic crypts were microdissected from frozen sections and genomic DNA amplified with PCR using primers specific for segment 3. The amplified DNA was transcribed in vitro and then translated. The resulting protein encoded by the amplified DNA was run on a gel and checked for truncated variants[36].

All crypts displayed the germline truncated form. Normal crypts also displayed the full length wild type protein product. Dysplastic crypts displayed an additional truncated form due to the somatic mutation generating the tumour. Importantly, many of the dysplastic crypts also displayed significant quantities of the wild-type product, indicating the presence of normal cells. Since these microdissected crypts were free of adherent stromal cells, these findings confirmed our observations with the antibody (adjacent sections from the same crypts were stained with the antibody to demonstrate the presence of APC-c-positive epithelial cells).

Importantly, all dysplastic crypts from the same tumour displayed the same somatic mutation[36]. This is consistent with the idea that the mutant cells are clonally related. Thus, the dysplastic epithelium appears to contain a dominant population of clonally related mutant cells and a secondary population of normal cells. It is also likely that the mutant and normal cells are clonally related (although more distantly so) since they presumably were derived from the same crypt[26-29] (see also Chapters 1 and 2). Our conclusions differ from those reached in a recent report giving evidence that most adenomas are polyclonal in the sense that different dysplastic crypts from the same tumour contain unrelated cells[40]. These authors found that all cells within single crypts were clonally related, but that neighbouring dysplastic crypts within the same tumour were occasionally unrelated. Their analysis was performed using tissues from an FAP patient who was also an XO/XY mosaic[40], and a Y chromosome probe was used to characterize crypt clonality. They would not have been able to detect the mixture of normal and mutant stem cells which we found because crypts would have been homogeneously XO or XY since childhood in their patient. The reason why we did not see evidence of polyclonality of the mutant population, which would have been expected from their conclusions, is not known. One possibility is that we did not study sufficient numbers of tumours, another is that many of the dysplastic crypts which they found to be of divergent clonality from the tumour may not have contained cells with *APC* mutations (they did not demonstrate *APC* status) and were actually derived from crypts other than that which gave rise to the tumour. Further study should resolve these issues.

The conclusions reached above from our findings were based on the assumption that the dominant mode of growth of ACF and adenomas is through a crypt-cycle like process involving crypt growth followed by crypt branching. Other possibilities exist. For example, it is plausible that mutant crypts grow by fusing with neighbouring normal crypts. Such a mechanism would explain the continued presence of normal stem cells within the dysplastic epithelium. However, in mildly dysplastic epithelium fusing crypts are rarely seen and, in fact, such merging crypts are usually considered an indication of severe dysplasia[38,39] (probably resulting from the accumulation of additional mutations in genes other than *APC*). Another possible mode of growth is diffusion of mutant stem cells into neighbouring crypts via the surface epithelium. Again such a mechanism could explain the continued presence of mixed crypts and offers an alternative explanation of our findings.

We also studied tissues from adenocarcinomas from FAP patients, and found that the carcinoma was uniformly APC-c negative (in contrast to the adjacent adeno-matous tissues)[36]. This finding suggests that the subsequent mutations leading to carcinoma have either altered the adhesive characteristics of the mutant cells allowing them to disperse away from the normal stem cells component, or that mutations have given the mutant cells a significant growth advantage allowing them to outgrow the normal cells.

References

1. Groden J, Thliveris A, Samovitz W et al. Identification and characterization of the familial adenomatous polyposis coli gene. Cell. 1991;66:589–600.
2. Jen J, Powell SM, Papadopoulous N et al. Molecular determinants of dysplasia in colorectal lesions. Cancer Res. 1994;54:5523–6.
3. Joslyn G, Carlson M, Thilveris A et al. Identification of deletion mutations and three new genes at the familial polyposis locus. Cell. 1991;66:601–13.
4. Kinzler KW, Nilbert MC, Su L-K et al. Identification of FAP locus genes from chromosome 5q21. Science. 1991;253:661–5.
5. Luongo C, Moser AR, Gledhill S, Dove WF. Loss of Apc* in intestinal adenomas from Min mice. Cancer Res. 1994;54:5947–52.
6. Nishisho I, Nakamura Y, Miyoshi Y et al. Mutations of chromosome 5q21 genes in FAP and colorectal cancer patients. Science. 1991;253:665–9.
7. Powell SM, Zilz N, Beazer-Barclay Y et al. APC mutations occur early during colorectal tumori-genesis. Nature. 1992;359:235–7.
8. Redston MS, Papadopoulos N, Caldas C, Kinzler KW, Kern SE. Common occurrence of APC and K-ras gene mutations in the spectrum of colitis-associated neoplasias. Gastroenterology. 1995; 108:383–92.
9. Smith AJ, Stern HS, Penner M et al. Somatic APC and K-ras mutations in aberrant crypt foci from human colons. Cancer Res. 1994;54:5527–30.
10. Su L-K, Kinzler KW, Vogelstein B et al. Multiple intestinal neoplasia caused by a mutation in the murine homolog of the APC gene. Science. 1992;256:668–70.
11. Bussey HJR. Familial Polyposis Coli. Baltimore: The Johns Hopkins University Press, 1975.
12. Roncucci L, Stamp D, Medline A, Cullen JB, Bruce WR. Identification and quantification of aberrant crypt foci and microadenomas in the human colon. Hum Pathol. 1991;22:287–94.
13. McLellan EA, Medline A, Bird RP. Sequential analysis of the growth and morphological charac-teristics of aberrant crypt foci: putative pre-neoplastic lesions. Cancer Res. 1991;51:5270–4.
14. Bjerknes M. A test of the stochastic theory of stem cell differentiation. Biophys J. 1986;49: 1223–7.
15. Totafurno J, Bjerknes M, Cheng H. The crypt cycle: Crypt and villus production in the intestinal epithelium. Biophys J. 1987;52:279–94.
16. Cheng H, Bjerknes M. Whole population cell kinetics and postnatal development of the mouse intestinal epithelium. Anat Rec. 1985;211:420–6.
17. Cheng H, Bjerknes M, Amar J, Gardiner G. Crypt production in normal and diseased human colonic epithelium. Anat Rec. 1986;216:44–8.
18. Bjerknes M, Cheng H, Hay K, Gallinger S. APC mutation and the crypt cycle in murine and human intestine. Am J Pathol. 1997; 150:833–9.
19. Bjerknes M. Simple stochastic theory of stem cell differentiation is not simultaneously consistent with crypt extinction probability and the expansion of mutated clones. J Theor Biol. 1994;168: 349–65.
20. Bjerknes M. Expansion of mutant stem cell populations in the human colon. J Theor Biol. 1996;178:381–5.
21. Bjerknes M. The crypt cycle and the asymptotic dynamics of the proportion of differently sized mutant crypt clones in the mouse intestine. Proc R Soc Lond B. 1995;260:1–6.

22. Reitmair AH, Cai J-C, Bjerknes M *et al.* MSH2 deficiency contributes to accelerated APC mediated intestinal tumorigenesis. Cancer Res. 1996;56:2922–6.
23. Moser AR, Pitot HC, Dove WF. A dominant mutation that predisposes to multiple intestinal neoplasia in the mouse. Science. 1990;247:322–4.
24. Levy DB, Smith KJ, Beazer-Barclay Y, Hamilton SR, Vogelstein B, Kinzler KW. Inactivation of both *APC* alleles in human and mouse tumors. Cancer Res. 1994;54:5953–58.
25. Moser AR, Shoemaker AR, Connelly CS *et al.* Homozygosity for the min allele of apc results in disruption of mouse development prior to gastrulation. Dev Dynamics. 1995;203:422–33.
26. Griffiths DFR, Davies SJ, Williams D, Williams GT, Williams ED. Demonstration of somatic mutation and crypt clonality by X-linked enzyme histochemistry. Nature. 1988;333:461–3.
27. Winton DJ, Blount MA, Ponder BAJ. A clonal marker induced by mutation in mouse intestinal epithelium. Nature. 1988;333:463–6.
28. Winton DJ, Ponder BAJ. Stem-cell organization in mouse small intestine. Proc R Soc Lond B. 1990;241:13–18.
29. Kusakabe M, Yokoyama M, Sakakura T, Nomura T, Hosick HL, Nishizuka Y. A novel methodology for analysis of cell distribution in chimeric mouse organs using a strain specific antibody. J Cell Biol. 1988;107:257–65.
30. Fearon ER, Hamilton SR, Vogelstein B. Clonal analysis of human colorectal tumors. Science. 1987;238:193–7.
31. Fearon ER, Vogelstein B. A genetic model for colorectal tumorigenesis. Cell. 1990;61:759–67.
32. Boland CR, Sato J, Appelman HD, Bresalier RS, Feinberg AP. Microallelotyping defines the sequence and tempo of allelic losses at tumour suppressor gene loci during colorectal cancer progression. Nature Med. 1995;1:902–9.
33. Tsao J, Shibata D. Further evidence that one of the earliest alterations in colorectal carcinogenesis involves APC. Am J Pathol. 1994;145:531–4.
34. Miyaki M, Konishi M, Kikuchi-Yanoshita R *et al.* Characteristics of somatic mutation of the adenomatous polyposis coli gene in colorectal tumours. Cancer Res. 1994;54:3011–20.
35. Powell SM, Petersen GM, Krush AJ *et al.* Molecular diagnosis of familial adenomatous polyposis. N Engl J Med. 1993;329:1982–7.
36. Bjerknes M, Cheng H, Kim H, Schnitzler M, Gallinger S. Clonality of dysplastic epithelium in colorectal adenomas from familial adenomatous polyposis patients. Cancer Res. 1997;57:355–61.
37. Miyoshi Y, Nagase H, Ando H *et al.* Somatic mutations of the *APC* gene in colorectal tumors: mutation cluster region in the *APC* gene. Human Molecular Genet. 1992;1:229–33.
38. Lev R. Adenomatous Polyps of the Colon. New York: Springer-Verlag, 1990.
39. Jass JR, Sobin LH. Histological Typing of Intestinal Tumours, 2nd edn. New York: Springer-Verlag, 1989.
40. Novelli MR, Williamson JA, Tomlinson IPM *et al.* Polyclonal origin of colonic adenomas in an XO/XY patient with FAP. Science. 1996;272:1187–90.

4
Towards gene correction for cystic fibrosis in intestinal stem cells

E. M. SLORACH and J. R. DORIN

INTRODUCTION

Treating diseases by putting recombinant genes into somatic cells is an appealing strategy. The simplistic concept is that for a recessive single gene disorder a normal copy of the defective gene in mutant cells will ameliorate the disease phenotype, even when the underlying biology of the disease may not be completely understood[1].

Cystic fibrosis (CF) is often considered one of the most accessible targets for somatic gene therapy: although pulmonary failure is the major cause of morbidity and mortality in early adulthood, the earliest manifestations of CF are localized in the intestinal tract[2]. Intestinal disease in CF presents at birth as intestinal blockage (meconium ileus) in 10–15% of patients. This defect can be corrected by surgery but later in life distal intestinal obstruction is a cause of abdominal swelling and pain. Patients suffer from malabsorption and malnutrition and are advised a high fat diet to compensate[3]. Eighty-five per cent of CF individuals have pancreatic insufficiency, and the routine taking of pancreatic supplements helps to counteract the malabsorption and malnutrition. As lung disease begins to take hold, however, the additional energy requirement intensifies the malnutrition deficit. The basic defect in CF is in chloride transport from the apical membrane of epithelial cells. In situ hybridization has revealed that the major site of the CF gene (*CFTR*; cystic fibrosis transmembrane conductance regulator) expression is in the crypt cells of the small intestine[4], which is consistent with CFTR being responsible for chloride ion secretion. The level of expression is low in the villi (site of chloride absorption) and decreases down the length of the intestine. A defect in CTR-mediated chloride conductance has been demonstrated in both the small and large intestine in vitro and in vivo in CF patients[5]. In CF the intestine is filled with a highly viscous mucus, which may disturb the motility of intestinal contents, lead to obstruction and create a barrier to absorption.

Clearly lung disease treatment must be the primary goal in CF, with intestinal disease being an important second target. However one important question that needs to be addressed is what level of gene correction is necessary to achieve a clinical effect?

HOW MUCH IS ENOUGH?

We have used the cystic fibrosis mouse models that have been created by disruption of the mouse *Cftr* gene by gene targeting into embryonic stem cells (ES cells) to address the issue of how much gene correction is required for phenotypic correction[6]. Homozygous *Cftr* mutant mice display a defect in cAMP-stimulated chloride ion transport[7], consistent with the disease in man. The phenotype in the intestine of mice expressing no CFTR or dysfunctional CFTR protein is one of goblet cell hyperplasia, intestinal obstruction and perforation[8]. This is very similar to the phenotype observed in 10–15% of CF patients who present with meconium ileus or gut blockage in the perinatal period[2].

Dysfunctional CFTR

CF patients who have a missense mutation (G551D) located in the first nucleotide binding fold of the CFTR protein produce a dysfunctional protein which is correctly localized to the apical membrane but produces cAMP-regulated chloride channels which show markedly reduced function. A key feature of this mutation is that CF patients carrying the G551D allele have a three-fold reduction in the incidence of meconium ileus[9]. We have generated a mouse carrying the human G551D mutation in the murine *Cftr* gene using a one step gene targeting procedure in mouse ES cells[10]. Mice with the G551D mutant protein show cystic fibrosis pathology but have a reduced risk of fatal intestinal blockage compared with mutant mice with no CFTR protein ('nulls')[8]. Only 8% of null mice survive to 35 days of age, compared with 27% of G551D homozygotes. G551D mice show greatly reduced CFTR-related chloride transport, equivalent to 4% of wild-type CFTR, and this implies that the reduced level of cAMP-mediated chloride transport is sufficient to have an effect on intestinal phenotype (survival).

How low can you go?

We have modulated the level of *Cftr* gene expression to demonstrate the relationship between CFTR activity and both ion transport and survival. For any recessive condition the unaffected phenotype of heterozygotes demonstrates that 50% of the normal level of gene expression is enough to prevent disease. A non-linear relationship between phenotype and gene activity is predicted by control analysis for any autosomal recessive inherited disease[11]. This is because the phenotype (flux) through a biochemical pathway is the result of a matrix of interrelated steps. Changes in any one step will thus affect the flow through all the adjacent intermediates. The net effect is that a change in any one component step will be buffered by the other components and minimize any alteration in the final output (phenotype). This explains why most genes which are part of a multistep pathway are recessive. We studied six genotypes of mice with different levels of *Cftr* gene

Table 1 CFTR activity and survival in Cftr mutant mice

Mutant mouse	CFTR activity (percentage of wild-type level)	Survival at 35 days (%)
+/+	100	100
$cftr^{tm1HGU}/+$	55	95
$cftr^{tm1UNC}/+$	50	95
$cftr^{tm1HGU}/cftr^{tm1HGU}$	10	95
$cftr^{tm1HGU}/cftr^{tm1UNC}$	5	95
$cftr^{tm1UNC}/cftr^{tm1UNC}$	0	8

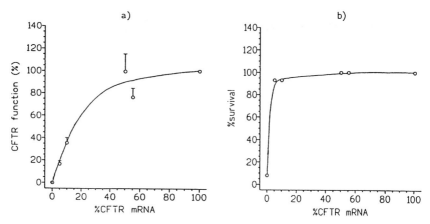

Figure 1 (a) The relationship between CFTR mRNA and CFTR function. Each point represents combined forskolin data derived from jejunum, caecum and rectum against Cftr mRNA levels particular for each genotype. (b) The relationship between Cftr mRNA and survival at 35 days

expression. These mice were generated by intercrossing mice carrying the $cftr^{tm1UNC}$ (replacement) allele[8] and mice carrying the $cftr^{tm1HGU}$ (insertional) allele, both created by ES cell gene targeting. The $cftr^{tm1UNC}$ is a complete knockout or null and the $cftr^{tm1HGU}$ allele is a slightly leaky mutation which expresses around 10% of the normal level of cftr mRNA as a result of exon skipping and aberrant splicing[12]. The message levels in the heterozygotes, homozygote and compound heterozygote mutants varied from 0 to 100% of wild-type CFTR levels (Table 1).

Electrophysiological measurements were made in three distinct parts of the gastrointestinal tract, where we have previously shown that the forskolin response principally relates to chloride secretion and reflects CFTR function[13]. In each of the intact tissues studied, whether in vivo or in vitro, very similar non-linear asymmetrical relationships were observed between the response to forskolin (stimulates cAMP) and cftr mRNA. The combined jejunal, caecal (in vitro) and rectal (in vivo) responses are graphically represented in Figure 1a. The response curve demonstrates that at low levels of Cftr mRNA (0–10% of wild-type) a small increase produces a large bioelectric response (0–30% of wild-type forskolin response). At high levels of message, however, there is a small change in chloride conductance (20%) for a large change in gene expression (50–100%).

Chloride conductance is a convenient and direct measure of CFTR function but of greater clinical relevance is to measure the net consequence on pathology. Figure 1b shows the consequence on survival (at 35 days) of increasing levels of *Cftr* mRNA. The relationship is distinctly non-linear and asymptotic and the symmetry is clearly exaggerated compared with the relationship between *Cftr* expression and chloride conductance (Figure 1a). We would predict that net phenotype (survival) is most likely at several additional (buffering) steps from chloride conductance, thus explaining the difference in the relationships[6]. Thus partial correction of the intestinal defect would be predicted to have a major effect on phenotype.

Inappropriate CFTR expression in the intestine

The hypothesis that partial gene correction in the gut will be sufficient is further corroborated by Zhou et al.[14], who expressed the human *CFTR* (h*CFTR*) gene in transgenic mice under the control of the rat intestinal fatty acid-binding protein (*FABP*) gene promoter. Transgenic mice carrying the transgene were crossed onto *cftr*[tm1UNC] homozygous mice. These mice would normally die around birth from intestinal blockage, display morphological changes including goblet cell hyperplasia and disruption of the crypt epithelial cell organization and accumulation of mucin in the lumen of the intestine[8]. The bitransgenic mice i.e. *cftr*[tm1UNC] homozygotes carrying the FABP-hCFTR transgene did not die at birth and in situ hybridization revealed that expression was present in the intestine of six founder lines. The human *CFTR* mRNA was most abundant in the intestinal epithelium of the ileum, jejunum and duodenum and less abundant in the colon and caecum. Importantly the transgene was expressed in the intestinal villi but not in the crypts of Lieberkühn, where the principal secretory activity of the small and large intestines resides. Endogenous murine *cftr* mRNA is expressed at high levels in the ileum, colon and jejunum of wild-type mice and, in common with man, the expression is localized to the crypt cells and decreases along the length of the villi. However short circuit measurements of tissue from the bitransgenic mice demonstrated a cAMP-stimulated chloride response in both jejunum and ileum which was approximately 30% of the level in wild-type mice. The conclusion must be, however, that the level of secretion that this aberrant expression pattern supports is sufficient to rescue the intestinal phenotype.

Gene correction to intestinal cells

Since the gene was cloned in 1989[15] a huge effort has been directed at introducing *CFTR* back into the respiratory epithelium. However the gene therapy vectors used at present have several limitations and the lack of success of the initial clinical trials undoubtedly reflects the fact that these are first generation gene therapy strategies[1]. Both adenovirus and DNA/cationic liposome vehicles have been used to treat patients[16-19], the approach being the introduction of DNA by transfection or transduction and expression of the recombinant *CFTR* gene under the control of a heterologous promoter. In vitro both these gene transfer vehicles can transfect cells at a high efficiency but, unfortunately, the transfection of ciliated epithelial cells in vivo appears to be extremely inefficient[20]. A further limitation is that the partial correction of the bioelectric defect in CF that has been reported is always transient[16,17,19].

We have attempted to introduce *CFTR* cDNA expression vectors into the intestinal epithelia of *cftr*[tm1HGU] mutant mice[21]. The *CFTR* cDNAs we used were under the control of three different promoters. The DNA was complexed with the cationic liposome DC–Chol/DOPE at a wt/wt ratio of 1:5 and each animal received 600 μg of plasmid delivered via a plastic tube inserted into the rectum. Methylene blue dye was delivered using the same apparatus and this demonstrated that delivery could be achieved to the rectum, colon, caecum and the distal ileum but not the jejunum. Electrophysiological analysis of treated animals 24 h after gene delivery revealed that cAMP-mediated chloride transport (stimulated by forskolin) did not alter in the jejunum but was increased by 20% in the distal ileum (in vitro) and the rectum (in vivo). Treatment also increased the response to carbachol (which produces chloride secretion through Ca^{2+}-mediated pathways) in the ileum, but again not in the jejunum. This is significant because in both CF subjects and the *cftr* mice calcium-linked chloride transport in the intestine is defective in addition to cAMP-mediated chloride transport[7]. In addition human *CFTR* mRNA was detected in the intestinal tissue of all treated but not untreated animals. The mRNA detection was not quantitative but our impression was that gene delivery by DNA liposome was highly variable between animals. Thus delivery of the human CFTR transgene to the intestine produced a transient and modest correction of the CF bioelectric defect whereas vector delivery by nebulization to the respiratory tract produced a large (50% of the deficit between wild type and *cftr*[tm1HGU] mice) effect.

PROBLEMS OF INTESTINAL GENE THERAPY IN VIVO

Several factors may be relevant in considering the difference in gene correction in vivo in the *cftr*[tm1HGU] mouse lung and intestine. Firstly the intestine may provide a simply less favourable environment for DNA/lipid transfection. Like the CF gut, the intestine of these mice is filled with mucus which may stop effective transfection. In addition the site of *CFTR* gene expression in the intestine is in the crypt cells, and these will be the most inaccessible. Long-term expression will only be achieved if intestinal crypt stem cells are transfected. The high cell turnover in the intestine is such that the entire villus epithelia is replaced every 3–5 days. The proliferating stem cells are located near the base of the crypts and therefore clearly even if these cells were transfected an episomal vector would be lost upon cell division very rapidly. One possible solution to this problem would be to transfect the stem cell population with an integrative vector such as a retrovirus. The potential worry here is of insertional mutation and, more importantly, the availability of a suitable promoter. In order to achieve the correct spatial and temporal pattern of *CFTR* expression the best solution would be to use a transgene driven by the endogenous gene promoter. Indeed position independent copy number dependent gene expression of several genes has been achieved in transgenic animals where the injected DNA is a large YAC insert which contains all the relevant sequence for correct gene expression[22]. However insert size limitations of the current gene therapy vectors means that large genomic regions cannot be included. In the future perhaps mini artificial chromosomes may be considered but that is not a reality at present.

The optimal approach therefore must be to use gene targeting technology to correct the chromosomal *CFTR* mutation so that gene expression is restored back to normal and, as discussed above, for a recessive disease, correction of one mutant allele will be sufficient for a normal phenotype in those cells. For a sustainable treatment however this requires gene targeting into stem cells ex vivo and then re-engraftment of the corrected cells to repopulate the diseased organ. Our gene targeting approach has concentrated on targeting the *Cftr* gene in the mutant mouse intestine. These mice provide the ideal test system for this strategy. Firstly precise clinical mutations e.g. ΔF508, G551D as well as the knockout *cftr* alleles have been created by gene targeting in the mouse. Secondly the mutant mice express a severe intestinal phenotype which is ideal to monitor functional correction.

DELIVERY OF DNA INTO INTESTINAL STEM CELLS

Experiments by Lau et al.[23] have shown that retroviral vectors can be used to deliver reporter genes to both the villus and crypt epithelium in vivo. Expression of the reporter genes can be detected up to 6 days after exposure to the retroviral vector, suggesting that it may be possible to infect intestinal stem cells.

Precise gene targeting however is not currently feasible in vivo since it requires not only the accurate delivery of DNA to stem cells, but homologous recombination to occur at the desired genomic site. Since random integration of DNA occurs at a much higher frequency than homologous recombination, selection of correctly targeted cells is necessary. This means an ex vivo approach must be taken whereby gene targeting and selection can take place in vitro before engraftment of correctly targeted cells. Del Buono et al.[24] have used a model of the developing intestine which involves the grafting of fetal intestinal endoderm within collagen gels prior to subcutaneous grafting, to show the successful delivery of a reporter gene to intestinal stem cells using a retroviral construct. Similarly, Patel et al.[25] have shown that, using an organoid culture and engraftment procedure, gene transfer into rat organoids can be achieved efficiently using an adenoviral vector. The organoids are incubated with the adenovirus prior to either primary culture or subcutaneous engraftment. Staining of cultures after 6 days reveals sustained expression of the marker gene whereas expression in the neomucosal grafts can be detected at least 14 days after infection, again suggesting successful gene transfer into stem cells.

The isolation and culture of a pure, or at least highly enriched population of intestinal stem cells would allow a greater understanding of the conditions required for successful gene transfer into pluripotent stem cells, as well as facilitating a more efficient approach to homologous recombination. This has been achieved with some success for the haemopoietic system due to the increasing number of markers available for haemopoietic stem cells. The identification of stem cell markers and a greater understanding of the signals required to maintain intestinal stem cells in their pluripotent state in vitro must be a priority for practical genetic manipulation of the intestinal epithelium.

INTESTINAL STEM CELL CULTURE

Primary culture of intestinal epithelium

Compared with other epithelial cell types, it has proved particularly difficult to grow epithelial cells from the small intestine in culture for any length of time. The establishment of immortal epithelial cell lines from the small intestine has also proved difficult with only a limited number of lines successfully generated so far, the majority of which are derived from fetal tissue. These problems relate to a lack of data on the nature of the various growth factors, cytokines, morphogens and survival signals necessary to maintain cell survival and proliferation in culture. There would also appear to be an inherent difficulty in maintaining survival of intestinal epithelial cells when removed from their natural environment. Indeed it has been shown in intestinal cell lines that inhibiting intercellular contact using antibodies directed against a specific integrin subunit induces apoptosis in these cells[26]. This makes sense when the fate of an intestinal epithelial cell is considered. These cells migrate rapidly along the crypt/villus axis until they reach the villus tip where the cells either undergo apoptosis or are extruded into the intestinal lumen. The nature of these cells makes the primary culture of intestinal stem cells a particularly difficult task. With this in mind, Evans et al.[27] developed a novel procedure for the primary culture of rat intestinal epithelium. It is this technique which we have used to establish primary cultures of mouse intestinal epithelium. The process involves the gentle dissociation of neonatal mouse small intestine using a collagenase/dispase mix followed by the isolation of small cell aggregates, termed organoids (Figure 2a), which contain a heterogeneous cell population of epithelia and various stromal cell types. The organoids are then cultured on collagen-coated tissue culture dishes. After 24 h cells can be seen proliferating out from adherent organoids. Using this technique, the cultures can survive for up to a month, which goes beyond most other attempts at primary culture. The success of this technique appears to lie in the maintenance of cell–cell and epithelial–stromal interactions, which are absent in cultures of pure populations of epithelial cells. Continued culture of these cells produces colonies of epithelial cells surrounded by stromal cells. By using relatively low quantities (2.5%) of fetal calf serum the stromal cell population can be kept to a minimum but with a consequent reduction in epithelial proliferation. Immunocytochemical staining of the mouse cultures has shown that the majority of cells express cytokeratin 18, a marker for simple epithelium (Figure 2b), and one of the four cytokeratins shown to be expressed in rodent intestinal epithelium[28]. Further characterization of the epithelial cell population reveals the presence of distinct colonies expressing alkaline phosphatase activity, suggestive of a terminally differentiated absorptive enterocyte phenotype (Figure 2c). None of the other three main epithelial cell types could be detected by histochemistry in culture, but we are also able to identify large colonies of what appear to be undifferentiated epithelium. Tait et al.[29] have used immunohistochemistry on rat primary cultures to show populations of smooth-muscle-like cells, myofibroblasts and endothelial cells also present within the cultures at a level of less than 10%.

Grafting of organoids and the generation of a neomucosa

Attempts to identify stem cell populations are severely limited by the fact that as yet no markers exist which are stem cell specific. This has led to various attempts to generate a functional assay for the presence of stem cells. In theory, if a population of cells can be shown to proliferate, produce the full range of differentiated multiple cell lineages found in the intestine and maintain the long-term presence of a proliferative undifferentiated stem cell population, then it can be assumed that stem cells must be present. Until recently, any attempts to generate an intestinal mucosa from dissociated cells have only been successful when using fetal intestinal endoderm along with a fetal mesenchymal support[30]. The use of embryonic endoderm, however, is inappropriate for our particular gene therapeutic approach. In addition, fetal intestinal endoderm is undifferentiated and pluripotent and therefore does not accurately represent intestinal epithelium from later developmental stages when the crypt/villus architecture is generated. Since the application of gene therapy will be directed towards children and adults, the isolation and maintenance of postnatal intestinal stem cells is a necessity. A major step forward was achieved by Tait et al.[31] who used the organoid isolation technique developed by Evans et al.[27] to generate a neomucosa from 20-day-old fetal rat organoids. By day 20 of development in the rat the crypt/villus architecture is already established and crypt stem cells are localized to a distinct niche. The organoids were maintained in culture for up to 4 days before grafting them along with fetal mesenchyme support, under the kidney capsule of adult nude mice. The neomucosa which was generated 14 days after engraftment contained crypt and villi structures which consisted of at least two cell types, namely columnar epithelium and goblet cells. The same group then made an important advance by showing that a neomucosa could be generated from the organoids of 6-day-old postnatal rats grafted subcutaneously into nude mice or isogenic adult rats[32]. After 14 days all four of the major intestinal epithelial cell types could be identified, along with expression of the digestive enzymes, alkaline phosphatase, lactase and sucrase. Further studies using this system revealed that the grafted tissue continued to develop normally with expression patterns and levels of digestive enzymes detected in a similar fashion to that found in intact age-matched intestine[33]. We have used this system to generate a neomucosa from mouse intestinal organoids grafted into immunodeficient *scid* mice. Sections made of the grafted material show a single layer of epithelium displaying a crypt/villus morphology, surrounding a central lumen (Figure 3a). Detection of alkaline phosphatase activity reveals localization to the apical membrane (Figure 3b) identical to that found in intact mouse small intestine (Figure 3c). Mucin-producing goblet cells can also be identified following PAS staining of the sectioned material (Figure 3d) and cells containing large granules consistent with Paneth cell morphology can be found at the base of the crypts. This system now provides us with a relatively simple assay for identifying the presence of intestinal stem cells.

GENE CORRECTION TO INTESTINAL STEM CELLS?

Is chromosomal gene mutation correction a realistic possibility for the intestine? The possibility of using homologous recombination to correct chromosomal

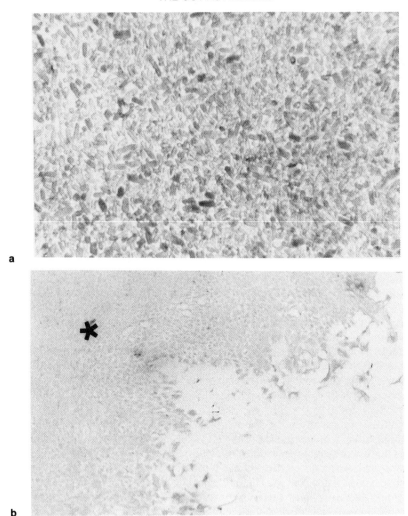

Figure 2 (a) Intestinal organoids isolated from 6 day old CBA mice obtained by enzymatic digestion of small intestine. (b) Primary culture of mouse intestinal organoid. Cells stained for the presence of cytokeratin 18 after 8 days in culture. Asterisk (*) denotes positively stained epithelial colony. (c) Primary cultures of mouse organoids stained for the presence of alkaline phosphatase activity (*) after 4 days in culture

gene mutation has always been an attractive but elusive possibility. Now that the propagation of small intestinal stem cells has been realized the potential of gene mutation correction should be considered in an enhanced light. Targeting the *CFTR* gene ex vivo at high frequency may not be an impossible task. Using insertional gene targeting vectors we can target the mouse *Cftr* gene in ES cells at a frequency of 1 in 6 transfected cells[34]. We are now extending this work to

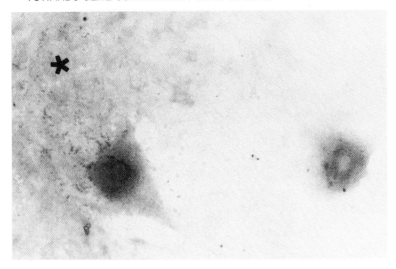

c

Figure 2 *Continued*

specifically target exon 10 of the *Cftr* gene with a vector that carries plasmid sequences flanked by *lox* sites so they can be removed after targeting with Cre recombinase[35]. Our major problem at present is effective transduction of the intestinal cells in culture. One possibility is to use replication-defective adeno-viruses[36], microinjection or improved lipid formulations. Kunzelmann et al.[37] recently reported using liposome- or polyamidoamine-mediated transfection of small fragments of genomic *CFTR* DNA to correct the ΔF508 mutation in trans-formed CF respiratory or pancreatic epithelial cells at a frequency of 1 in 100. Even more encouraging is data from Cole-Strauss et al.[38], who report correction of the mutation in the haemoglobin HB^S allele in lymphoblastoid cells. Using lipofection of a chimeric oligonucleotide composed of DNA and modified RNA residues which spanned the mutation region, they achieved a correction frequency of 20%. As factors which influence homologous recombination are identified and stem cell culture and transfection improves, gene mutation correction will undoubtedly move into a realistic arena with the intestine being one of the first players.

Acknowledgements

This work was funded in part by the Medical Research Council and the Cystic Fibrosis Research Trust, UK. EMS is a CFRT postgraduate student. Thanks to Charles Campbell and Hitendra Patel for all their help in establishing intestinal organoid culture, and Dr Eric Alton and Steve Smith for electrophysiological analysis and discussion. Thanks also to Prof. Dairo Porteous and the members of the Edinburgh CF group.

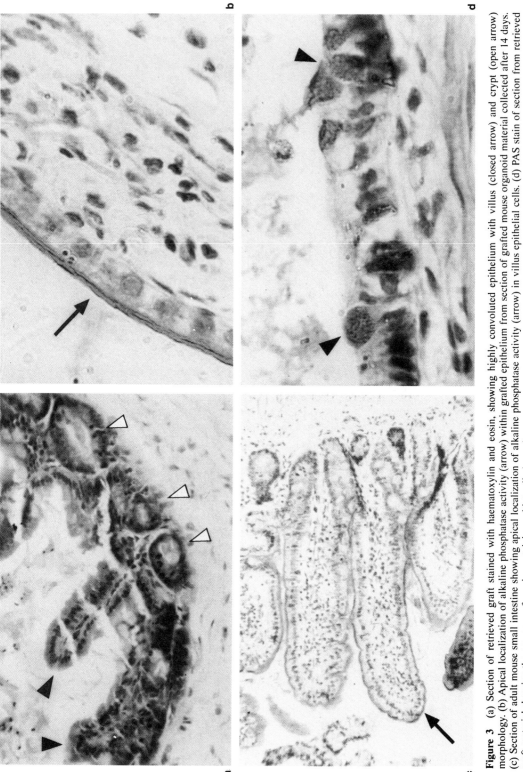

Figure 3 (a) Section of retrieved graft stained with haematoxylin and eosin, showing highly convoluted epithelium with villus (closed arrow) and crypt (open arrow) morphology. (b) Apical localization of alkaline phosphatase activity (arrow) within grafted epithelium from section of grafted mouse organoid material collected after 14 days. (c) Section of adult mouse small intestine showing apical localization of alkaline phosphatase activity (arrow) in villus epithelial cells. (d) PAS stain of section from retrieved graft material showing the presence of mucin containing goblet cells (arrow).

References

1. Dorin JR. Somatic gene therapy: Optimism tempered by reality. Br Med J. 1996;312:323–4.
2. Boat TF, Welsh MJ, Beaudet AL. Cystic fibrosis. In: Scriver CR, Beaudet AL, Sly WS, Valle D, editors. The Metabolic Locus of Inherited Disease. 6th edn. New York: McGraw Hill Inc; 1989: 2649–80.
3. Dodge JA, O'Rawe AM. Energy requirement in cystic fibrosis. In: Dodge JA, Brock DJH, Widdicombe JH, editors. Cystic Fibrosis: Current Topics. Chichester: John Wiley & Sons Ltd; 1994:236–54.
4. Trezise AEO, Buchwald M. In vivo cell-specific expression of the cystic fibrosis transmembrane conductance regulator. Nature. 1991;46:275–9.
5. Sinaasappel M. Present and future treatment modalities for gastrointestinal diseases in cystic fibrosis. Neth J Med. 1995;46:275–9.
6. Dorin JR, Farley R, Webb S et al. A demonstration using mouse models that successful gene therapy for cystic fibrosis requires only partial gene correction. Gene Ther. 1996;3:797–801.
7. Dorin JR, Alton EWFW, Porteous DJ. Mouse models for cystic fibrosis. In: Dodge JA, Brock DJH, Widdicombe JH, editors. Cystic Fibrosis: Current Topics. Chichester: John Wiley & Sons; 1994:3–31.
8. Snouwaert JN, Brigman KK, Latour AM et al. An animal model for cystic fibrosis made by gene targeting. Science. 1992;257:1083–8.
9. Hamosh A, King TM, Rosenstein BJ et al. Cystic fibrosis patients bearing both the common missense mutation Gly-Asp at codon 551 and the delta F508 mutation are clinically indistinguishable from deltaF508 homozygotes except for decreased risk of meconium ileus. Am J Hum Genet. 1992;51:245–50.
10. Delaney SJ, Alton EWFW, Smith SN et al. Cystic fibrosis mice carrying the missense mutation G551D replicate human genotype-phenotype correlations. EMBO J. 1996;15:955–63.
11. Kascer H, Burns J. Molecular basis of dominance. Genetics. 1981;97:638–66.
12. Dorin JR, Stevenson BJ, Fleming S, Alton EWFW, Dickinson P, Porteous DJ. Long-term survival of the exon 10 insertional cystic fibrosis mutant mouse is a consequence of low level residual wild-type CFTR gene expression. Mamm Genome. 1994;5:465–72.
13. Smith SN, Steel DM, Middleton PG et al. Bioelectric characteristics of the exon 10 insertional cystic fibrosis mouse: comparison with humans. Am J Physiol. 1995;268:C297–307.
14. Zhou L, Dey CR, Wert SE, DuVall MD, Frizzell RA, Whitsett JA. Correction of lethal intestinal defect in a mouse model of cystic fibrosis by human CFTR. Science. 1993;266:1705–8.
15. Rommens JM, Iannuzzi MC, Kerem B-S et al. Identification of the cystic fibrosis gene: chromosome walking and jumping. Science. 1989;245:1059–65.
16. Caplen NJ, Alton EWFW, Middleton PG et al. Liposome-mediated CFTR gene transfer to the nasal epithelium of patients with cystic fibrosis. Nature Med. 1995;1:39–46.
17. Zabner JL, Couture A, Smith AE, Welsh MJ. Correction of cAMP-stimulated fluid secretion in cystic fibrosis airway epithelia: efficiency of adenovirus-mediated gene transfer in vitro. Hum Gene Ther. 1994;5:585–93.
18. Crystal RG, McElvaney NG, Rosenfeld MA et al. Administration of an adenovirus containing human CFTR cDNA to the respiratory tract of individuals with cystic fibrosis. Nature Genet. 1994;8:42–51.
19. Knowles MR, Hohneker KW, Zhaoqing Z et al. A controlled study of adenoviral-vector-mediated gene transfer in the nasal epithelium of patients with cystic fibrosis. N Engl J Med. 1995;333: 823–31.
20. Grubb BR, Pickles RJ, Ye H et al. Inefficient gene transfer by adenovirus vector to cystic fibrosis airway epithelia of mice and humans. Nature. 1994;371:802–6.
21. Alton EWFW, Middleton PG, Caplen NJ et al. Non-invasive liposome-mediated gene delivery can correct the ion transport defect in cystic fibrosis mutant mice. Nature Genet. 1993;5:135–42.
22. Schedl A, Montoliu L, Kelsey G, Schutz G. A yeast artificial chromosome covering the tyrosinase gene confers copy number-dependent expression in transgenic mice. Nature. 1993;362:258–61.
23. Lau C, Soriano H, Ledley FD et al. Retroviral gene transfer into the intestinal epithelium. Hum Gene Ther. 1995;6:1145–51.
24. del Buono R, Mandir N, Wright NA. Approaches to gene therapy in the gut: retrovirus mediated gene transfer in a model of gastrointestinal development. Gastroenterology. 1994;106:381.
25. Patel HRH, Brierley CH, Burchell B et al. Transplantation of small intestinal stem cells after genetic modification. Gastroenterology. 1995;108:A1238.

26. Bates RC, Buret A, van Helden DF, Horton MA, Burns GF. Apoptosis induced by inhibition of intercellular contact. J Cell Biol. 1994;125:403–15.
27. Evans GS, Flint N, Somers AS, Eyden B, Potten CS. The development of a method for the preparation of rat intestinal epithelial cell primary cultures. J Cell Sci. 1992;101:219–31.
28. Flint N, Pemberton PW, Lobley RW, Evans GS. Cytokeratin expression in epithelial cells isolated from the crypt and villus regions of the rodent small intestine. Epithelial Cell Biol. 1994;3:16–23.
29. Tait IS, Flint N, Evans GS, Potten CS, Hopwood D, Campbell FC. Progress with small bowel enterocyte culture and transplantation. Transplant Proc. 1992;24:1061–4.
30. Kedinger M, Simon-Assmann PM, Lacroix B, Marxer A, Hauri HP, Haffen K. Fetal gut mesenchyme induces differentiation of cultured intestinal endodermal and crypt cells. Dev Biol. 1986;113:474–83.
31. Tait IS, Evans GS, Kedinger M, Flint N, Potten CS, Campbell FC. Progressive morphogenesis in vivo after transplantation of cultured small bowel epithelium. Cell Transplant. 1994;3:33–40.
32. Tait IS, Flint N, Campbell FC, Evans GS. Generation of neomucosa in vivo by transplantation of dissociated rat postnatal small intestinal epithelium. Differentiation. 1994;56:91–100.
33. Tait IS, Penny JI, Campbell FC. Does neomucosa induced by small bowel stem cell transplantation have adequate function? Am J Surg. 1995;169:120–5.
34. Dickinson P, Kimber W, Kilanowski F, Stevenson B, Porteous DJ, Dorin JR. High frequency gene targeting using insertional vectors. Hum Mol Genet. 1993;2:1299–302.
35. Lakso M, Sauer B, Mosinger B et al. Targeted oncogene activation by site-specific recombination in transgenic mice. Proc Natl Acad Sci USA. 1992;89:6232–6.
36. Fujita A, Sakagami K, Kanegae Y, Saito I, Kobayashi I. Gene targeting with a replication-defective adenovirus vector. J Virol. 1995;69:6180–90.
37. Kunzelmann K, Legendre J, Knoell DL, Escobar LC, Xu Z, Gruenert DC. Gene targeting of CFTR DNA in CF epithelial cells. Gene Ther. 1996;3:859–67.
38. Cole-Strauss A, Kyonggeun Y, Xiang Y et al. Correction of the mutation responsible for sickle cell anemia by an RNA-DNA oligonucleotide. Science. 1996;273:1386–9.

Section II
Growth and development

5
Gastrointestinal development: an overview

S. J. HENNING

INTRODUCTION

For many years, research in the field of gastrointestinal development has leaned heavily on rodent models. Much of the central work in the 1960s to 1980s utilized laboratory rats, and more recently, mice have come into favour because they are more amenable to genetic manipulation. Pigs have also constituted an important large animal model whose physiology is in many ways more similar to that of humans. Inevitably, because of the much greater costs of procurement and mainten-ance, fewer studies are performed in pigs than in rodents. Ultimately, a goal of all research in animal models is to throw light on the human condition, and in this regard, the field of gastrointestinal development is at an exciting stage. Because of technological developments, some of the major findings from animal models can now be investigated directly in human infants. Unfortunately, due to space limitations, the current review will focus primarily on studies in rodents, with only brief allusions to parallel findings in pigs and humans. Readers are referred elsewhere to more comprehensive coverage of the topic of gastrointestinal develop-ment in pigs and humans[1].

SUMMARY OF GASTROINTESTINAL DEVELOPMENT

In laboratory rodents the entire gastrointestinal tract displays two major phases of development. First, there is the late gestational phase in which virtually all organs of the gastrointestinal tract undergo morphological maturation. During this phase, functional maturation tends to be limited to the expression of proteins required for the digestion and absorption of the components of milk. The second phase of maturation begins during the third postnatal week, coincident with the onset of weaning. At this time, morphological changes are relatively minor, but dramatic functional changes occur as the entire gastrointestinal tract acquires proteins required for digestion and absorption of solid food. Complete details of

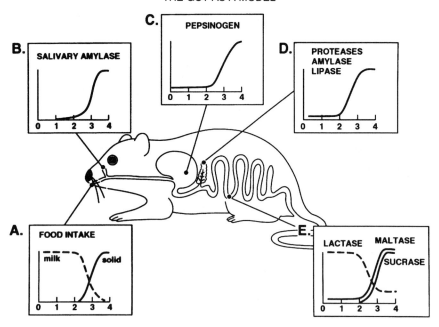

Figure 1 Representative changes throughout the rodent gastrointestinal tract during the third and fourth postnatal weeks. All panels show postnatal ages in weeks on the axis and the designated function on the ordinate. (A) Time course of weaning. (B) Parotid amylase as an example of salivary maturation. (C) Changes in content of pepsinogen in gastric mucosa. (D) General pattern of pancreatic maturation as assessed by activities of trypsin, chymotrypsin, amylase and lipase in intestinal lumen. (E) Patterns of maturation in the small intestine illustrated by changing expression of brush border disaccharidases. Drawn from data shown in Ref. 2

these changes can be found elsewhere[1,2], but examples from throughout the tract are shown in Figure 1.

In the small intestine, examples of functions that appear during late gestation can be classified according to their roles in digestion and absorption of the macronutrients of milk. Thus, with respect to carbohydrate, lactase-phlorizin hydrolase (LPH) expression is activated[1,3], as is the sodium-dependent glucose cotransporter (SGLT-1), which transports both the glucose and galactose moieties released as a result of LPH action on milk lactose[4]. As lipid is the major energy source of milk, it is not surprising that proteins involved with absorption and transport of lipid are expressed at birth as a result of activation of their respective genes in the prenatal period. Examples from this category include both intestinal and liver fatty acid binding proteins (I-FABP and L-FABP) as well as various apolipoproteins including apo A-1, apo A-IV and apoB[1]. With respect to protein digestion and absorption, the lack of gastric and pancreatic proteases (Figure 1) is associated with a high capacity for pinocytotic absorption of intact proteins in the small intestine[1,2]. Despite this special mechanism, amino acid transporters appear to be fully expressed by the time of birth[1].

At the time of weaning, it is the carbohydrate component of diet that changes most dramatically (from lactose to starch and sucrose). This change is associated with the maturation of both digestive and absorptive capacities for the carbohydrates of the solid diet. Examples of proteins whose expression increases markedly at this time are sucrase-isomaltase (SI), maltase-glucoamylase (MGA), trehalase and GLUT-5, the fructose transporter[1]. For those that have been studied at the mRNA level, namely SI, trehalase and GLUT-5, the changes in functional activity are reflected by changes of gene expression[1,5,6]. As noted above, most proteins involved in absorption and transport of triglycerides and amino acids are expressed from birth onward. Thus, when gastric and pancreatic hydrolases for dietary lipid and protein mature (see Figure 1), the adult patterns of digestion and absorption of these macronutrients are complete. The only significant intestinal change associated with lipid digestion and absorption at the time of weaning is the marked increase in the expression of proteins involved in the ileal absorption of bile acids, namely the apical transporter[7] and the cytosolic bile acid binding protein[8], also known as ileal lipid binding protein[9].

Although the major changes in the small intestine during the third postnatal week reflect the acquisition of mature digestive and absorptive capacities, certain functions peculiar to the suckling phase decline at this time. The most notable example of a declining function is lactase hydrolysis associated with decreased levels of LPH enzyme. The latter is reflective of changes of various parameters including transcription, translation and protein turnover[1,3]. The recent demonstration that a *cis*-acting element of the LPH gene is associated with hypolactasia in humans[10] represents one of the exciting extensions of knowledge from animal models to humans. Another example of a function that declines at the time of weaning is the capacity for pinocytotic uptake of intact proteins[1,2]. Molecular details of this interesting cellular change have not yet been elucidated.

REGULATION OF INTESTINAL ONTOGENY

Detailed analysis of this extensive topic is beyond the scope of this review, and readers are referred elsewhere[1,2]. My main goal here is to present the concept that, as for other critical organ systems, normal maturation of intestinal function has evolved a multiplicity of alternative control mechanisms. Although the term 'functionally redundant' has come into common parlance, Hochgeschwender and Brennan[11] have pointed out that this term is misleading in the context of evolution. Specifically, although certain control mechanisms may appear to be redundant when studied in laboratory rodents, these mechanisms in fact may have conferred adaptive advantages when organisms were under selective pressure. Thus, for the purpose of the current discussion, the term 'multiplicity' is proposed as being more appropriate than 'redundancy'. Selected examples of such multiplicity are given below.

Studies in C/EBPα-deficient mice

CCAAT enhancer binding protein-alpha (C/EBPα) is a transcription factor which appears to play a causal role in differentiation of a number of tissues[12,13]. In the small intestine, expression of C/EBPα increases prenatally[14] coincident with the onset of expression of genes such as LPH, I-FABP, L-FABP, apo A-IV, apoB, etc. (see above). Since several of these genes have been reported to have C/EBP sites in their promoters, we decided to capitalize on the existence of a C/EBPα-deficient mouse[15] to determine whether C/EBPα is essential in the developmental onset of transcription of this group of genes. Thus, RNA was extracted from intestines of newborn C/EBPα-deficient (−/−) mice and their heterozygote (+/−) and wild-type (+/+) littermates, and levels of mRNA for LPH, SGLT-1, GLUT-2, I-FABP, apoB and apo A-IV were quantified by Northern blotting[16]. To our surprise, none of the mRNAs were reduced in the −/− mice. Since other members of the C/EBP family recognize the same DNA binding element[17], the most obvious explanation for these findings is that in the absence of C/EBPα, one of the other isoforms serves an alternative regulatory function.

Glucocorticoids versus intrinsic timing

As reviewed elsewhere[1], several elegant studies using fetal intestine isografted into adult hosts have shown that functional changes which normally occur in the intestinal epithelium during the third postnatal week will occur in the absence of specific ontogenic signals from either the lumen or the circulation. This has led to the concept that one or more timing mechanisms are intrinsic to the intestinal mucosa[1], or, in other words, that intestinal maturation is 'hard-wired'[18]. The question of whether there is a single, master timing mechanism or separate mechanisms for each gene represents an exciting area of current and future research. The cellular location of this mechanism (or these mechanisms) is also a topic of substantial interest. Recent work by Duluc et al.[19] indicates that, at least for the decline of lactase expression, the timing mechanism is within the endoderm and is presumably a function of the epithelial stem cells. Extension of such investigations to other aspects of intestinal development is eagerly awaited.

In addition to intrinsic timing, there is also extensive evidence that glucocorticoids are involved in the functional maturation of the intestinal epithelium[1,2,20]. Circulating levels of endogenous glucocorticoid surge just prior to the enzymatic changes[2]. However, ablation of this surge by adrenalectomy alters the rate of change, but not the timing of the initiation of change (see Figure 2). On the other hand, precocious administration of exogenous glucocorticoid during the first or second postnatal week elicits precocious maturation[1,2,20,21]. Recent evidence suggests that the molecular pathway of precocious maturation is distinct from that of normal (intrinsic) maturation[22,23]. We speculate that this duality of control may have conferred a selective advantage during evolution. Specifically, the stress of loss of the mother (thus, the milk supply) would cause a precocious surge of glucocorticoid in the offspring, thereby eliciting precocious intestinal maturation, which would allow an early switch to solid food. Thyroxine almost certainly contributes to this multiplicity of controls in the sense that its presence greatly enhances the ability of the intestine to respond to glucocorticoids[24].

In species such as pigs and humans, in which the intestinal epithelium is almost fully mature at birth[1], there may be an analogous duality between intrinsic timing mechanisms and glucocorticoids. Human intestine, just like rodent intestine, has been shown to undergo at least some aspects of maturation when xenografted into mice[25–27], indicating the presence of intrinsic timing. To our knowledge, analogous studies with pig intestine have not been reported. On the other hand,

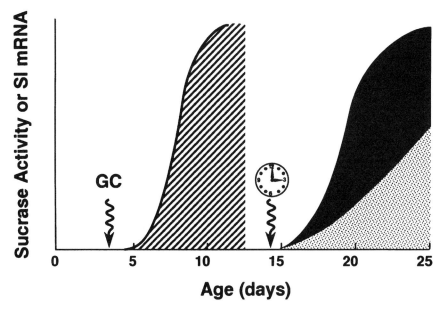

Figure 2 Pictorial representation of the influence of glucocorticoids as compared with an intrinsic timing mechanism on developmental changes of sucrase-isomaltase (SI) expression in rat small intestine. Dark curve shows normal development; stippled curve shows effect of adrenalectomy, i.e. glucocorticoid-independent maturation. This is believed to be initiated by an intrinsic timing mechanism (shown as 'clock'). Hatched curve shows precocious induction by exogenous glucocorticoids (GC). Drawn from data in Ref. 21 and information reviewed in Refs 1, 2 and 20

there is good evidence that glucocorticoids can enhance maturation in pig intestine[1]. Recent studies using the triple lumen perfusion technique in preterm human infants have shown that infants born to mothers who received prenatal glucocorticoids have significantly more mature intestinal function[28]. In the term infant, the surge of cortisol accompanying normal delivery may well be critical in gut maturation. Support for this suggestion comes from studies by Sangild et al.[29], who compared gut maturation in pigs delivered vaginally (when there is a large surge of cortisol) with that in animals delivered by Caesarean section (where there is only a modest rise of cortisol). Representative data from these studies are shown in Figure 3. Thus, in early maturing species, just as in altricial species like laboratory rodents, the stress/glucocorticoid effect on intestinal maturation may constitute an important auxiliary control mechanism.

Role of EGF and TGF-α in intestinal growth and development

Epidermal growth factor (EGF) and transforming growth factor-α (TGF-α) are the two most studied members of a family of growth factors that now includes a total of five distinct peptides[30,31]. In adult animals, the major role of EGF and TGF-α in the gastrointestinal tract appears to be in stimulating repair after mucosal

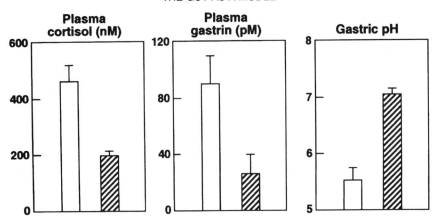

Figure 3 Effect of mode of delivery on plasma cortisol and gastric maturation in preterm pigs. Fifteen days before term, pregnant sows were either induced to deliver vaginally (open column) or were subjected to Caesarean section (hatched column). Panels show data for cortisol and amidated (bioactive) gastrin in plasma of the piglets as well as pH of their gastric fluid. Drawn from data in Ref. 29

injury[31,32]. During ontogeny, they also seem to be important for mucosal growth[33,34]. Koldovsky has recently reviewed the evidence in favour of a specific role for EGF in the postnatal growth of the rodent small intestine. Critical elements of the evidence include first, EGF is abundant in milk and can be absorbed intact during the suckling period; second EGF receptors are present in the intestinal epithelium from birth onward; and third, when luminal EGF is increased or decreased during the suckling period, intestinal growth is stimulated and inhibited, respectively[33]. The fact that the EGF receptor is localized on the basolateral surface of enterocytes at all stages of development[33,35] emphasizes the importance of the permeability of the suckling gut in allowing milk EGF to exert its growth-stimulating effect[35]. Interestingly, the endogenous expression of EGF in the intestine is low during the suckling period and increases after weaning[36]. Conversely, TGF-α which is not present in rat milk, is expressed at high levels in the crypts of both suckling and adult rats[36]. Moreover, a role for TGF-α in the regulation of intestinal growth is consistent with the intestinal hyperplasia observed in transgenic mice which over-express TGF-α[30]. Since EGF and TGF-α are known to utilize the same receptor[30], the idea that they represent another example of multiplicity of controls is obvious. Specifically, it can be argued that during the suckling period, endogenous production of TGF-α in the intestinal epithelium serves as an alternative growth regulator for the scenario in which normal quantities of EGF are not present in mother's milk.

Recent data from a number of interesting mice generated by gene targeting suggest that the multiplicity may extend beyond EGF and TGF-α to other ligands in the family and/or to other receptors within the EGF receptor family. In view of the duality already noted between milk EGF and endogenous TGF-α, it is not surprising that intestinal growth is not affected in TGF-α-null animals[37,38]. However, based on the present dogma of a shared receptor, it is surprising that when the gene for the EGF receptor was subjected to a targeted disruption[39–41], two of the three lines of mice that survived postnatally showed no intestinal phenotype[40,41]. The third[39] had evidence of shorter and fewer villi and of mucosal ulceration. An important point to note, however, is that the survival of these receptor-null mice was critically dependent on the genetic background. Animals from certain backgrounds (notably CF-1 and 129/sv) all died in utero[40,41]. It is possible that these strains have reduced levels of alternative growth factor/receptor systems and thus are much more sensitive to the loss of stimulation by EGF and TGF-α through the EGF receptor. Intestine-specific disruption of the receptor would be necessary to investigate this suggestion.

Clearly, elucidation of the complete details of the EGF/TGF-α influences on intestinal growth and development is a fertile area of research. In addition to the questions posed above, other matters of interest include the physiological significance of the rise in abundance of EGF receptor in the intestine at the time of weaning[42]; whether the numerous reports of precocious intestinal maturation following systemic administration of EGF to suckling rodents[1,34,43] represent physiological as opposed to pharmacological actions (see Ref. 33 for good definition of 'physiological'); and whether the different substrates that have been identified for the EGF receptor tyrosine kinase in the developing intestine[42,44] are indicative of distinct signal transduction pathways for effects on differentiation as compared with effects on proliferation.

METHODS TO STUDY INTESTINAL GROWTH AND DEVELOPMENT

In reviewing the methods that have been and will be important in furthering our understanding of this complex area, it is important to keep in mind that in the intestine, developmental changes are superimposed on a constant pattern of proliferation, differentiation and apoptosis within the epithelium. Moreover, this dynamic cell population is organized in a complex architecture having intimate relationships with the underlying matrix and, in turn, with the stromal cells of mesenchymal origin (see Chapter 13). In view of these complexities, it is not surprising that no one has yet successfully recapitulated intestinal development in vitro. Although numerous rodent intestinal cell lines have now been generated, none is capable of mimicking the changes of gene expression seen in the developing intestine in vivo. Thus, although valuable for studying basic processes such as proliferation, migration, intracellular processing, etc., these cell lines have found little place in studies designed to understand the regulation of intestinal development.

In the absence of amenable in vitro systems, investigators have been forced to rely upon a variety of in vivo approaches. Many of these approaches already have been mentioned in the preceding sections. For example, in assessing roles of hormones and growth factors, investigators typically began with classical addition and ablation experiments[1,2,20,33,34]. The ability to graft fetal intestine from rodents (reviewed in Ref. 1) and then humans[25–27] represented important advances. Further refinements of the grafting technique allowed it to be used on various combinations of endoderm and mesoderm from the gastrointestinal tract[1,19] and thus to identify their respective roles in gut maturation. Likewise, the use of aggregation chimeras[1,45] (see also Chapter 1) greatly advanced our understanding of the behaviour of intestinal stem cells during the developmental period and in adulthood.

Since the initial studies in the late 1980s, regulation of gene expression in the developing intestine has been analysed extensively using transgenic mice[1,45] (see also Chapters 19 and 21). The 1990s have seen the advent of two very elegant techniques, namely the transgenic/chimeric approach, which allows examination of either increased or decreased expression of a given gene within a limited cell population of the epithelium[46], and the use of homologous recombination in embryonic stem cells to generate mice with targeted gene disruptions (see examples above). A further combination of transgenic and targeting technologies now makes it at least theoretically possible to generate tissue-specific[47] and/or inducible[48] gene disruptions. To our knowledge, this particular approach has not yet been applied to the developing intestine, although such application is certainly imminent and exciting. Likewise, the advent of gene replacement[49], which allows investigators to determine whether two genes can substitute for each other, will provide an elegant approach to some of the issues raised earlier in this review regarding the multiplicity of alternative controls of intestinal development.

While many of the recent approaches discussed above are applicable only in mice, there also have been significant advances in techniques for studying human intestinal development. Particularly notable is the use of reverse transcription–polymerase chain reaction (RT–PCR) on biopsy samples to study gene expression in the developing small intestine[50,51]. Even less invasive is the use of double or triple lumen perfusion to study both digestive and absorptive functions in the human infant, including the preterm infant[52,53]. An exciting possibility is raised by the recent demonstration that RNA can be extracted from desquamated epithelial cells collected during triple lumen perfusion (R.J. Shulman, personal communication). This, combined with existing RT–PCR methods[51], should allow repetitive sampling in individual infants and thus, for the first time, offer the possibility of documenting longitudinal changes in gene expression in the developing human intestine.

Returning to the rodent model, 3–4 years ago we were struck by the fact that all the new technologies (transgenic, chimeric, chimeric/transgenic and gene targeting) rested on manipulations made very early in development (specifically, the fertilized egg in the case of transgenics and the blastocyst in the case of chimeras and gene targeting). In view of this tight temporal limitation, we proposed that there may be significant advantages to a new type of genetic engineering that could be applied at any time during development. To this end we initiated a series of experiments designed to investigate the feasibility of luminal delivery of genes to intestinal stem cells. In order to achieve continued expression, we reasoned that the gene of interest not only needed to be delivered to the stem cells, but also needed to integrate into the host chromosome. As retroviruses currently are the only vector that achieve the latter, they seemed the obvious vehicle for gene delivery. Our detailed experience with this methodology to date is reviewed elsewhere[54,55]. Suffice it to say here that successful gene transfer has been achieved, although presently the overall efficiency of the process is very low. Ongoing studies are designed to improve the efficiency in the belief that it indeed would be a useful addition to the arsenal of technologies available for the study of intestinal development. Particular advantages compared with other approaches are that genes could be introduced any time from fetal life onward; that gene transfer can be purposefully directed to any region along the length of the gastrointestinal tract; because only the targeted segment is modified, the remaining intestine serves as the normal control; since the remaining intestine is normal, manipulations that disrupt digestion or absorption in the experimental segment will not compromise the overall nutrition of the animal; unlike transgenics and gene targeting, the procedure for retrovirally mediated gene transfer does not require specialized equipment (e.g. for microinjection); and finally, this technology should be equally applicable in all species, including humans. The latter points to another important application, namely the potential for using the intestinal epithelium as a site for somatic gene therapy. This topic is discussed in detail elsewhere[54].

SUMMARY

Some 20 years ago, intestinal development appeared to be a relatively simple process with a limited number of definitive control mechanisms[20]. Now it is clear that mammals have evolved multiple layers of alternative control mechanisms. Unravelling these, particularly at the molecular level, has only just begun and presents an enormous challenge for the future. Likewise, the continual use of knowledge generated in rodents to push the frontiers of research in human intestinal development is of great importance. Although there are now many new and elegant approaches for use in both animal models and humans, additional techniques still should be pursued in the confidence that new methods almost always yield new insights. The latter is certainly attested by numerous examples throughout this exciting and timely symposium.

Acknowledgements

Original research in this review was supported by NIH grant numbers R37-HD14094 and R01-DK44646. The individuals who contributed to these studies can be found in the relevant references. On the EGF/TGF-α topic the author gratefully acknowledges helpful discussions with Drs Otakar Koldovsky, Brent Polk, David Lee, Robert Coffey and John Thompson. I also thank Lucy L. Leeper for help with references and for critical comments on the manuscript.

Dedication

This paper is dedicated to the memory of two colleagues who passed away during this last year. Both were pioneers in critical eras of research on intestinal development. The first, Dr Norman Kretchmer, generated much of the earliest data regarding sucrase and lactase development and the influence of glucocorticoids (reviewed in Ref. 20). He served as my postdoctoral mentor and remained a close colleague and staunch supporter throughout my career. He not only was responsible for introducing me to the field of intestinal development, but also stimulated me to think about general questions regarding the evolutionary significance of control mechanisms. The second, Dr Edward H. Birkenmeier, was responsible for mapping a number of intestinal and hepatic genes and for generating the first transgenic mice designed to investigate intestinal gene expression (reviewed in Ref. 1). He was a valued collaborator and friend who was particularly generous with his time and materials and who was always willing to help us, especially during the early days of our forays into molecular aspects of intestinal development.

References

1. Henning SJ, Rubin DC, Shulman RJ. Ontogeny of the intestinal mucosa. In: Johnson LR, editor. Physiology of the Gastrointestinal Tract, 3rd edn. New York: Raven Press, 1994:571–610.
2. Henning SJ. Postnatal development: coordination of feeding, digestion, and metabolism. Am J Physiol. 1981;241:G199–214.
3. Montgomery RK, Büller HA, Rings EHHM, Grand RJ. Lactose intolerance and the genetic regulation of intestinal lactase-phlorizin hydrolase. FASEB J. 1991;5:2824–32.
4. Wright EM, Turk E, Zabel B, Mundlos S, Dyer J. Molecular genetics of intestinal glucose transport. J Clin Invest. 1991;88:1435–40.
5. Galand G, L'Horset F, Longis Y, Perret C. Trehalase gene expression during postnatal development of rabbit intestine and kidney: effects of glucocorticoids. Am J Physiol. 1995;269:G833–41.
6. Rand EB, DePaoli AM, Davidson NO, Bell GI, Burant CF. Sequence, tissue distribution, and functional characterization of the rat fructose transporter GLUT5. Am J Physiol. 1993;264: G1169–76.
7. Shneider BL, Dawson PA, Christie D-M, Hardikar W, Wong MH, Suchy FJ. Cloning and molecular characterization of the ontogeny of a rat ileal sodium-dependent bile acid transporter. J Clin Invest. 1995;95:745–54.
8. Gong Y-Z, Kato T, Schwartz DA, Norris JS, Wilson FA. Ontogenic and glucocorticoid-accelerated expression of rat 14 kDa bile acid-binding protein. Anat Rec. 1996;245:532–8.
9. Sacchettini JC, Hauft SM, Van Camp SL, Cistola DP, Gordon JI. Developmental and structural studies of an intracellular lipid binding protein expressed in the ileal epithelium. J Biol Chem. 1990;265:19199–207.
10. Wang Y, Harvey CB, Pratt WS et al. The lactase persistence/non-persistence polymorphism is controlled by a cis-acting element. Hum Mol Genet. 1995;4:657–62.
11. Hochgeschwender U, Brennan MB. Redundant genes? Nature Genet. 1994;8:219–20.
12. Darlington GJ, Wang N, Hanson RW. C/EBPα: a critical regulator of genes governing integrative metabolic processes. Curr Opin Genet Dev. 1995;5:565–70.
13. Umek RM, Friedman AD, McKnight SL. CCAAT-enhancer binding protein: a component of a differentiation switch. Science. 1991;251:288–92.
14. Birkenmeier EH, Gwynn B, Howard S et al. Tissue-specific expression, developmental regulation, and genetic mapping of the gene encoding CCAAT/enhancer binding protein. Genes Dev. 1989;3:1146–56.
15. Wang N, Finegold MJ, Bradley A et al. Impaired energy homeostasis in C/EBPα knockout mice. Science. 1995;269:1108–12.
16. Oesterreicher TJ, Leeper LL, Darlington GJ, Henning SJ. Mice lacking C/EBPα show normal perinatal expression of various intestinal mRNAs. Gastroenterology. 1996;110:A826.
17. Cao Z, Umek RM, McKnight SL. Regulated expression of three C/EBP isoforms during adipose conversion of 3T3/L1 cells. Genes Dev. 1991;5:1538–52.
18. Diamond JM. Hard-wired local triggering of intestinal enzyme expression. Nature. 1986;324: 408.
19. Duluc I, Freund J-N, Leberquier C, Kedinger M. Fetal endoderm primarily holds the temporal and positional information required for mammalian intestinal development. J Cell Biol. 1994; 126:211–21.
20. Henning SJ, Kretchmer N. Development of intestinal function in mammals. Enzyme. 1973;15: 3–23.

21. Nanthakumar NN, Henning SJ. Ontogeny of sucrase-isomaltase gene expression in rat intestine: responsiveness to glucocorticoids. Am J Physiol. 1993;264:G306–11.
22. Nanthakumar NN, Henning SJ. Distinguishing normal and glucocorticoid-induced maturation of intestine using bromodeoxyuridine. Am J Physiol. 1995;268:G139–45.
23. Tung JY, Traber PG. Molecular mechanisms of sucrase-isomaltase (SI) gene transcription during intestinal development. Gastroenterology. 1996;110:A846.
24. McDonald MC, Henning SJ. Synergistic effects of thyroxine and dexamethasone on enzyme ontogeny in rat small intestine. Pediatr Res. 1992;32:306–11.
25. Winter HS, Hendren RB, Fox CH et al. Human intestine matures as nude mouse xenograft. Gastroenterology. 1991;100:89–98.
26. Shmakov AN, Morey AL, Ferguson DJP, Fleming KA, O'Brien JA, Savidge TC. Conventional patterns of human intestinal proliferation in a severe-combined immunodeficient xenograft model. Differentiation. 1995;59:321–30.
27. Savidge TC, Morey AL, Ferguson DJP, Fleming KA, Shmakov AN, Phillips AD. Human intestinal development in a severe-combined immunodeficient xenograft model. Differentiation. 1995;58: 361–71.
28. Shulman RJ, Schanler RJ, Heitkemper MA. Antenatal glucocorticoids decrease intestinal permeability in low birth weight infants. Pediatr Res. 1994;35:255A.
29. Sangild PT, Hilsted L, Nexo E, Fowden AL, Silver M. Vaginal birth vs elective Caesarean section: effects on gastric function in the neonate. Exp Physiol. 1995;80:147–57.
30. Lee DC, Fenton SE, Berkowitz EA, Hissong MA. Transforming growth factor α: expression, regulation, and biological activities. Pharmacol Rev. 1995;47:51–85.
31. Barnard JA, Beauchamp RD, Russell WE, Dubois RN, Coffey RJ. Epidermal growth factor-related peptides and their relevance to gastrointestinal pathophysiology. Gastroenterology. 1995; 108:564–80.
32. Playford RJ, Wright NA. Why is epidermal growth factor present in the gut lumen? Gut. 1996; 38:303–5.
33. Koldovsky O. The potential physiological significance of milk-borne hormonally active substances for the neonate. J Mam Gland Biol Neoplasia. 1996;1:317–22.
34. Xu R-J. Development of the newborn GI tract and its relation to colostrum/milk intake: a review. Reprod Fertil Dev. 1996;8:35–48.
35. Thompson JF, van den Berg M, Stokkers PCF. Developmental regulation of epidermal growth factor receptor kinase in rat intestine. Gastroenterology. 1994;107:1278–87.
36. Dvorak B, Holubec H, LeBouton AV, Wilson JM, Koldovsky O. Epidermal growth factor and transforming growth factor-α mRNA in rat small intestine: in situ hybridization study. FEBS Lett. 1994;352:291–5.
37. Luetteke NC, Qiu TH, Peiffer RL, Oliver P, Smithies O, Lee DC. TGFα deficiency results in hair follicle and eye abnormalities in targeted and waved-1 mice. Cell. 1993;73:263–78.
38. Mann GB, Fowler KJ, Gabriel A, Nice EC, Williams RL, Dunn AR. Mice with a null mutation of the TGFα gene have abnormal skin architecture, wavy hair, and curly whiskers and often develop corneal inflammation. Cell. 1993;73:249–61.
39. Miettinen PJ, Berger JE, Meneses J et al. Epithelial immaturity and multiorgan failure in mice lacking epidermal growth factor receptor. Nature. 1995;376:337–41.
40. Threadgill DW, Dlugosz AA, Hansen LA et al. Targeted disruption of mouse EGF receptor: effect of genetic background on mutant phenotype. Science. 1995;269:230–4.
41. Sibilia M, Wagner EF. Strain-dependent epithelial defects in mice lacking the EGF receptor. Science. 1995;269:234–8.
42. Polk DB. Ontogenic regulation of phospholipase C-γ1 activity and expression in the rat small intestine. Gastroenterology. 1994;107:109–16.
43. Foltzer-Jourdainne C, Garaud J-C, Nsi-Emvo E, Raul F. Epidermal growth factor and the maturation of intestinal sucrase in suckling rats. Am J Physiol. 1993;265:G459–66.
44. Polk DB. Shc is a substrate of the rat intestinal epidermal growth factor receptor tyrosine kinase. Gastroenterology. 1995;109:1845–51.
45. Gordon JI, Schmidt GH, Roth KA. Studies of intestinal stem cells using normal, chimeric, and transgenic mice. FASEB J. 1992;6:3039–50.
46. Wong MH, Hermiston ML, Syder AJ, Gordon JI. Forced expression of the tumor suppressor adenomatosis polyposis coli protein induces disordered cell migration in the intestinal epithelium. Proc Natl Acad Sci USA. 1996;93:9588–93.

47. Gu H, Marth JD, Orban PC, Mossmann H, Rajewsky K. Deletion of a DNA polymerase β gene segment in T cells using cell type-specific gene targeting. Science. 1994;265:103–6.
48. Kühn R, Schwenk F, Aguet M, Rajewsky K. Inducible gene targeting in mice. Science. 1995; 269:1427–9.
49. Hanks M, Wurst W, Anson-Cartwright L, Auerbach AB, Joyner AL. Rescue of the *En-1* mutant phenotype by replacement of *En-1* with *En-2*. Science. 1995;269:679–82.
50. Nichols BL, Dudley MA, Nichols VN *et al.* Effects of malnutrition on expression and activity of lactase in children. Gastroenterology. 1997;112:742–51.
51. Wang Y, Harvey C, Rousset M, Swallow DM. Expression of human intestinal mRNA transcripts during development: analysis by a semiquantitative RNA polymerase chain reaction method. Pediatr Res. 1994;36:514–21.
52. Shulman RJ, Feste A, Ou C. Absorption of lactose, glucose polymers, or combination in premature infants. J Pediatr. 1995;127:626–31.
53. Stathos TH, Shulman RJ, Schanler RJ, Abrams SA. Effects of carbohydrates on calcium absorption in premature infants. Pediatr Res. 1996;39:666–70.
54. Henning SJ. Gene transfer into the intestinal epithelium. Adv Drug Del Rev. 1995;17:341–7.
55. Jacomino M, Lau C, James SZ, Shukla P, Henning SJ. Gene transfer into fetal rat intestine. Hum Gene Ther. 1996;7:1757–62.

6
Recent insights into roles for EGF receptor ligands in epithelial cell systems

R. J. COFFEY, R. CHINERY, J. BARNARD, L. GANGAROSA,
N. SIZEMORE and P. J. DEMPSEY

INTRODUCTION TO THE EGFR FAMILY AND THEIR LIGANDS

The full complement of mammalian EGF receptors (EGFRs) and their cognate ligands are depicted in Figure 1. These are also referred to as *human EGFR* homologues (HER 1–4). The greatest degree of homology is found in the cytoplasmic tail of these receptors[1]. Epidermal growth factor (EGF), transforming growth factor-α (TGF-α), amphiregulin (AR), heparin-binding EGF-like growth factor (HB-EGF), betacellulin (BTC) and epiregulin[2] all bind to the EGFR (for review, see Ref. 5). It is generally accepted that binding of ligand to receptor induces receptor oligomerization, activation of intrinsic tyrosine kinase activity and tyrosine autophosphorylation that probably represents transphosphorylation by the kinase onto tyrosine residues on its oligomerized partner[3]. Substrates with Src-homology-2 (SH2) domains are recruited to these tyrosine phosphorylated species and signal transduction cascades are initiated[4]. Sites for substrate binding are more permissive for the EGFR than platelet-derived growth factor receptor (PDGF) receptor, in which SH2-bearing proteins bind to specific tyrosine phosphorylated residues. Although receptor oligomerization is thought to initiate signalling, it should be pointed out that signalling by a monomeric EGFR has not been excluded formally[6].

Neu differentiation factor (NDF) and heregulins bind to ErbB3 and ErbB4[7,8]. Dimeric BTC has been reported to bind to ErbB4[9]. No ligand has been demonstrated conclusively to bind directly to ErbB2.

Data are accumulating in support of a complex pattern of cross-talk among EGFRs. Cross-talk may take the form of transactivation and/or heterodimer formation[7,10–15]. This adds complexity and diversity to signalling pathways. The heterodimer pairs that have been identified are listed in Figure 1. For example, EGF activates phosphatidylinositol 3-kinase indirectly by heterodimerization of EGFR with ErbB-3[16,17]. Recent studies have shown differential activation of ErbB

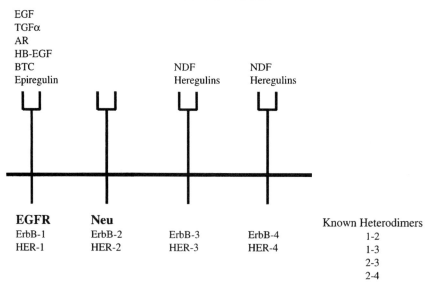

Figure 1   Summary of ErbB protein tyrosine kinase family members and their ligands

receptors by EGF-related peptides which may account for subtle variation in biological activity within the EGF family[18].

We have addressed the phenomenon of cross-talk indirectly in vivo by generating MMTV-TGF-α and MMTV-c-neu bigenic mice[19]. Virgin MMTV c-neu mice and MMTV-TGF-α monogenic mice develop spontaneous mammary tumours at approximately 9 and 12 months of age, respectively. Virgin bigenic mice exhibit a dramatic temporal acceleration of mammary tumour formation, with 50% of these bigenic mice developing multiple mammary tumours by 6 months of age. We have previously shown that the EGFR is up-regulated in MMTV-TGF-α tumour and peritumoral mammary tissue[20,21]. This accelerated tumour formation in bigenic mice is suspected to be due to cross-talk between EGFR and neu; however, we have not been able to demonstrate a physical association between these two receptors. These studies do not allow us to ascertain whether this temporal acceleration of mammary tumours is due to amplification of normal signalling or recruitment of unique signalling pathways.

We have recently reviewed characteristic features of EGFR ligands[5]. They are produced as high molecular weight glycoproteins that are inserted into the plasma membrane and then acted upon by as yet uncharacterized proteolytic enzymes to produce the mature soluble growth factor. The mature peptides share the exact spacing of six cysteine residues which result in three disulphide bonds providing the secondary structure for these ligands that allows binding to the EGFR. Several features of these ligands merit emphasis. EGF contains nine EGF-like repeats, whereas the other ligands only contain one EGF repeat. Mature AR and HB-EGF, as well as proEGF[22], bind to heparin. As mentioned above, dimeric BTC is also reported to bind to ErbB4[9]. HB-EGF is the first member of this family of ligands that has been reported to be a receptor; transmembrane HB-EGF serves as the receptor for the B fragment of diphtheria toxin and thus serves as this toxin's portal of cell entry[23]. Cellular toxicity following administration of diphtheria toxin has been used by investigators to provide indirect evidence for HB-EGF production by that cell[24]. It is not known whether any of the other ligands may lso serve as receptors. Derynck and co-workers have suggested that there may be reverse signalling by membrane-bound TGF-α that is regulated by the terminal eight amino acids in the cytoplasmic tail of TGF-α[25].

AUTO- AND CROSS-INDUCTION OF EGFR LIGANDS

Our laboratory is interested in the pathogenesis of intestinal neoplasia. Initial studies have focused on the growth regulation of non-transformed intestinal epithelial cells to understand better the progression to disordered growth control which is a hallmark of malignant transformation. We have chosen RIE-1 cells as a model system; this non-transformed, diploid cell line was derived from rat small intestine by Brown and co-workers[26]. These investigators showed that EGF stimulated growth of these cells. We have demonstrated that TGF-α stimulates mitogenesis with a peak of DNA replication at $18-20$ h after peptide delivery[27]. In previous studies of secondary cultures of human keratinocytes, we reported that TGF-α induces its own expression and described the phenomenon of auto-induction[28]. More extensive experiments have been performed in RIE-1 cells[29]. Confluent cells, serum-deprived for 3 days and then treated with TGF-α, were harvested at various times following treatment, poly(A) RNA was isolated and northern blots hybridized to cDNA probes for all of the EGFR ligands except epiregulin. After normalization to the constitutively expressed 1B15, we observed that TGF-α induced its own expression, albeit weakly, at 4 h. There was a striking, rapid induction of AR and HB-EGF, peaking at 8 h with a return to baseline by 12 h. BTC was intermediate in its temporal pattern of expression between the early induction of AR and HB-EGF and the later induction of TGF-α.

Figure 2 depicts some of the genes that are known to be induced by treatment of RIE-1 cells with TGF-α. Immediate early genes such as *COX-2, c-myc, zif268* and *nup475* are induced. The early, transcriptional induction of AR and HB-EGF and their enhanced expression in the presence of cycloheximide qualifies them as immediate early genes. We speculate that the early induction of AR and HB-EGF, as well as possibly the later induction of BTC and TGF-α, may contribute to the enhanced mitogenesis observed following exogenous TGF-α administration. A prediction of this model is that blockade of AR and HB-EGF production would result in attenuation of TGF-α-stimulated mitogenesis (Figure 3). Preliminary results with AR and HB-EGF antisense oligonucleotides are encouraging, but confirmation of this hypothesis will require more definitive studies using stably transfected AR and HB-EGF antisense RIE-1 cells.

ROLE OF EGFR SIGNALLING IN *ras*TRANSFORMATION

We recently have observed that RIE-1 cells infected with activated *H*- and *K-ras*, but not *raf*, cDNA constructs are transformed as determined by morphological transformation, growth in soft agar and the rapid appearance of tumours in nude

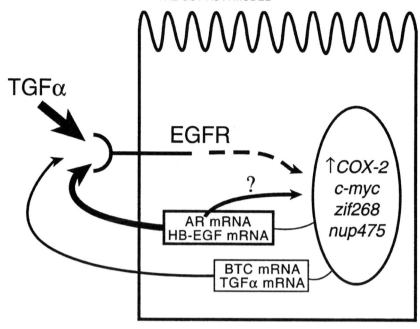

Figure 2 Selected genes induced by exogenous TGF-α administration to RIE-1 cells. There is early (30 min) and intense induction of AR and HB-EGF mRNA transcripts. There is later and weaker induction of BTC and TGF-α signals. The peptides are secreted and able to bind to the EGFR. It has been suggested, but not proven, that AR may not exit the cell and move to the nucleus

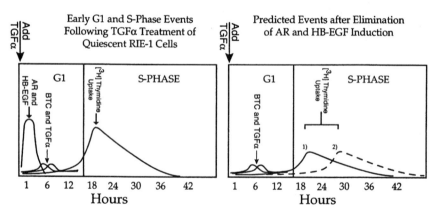

Figure 3 Proposed model of role of endogenous AR and HB-EGF in TGF-α-stimulated mitogenesis. It is postulated that blockade of AR and HB-EGF would result in (1) attenuation and/or (2) delay of DNA replication in RIE-1 following TGF-α administration

mice[30]. Both Ras and Raf RIE-1 cells exhibit equivalent Raf kinase activity. In contrast, both activated *ras* and *raf* cDNA constructs transform NIH-3T3 fibroblasts. These results support the contention that mechanisms underlying transformation of fibroblasts and epithelial cells differ. This is not altogether surprising

Table 1 Polarizing epithelial cell lines

Dog	Pig	Human
MDCK	LLCPK	Caco-2
		T-84
		HCA-7 (Colony 29)

in that there are clear differences in the growth regulation of these two cell types. For example, PDGF receptors are present on fibroblasts but are reported to be absent on epithelial cells. TGF-β stimulates the growth of fibroblasts, whereas it is a potent growth inhibitor for epithelial cells. These results also indicate that signalling through the Raf MAP kinase signalling pathway is not sufficient for epithelial cell transformation, and suggests that Ras mediates its transforming effects, at least in part, through alternate pathway(s).

Studies have been directed toward elucidating the biochemical and molecular basis for Ras-mediated transformation[31]. Activated *ras-*, *raf-* and v-*src*-infected RIE-1 cells were compared. We focused on production of EGFR ligands since Ras-conditioned medium was able to morphologically transform parental RIE-1 cells and exogenous TGF-α caused similar morphological effects. Activated Ras, but not Raf or v-Src, RIE-1 cells exhibited increased TGF-α, AR and HB-EGF mRNA expression and a marked increase in TGF-α peptide levels in Ras-conditioned media and lysates. Furthermore, studies using a specific EGFR tyrosine kinase inhibitor PD153035 indicated that EGFR signalling contributes significantly to the Ras transformed phenotype. This compound inhibits soft agar growth of H- and K-Ras-, but not v-Src-, transformed RIE-1 cells. PD153035, and to a lesser extent a TGF-α neutralizing antibody, are able to block the ability of Ras-conditioned medium to transform parental RIE-1 cells. Finally, the compound is able to cause morphological reversion of Ras-transformed RIE-1 cells but exhibits no effect on v-Src-transformed RIE-1 cells. Thus, Ras transformation is dependent, at least in part, on EGFR signalling, whereas signalling through this receptor does not appear to be required for Src transformation.

TRAFFICKING OF TGF-α AND EGF IN POLARIZED EPITHELIAL CELLS

In vivo, epithelial cells grow as a polarized monolayer with discrete apical and basolateral surfaces separated by tight junctions[32,33]. Thus, in vitro models used in the study of colonic neoplasia are best designed using polarized colonic epithelial cells. A limited number of epithelial cells will grow as a uniform polarizing monolayer when cultured on Transwell filters. These are listed in Table 1. Initially, we used polarized MDCK cells to examine the trafficking and processing of EGFR ligands. MDCK cells are derived from canine kidney epithelial cells and, like all polarized epithelial cells, the EGFR is confined to the basolateral surface. Parent MDCK cells express little, if any, of the EGFR ligands. We have used constitutive and inducible promoters to direct expression of full-length human TGF-α cDNAs. Both wild-type and membrane-fixed constructs were used in transfection experiments. The results are depicted in Figure 4A.

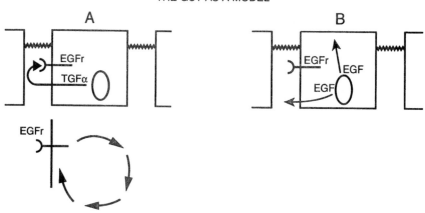

Figure 4 Summary of trafficking of TGF-α (A) and EGF (B) in polarized MDCK cells. See text for details

TGF-α is targeted preferentially to the basolateral compartment of polarized MDCK cells[34]. The ratio of basolateral to apical cell surface TGF-α as determined by cell surface immunoprecipitations is greater than 20:1. A novel motif has been identified in the cytoplasmic tail of TGF-α that confers this basolateral targeting (P.J. Dempsey and R.J. Coffey, unpublished observation). TGF-α is delivered to the compartment in which the EGFR resides and is rapidly bound. These cells can be induced to produce approximately 20 ng TGF-α/10[6] cells over 24 h and exhibit approximately 40000–60000 basolateral EGFRs. However, immunoreactive TGF-α was only detected in the basolateral medium following addition of an EGFR neutralizing monoclonal antibody. Therefore, the EGFR has a great avidity and capacity to take up secreted TGF-α. In fact, we have shown, in collaborative studies with Steve Wiley at the University of Utah, that EGFRs in epithelial cells recycle 10–20 times compared to 2–3 times in fibroblasts. Thus, TGF-α functions as an autocrine peptide in these polarized epithelial cells since it is directed preferentially to the specific compartment in which EGFRs reside, is cleaved at the basolateral cell surface and rapidly binds to basolateral EGFRs. A corollary point is that TGF-α is unlikely to act in a paracrine manner in this system since it is so efficiently consumed by the cells that produce it.

EGF is processed differentially from TGF-α (Figure 4B)[35]. Under steady-state conditions, EGF immunofluorescence is detected predominantly at the apical surface. However, biochemical studies reveal that EGF is delivered equally to the apical and basolateral surface. EGF accumulates at the apical surface, whereas it is cleaved rapidly from the basolateral surface, and is secreted into the basolateral medium as a 170 kDa high molecular weight precursor. However, this high molecular weight form of EGF does not interact with EGFRs in polarized MDCK cells. Thus, preferential cleavage at one cell surface is a novel mechanism of achieving differential cell surface localization of a protein.

Differential sorting, processing and receptor utilization of TGF-α and EGF provide insights into their diverse activities and may, in part, address the apparent redundancy of this family of peptides.

EGFR REGULATION OF COX-2 AND PGs IN HUMAN COLON CANCER CELLS

We have exploited the ability of two human colon cancer cell lines, HCA-7 Colony 29 (HCA-7) and Caco-2, to polarize in order to examine EGFR regulation of the enzyme cyclooxygenase-2 (COX-2) and the release of its prostaglandin (PG) products. COXs are key enzymes in the conversion of arachidonic acid to PGs and other eicosanoids. Two isoforms of this enzyme have been characterized. COX-1 is expressed constitutively in most cells; a second inducible form known as COX-2 also has been identified. Epidemiological data have shown that chronic consumers of aspirin exhibit a 50% reduction in colorectal cancer mortality. Aspirin acts as a 'suicide inhibitor' of COXs by irreversible, covalent binding to specific serine residues on the two enzymes. We reasoned that if aspirin was acting to reduce colorectal mortality then expression of one of these enzymes might be increased in malignant colorectal tissues. In fact, studies undertaken in collaboration with the lab of Ray DuBois found that 86% of human colorectal cancers exhibit a 2–50-fold increase in steady state COX-2 mRNA expression by northern blot, compared with adjacent normal mucosa[36]. In addition, the COX-2 transcript is increased in a subset of adenomatous polyps. No differences were observed in the intensity of COX-1 expression between normal and malignant colorectal tissue. Subsequent studies have demonstrated that COX-2 immuno-reactivity is confined to epithelial cells within malignant tissue, and that COX-2 is not detectable in normal tissue[37]. Recent genetic studies in mice have confirmed an important role for COX-2 expression in the pathogenesis of colorectal cancer[38].

These observations emphasize the importance of defining potential autocrine and paracrine pathways for regulation of gastrointestinal epithelial cell growth by COX. Signalling through the EGFR induces COX-2 expression[39] and up-regulated expression of COX-2 results in a tumorigenic phenotype in RIE-1 cells[40], suggesting that growth factor and COX-related signalling pathways intersect to regulate cellular proliferation. We have explored this interaction using the above mentioned human colorectal cancer cell lines. HCA-7 cells were derived from a human well-differentiated adenocarcinoma of the rectum[41,42]. The cells are structurally polarized and form domes. We have found that HCA-7 cells, like Caco-2 cells, functionally polarize when cultured on Transwell filters. HCA-7 cells produce PGs when cultured as a flat monolayer on plastic. PGE_2, $PGF_{2\alpha}$, PGD_2 and thromboxane are the major PGs produced. Prostacyclin is not produced. Caco-2 cells express little, if any, COX-2 and PGs are not detected in medium conditioned by these cells. We examined the effect of TGF-α added selectively to the apical or basolateral compartment on vectorial release of PGs when HCA-7 cells were cultured as a polarizing monolayer on Transwell filters. PG levels increased only when TGF-α was added to the EGFR-bearing basolateral compartment. This increase was dose- and time-dependent and was detected only in the basolateral medium. We have also observed that basolateral, but not apical, administration of TGF-α results in a marked increase in DNA replication. Of interest, TGF-α increases COX-2, but not COX-1, protein as assayed by Western blot and results in the unexpected appearance of COX-2 protein in the nucleus by immunofluorescence using confocal microscopy[43].

The detection of PGs in the basolateral medium of untreated HCA-7 cells led us

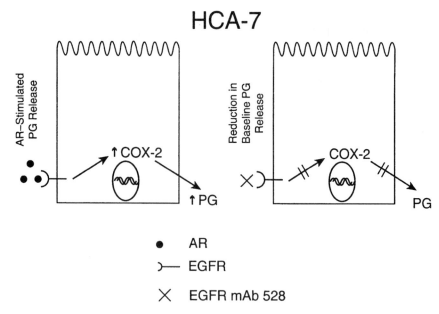

Figure 5 Summary of EGFR regulation of COX-2 and PGs in polarized HCA-7 cells. See text for details

to examine the mechanism underlying these baseline PG levels. EGFR blockade using a neutralizing antibody to the EGFR resulted in a dose-dependent decrease in COX-2 immunoreactivity, basolateral PG levels and DNA replication. AR, the most abundant EGFR ligand expressed by HCA-7 cells, is delivered to the basolateral surface and is secreted into the basolateral medium. Furthermore, administration of AR and EGFR neutralizing antibodies to the basolateral medium results in dose-dependent decreases in mitogenesis. Thus, autocrine signalling through the EGFR contributes to COX-2 production, basolateral release of PGs, and mitogenesis in a well-differentiated polarizing human colon cancer cell line (Figure 5). As mentioned above, polarized Caco-2 cells express little, if any, COX-2, and Caco-2 cells genetically engineered to constitutively over-express COX-2 are unable to polarize. This finding is of interest based on the observation that RIE-1 cells which over-express COX-2 exhibit downregulation of E-cadherin[40], and suggests that constitutive over-expression of COX-2 may lead to a loss of polarity and a more invasive phenotype by this mechanism.

SUMMARY

As outlined in this brief review, the increasing appreciation of the complexity of the EGFR family and the EGF-related peptide family has resulted in new opportunities for the study of normal and aberrant gastrointestinal epithelial cell growth. It is clear that understanding cross-talk between receptors and cross-talk between ligands will explain variation in biological activity. New model systems for the study of epithelial growth using polarized cells have greatly increased our ability to address more relevant hypotheses for understanding growth regulation in vivo.

Acknowledgements

This work was supported by NCI CA46413 and a Veterans Association Merit Review grant. RJC is a Veterans Association Clinical Investigator. RJC acknowledges the generous support of the Peter Powell Memorial Fund.

References

1. Earp H, Dawson T, Li X, Yu H. Heterodimerization and functional interaction between EGF receptor family members: A new signaling paradigm with implications for breast cancer research. Breast Cancer Res Treat. 1995;35:115–32.
2. Toyoda H, Komurasaki T, Uchida D et al. Epiregulin: a novel epidermal growth factor with mitogenic activity for rat primary hepatocytes. J Biol Chem. 1995;270:7495–500.
3. Ullrich A, Schlessinger J. Signal transduction by receptors with tyrosine kinase activity. Cell. 1990;61:203–12.
4. Pawson T. Protein modules and signalling networks. Nature. 1995;373:573–80.
5. Barnard J, Beauchamp R, Russell W, DuBois R, Coffey R. Epidermal growth factor-related peptides and their relevance to gastrointestinal pathophysiology. Gastroenterology. 1995;108: 564–80.
6. Carraway K, Cerione R. Inhibition of epidermal growth factor receptor aggregation by an anti-body directed against the epidermal growth factor receptor extracellular domain. J Biol Chem. 1993;268:23860–7.
7. Tzahar E, Waterman H, Chen X et al. A hierarchical network of interreceptor interactions deter-mines signal transduction by neu differentiation factor/neuregulin and epidermal growth factor. Mol Cell Biol. 1996;16:5276–87.
8. Carraway K, Sliwkoski M, Akita R et al. The erbB-3 gene product is a receptor for heregulin. J Biol Chem. 1994;269:14303–6.
9. Riese D, Bermingham Y, vanRaaij T, Buckley S, Plowman G, Stern D. Betacellulin activates the epidermal growth factor receptor and erbB-4, and induces cellular response patterns distinct from those stimulated by epidermal growth factor or neuregulin-β. Oncogene. 1996;12:345–53.
10. Riese D, vanRaaij T, Plowman G, Andrews G, Stern D. The cellular response to neuregulins is governed by complex interactions of the erbB receptor family. Mol Cell Biol. 1995;15:5770–6.
11. Riese D, Kim E, Elenius K et al. The epidermal growth factor receptor couples transforming growth factor alpha, heparin-binding epidermal growth factor-like factor, and amphiregulin to Neu, ErbB-3, and ErbB-4. J Biol Chem. 1996;271:20047–52.
12. Carraway K, Cantley L. A neu acquaintance for erbB-3 and erbB-4: A role for receptor hetero-dimerization in growth signaling. Cell. 1994;78:5–8.
13. Sliwkowski M, Schaefer G, Akita R et al. Coexpression of erbB2 and erbB3 proteins reconstitutes a high affinity receptor for heregulin. J Biol Chem. 1994;269:14661–6.
14. Wada T, Qian X, Greene M. Intermolecular association of the p185^{neu} protein and EGF receptor modulates EGF receptor function. Cell. 1990;61:1339–47.
15. Murali R, Brennan P, Kieber-Emmons T, Greene M. Structural analysis of p185c-neu and epidermal growth factor receptor tyrosine kinases: Oligomerization of kinase domains. Proc Natl Acad Sci USA. 1996;93:6252–7.
16. Soltoff S, Carraway K, Prigent S, Gullick W, Cantley L. ErbB3 is involved in activation of phos-phatidylinositol 3-kinase by epidermal growth factor. Mol Cell Biol. 1994;14:3550–8.
17. Fedi P, Pierce J, DiFiore P, Kraus M. Efficient coupling with phosphatidylinositol 3-kinase, but not phospholipase Cγ or GTPase-activating protein, distinguishes ErbB-3 signalling from that of other ErbB/EGFR family members. Mol Cell Biol. 1994;14:492–500.
18. Beerli R, Hynes N. Epidermal growth factor-related peptides activate distinct subsets of ErbB receptors and differ in their biological activities. J Biol Chem. 1996;271:6071–6.
19. Muller W, Arteaga C, Muthuswamy S et al. Synergistic interaction of the Neu protooncogene and

TGFα in the development of mammary neoplasia in transgenic mice. Mol Cell Biol. 1996; 19:5726–36.

20. Matsui Y, Halter S, Holt J, Hogan BM, Coffey R. Development of mammary neoplasia and neo-plasia in MMTV-TGFα transgenic mice. Cell. 1990;61:1147–55.
21. Halter S, Dempsey P, Matsui Y et al. Distinctive patterns of hyperplasia in MMTV-TGFα trans-genic mice: characterization of mammary gland and skin proliferations. Am J Pathol. 1992;140: 1131–46.
22. Parries G, Chen K, Misono K, Cohen S. The human urinary epidermal growth factor (EGF) precursor. Isolation of a biologically active 160-kilodalton heparin-binding pro-EGF with a truncated carboxyl terminus. J Biol Chem. 1995;270:27954–60.
23. Naglich J, Metherall J, Russell D, Eidels L. Expression cloning of a diphtheria toxin receptor: identity with a heparin-binding EGF-like growth factor precursor. Cell. 1992;69:1051–61.
24. Mitamura T, Higashiyama S, Taniguchi N, Klagsbrun M, Mekada E. Diphtheria toxin binds to the epidermal growth factor (EGF)-like domain of human heparin-binding EGF-like growth factor/ diphtheria toxin receptor and inhibits specifically its mitogenic activity. J Biol Chem. 1995;270: 1015–9.
25. Shum L, Turck C, Derynck R. Cysteines 153 and 154 of transmembrane transforming growth factor alpha are palmitoylated and mediate cytoplasic protein association. J Biol Chem. 1996; 271:28502–8.
26. Blay J, Brown K. Functional receptors for epidermal growth factor in an epithelial-cell line derived from the rat small intestine. Biochem J. 1985;225:84–94.
27. DuBois R, Bishop P, Graves-Deal R, Coffey R. Transforming growth factor α regulation of two zinc finger containing immediate early response genes in intestinal epithelial cells. Cell Growth Differ. 1995;6:523–9.
28. Coffey R, Derynck R, Wilcox C et al. Production and autoinduction of transforming growth factor α in human keratinocytes. Nature. 1987;328:817–20.
29. Barnard J, Graves-Deal R, Pittelkow M et al. Auto- and cross induction within the mammalian epidermal growth factor-related peptide family. J Biol Chem. 1994;269:22817–22.
30. Oldham S, Clark G, Gangarosa L, Coffey R, Der C. Activation of the Raf/MAP kinase cascade is not sufficient for Ras transformation of RIE epithelial cells. Proc Natl Acad Sci USA. 1996; 93:6924–8.
31. Gangarosa L, Dempsey P, Damstrup L, Barnard J, Coffey R. Transforming growth factor alpha. Bailliere's Clin Gastroenterol. 1996;10:49–65.
32. Drubin D, Nelson W. Origins of cell polarity. Cell. 1996;84:335–44.
33. Mostov K, Cardone M. Regulation of protein traffic in polarized epithelial cells. BioEssays. 1995;17:129–38.
34. Dempsey P, Coffey R. Basolateral targeting and efficient consumption of transforming growth factor-α when expressed in Madin-Darby canine kidney cells. J Biol Chem. 1994;269:16878–89.
35. Dempsey P, Miese K, Coffey R. Human EGF precursor is not sorted in polarized MDCK cells but accumulates at the apical membrane due to increased basolateral proteolytic activity. J Cell Biol. Submitted.
36. Eberhart CE, Coffey RJ, Radhika A, Giardiello FM, Ferrenbach S, DuBois RN. Up-regulation of cyclooxygenase 2 gene expression in human colorectal adenomas and adenocarcinomas. Gastroenterology. 1994;107:1183–8.
37. Sano H, Kawahito Y, Wilder RL et al. Expression of cyclooxygenase-1 and -2 in human colorectal cancer. Cancer Res. 1995;55:3785–9.
38. Oshima M, Dinchuk J, Kargman S et al. Suppression of intestinal polyposis in Apc$^{\Delta716}$ knockout mice by inhibition of cyclooxygenase 2 (COX-2). Cell. 1996;87:803–9.
39. DuBois R, Awad J, Morrow J, Roberts LR, Bishop P. Regulation of eicosanoid production and mito-genesis in rat intestinal epithelial cells by transforming growth factor-α and phorbol ester. J Clin Invest. 1994;93:493–8.
40. Tsujii M, DuBois RN. Alterations in cellular adhesion and apoptosis in epithelial cells over-expressing prostaglandin endoperoxide synthase-2. Cell. 1995;83:493–501.
41. Kirkland S. Dome formation by a human colonic adenocarcinoma cell line (HCA-7). Cancer Res. 1985;45:3790–5.
42. Marsh K, Stamp G, Kirkland S. Isolation and characterization of multiple cell types from a single human colonic carcinoma: tumourigenicity of these cell types in a xenograft system. J Pathol. 1993;170:441–50.
43. Coffey R, Hawkey C, Damstrup L et al. EGF receptor activation induces nuclear targeting of COX-2, basolateral release of prostaglandins and mitogenesis in polarizing colon cancer cells. Proc Natl Acad Sci USA. 1997;94:657–62.

7
Paba-peptide hydrolase: just another digestive enzyme?

E. E. STERCHI

INTRODUCTION

The apical plasma membrane of epithelial cells from small intestine is rich in exo- and endopeptidases. The enzyme referred to here as Paba-peptide hydrolase (PPH) was discovered in the early 1980s as an activity hydrolysing N-benzoyl-L-tyrosyl-p-aminobenzoic acid (PABA-peptide), a chymotrypsin substrate used in the clinical evaluation of exocrine pancreas function (Figure 1)[1,2]. PPH is localized to the microvillus membrane of epithelial cells from small intestine and cleaves a number of biologically active peptides including bradykinins, angiotensins, substance P and insulin B-chain[3]. A similar enzyme activity named meprin was isolated from rodent kidney[4-6]. Characterization of the rodent and human enzymes showed very similar biochemical properties[3,5,7]. Two types of subunits, α and β, with molecular weights between 90 and 110 kDa were identified which form disulphide-linked homo- or heterooligomers[3,5,7,8].

In 1991 partial clones of human intestinal N-benzoyl-L-tyrosyl-p-aminobenzoic acid hydrolase (PPH) and mouse kidney meprin were isolated and characterized[9]. The enzymes showed over 80% identity in the N-terminal amino acid sequence (192 residues). Comparison of the deduced sequences with protein databases showed similarities with a digestive protease from freshwater crayfish (*Astacus astacus*) and the N-terminal domain of a human bone morphogenetic protein (BMP-1). Alignments showed that human PPH and mouse meprin were approximately 30% identical with astacin and BMP-1. Thirty-seven amino acid residues, including three cysteines, were strictly conserved in all four proteins in a domain equivalent to the complete 200 amino acid residue sequence of the astacus protease. All four proteins were further shown to contain a zinc-binding motif (HEXXH) within an extended sequence of HEXXHXXGFXHE, which established their identification as metalloendopeptidases. A developmentally regulated protein from frog, UVS-2, was also shown to have sequence identity with these metalloendopeptidases. These data provided strong evidence for an evolutionary relationship among these proteins and the name 'astacins' was proposed for this family of metalloendopeptidases.

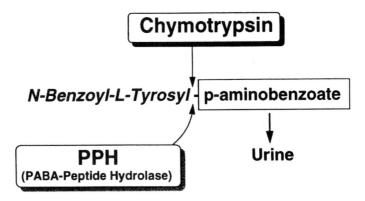

Figure 1 Principle of the Paba-test for exocrine pancreas function. *N*-Bz-L-tyrosyl-*p*-aminobenzoic acid (Paba-peptide) has been designed as a substrate for chymotrypsin. Oral administration of Paba-peptide is followed by recovery/quantification of *p*-aminobenzoic acid in a 6 h urine pool after hydrolysis of the substrate in the gut by pancreatic chymotrypsin. Normal exocrine pancreatic function results in recovery of up to 70% of the given dose of hydrolysed Paba-peptide. Recovery is diminished in impaired exocrine pancreatic function. Paba-peptide is also hydrolysed by PPH

MOLECULAR STRUCTURE OF PPH

The full-length sequences of the α subunit of mouse and rat kidney meprin and of human intestinal PPH were reported in the early 1990s[10-12]. The human enzyme is 75% identical to mouse and 78% identical to rat α subunit respectively. This was followed by the identification of full-length sequences of the rodent β sub-units[13,14], and the human β subunit (Genbank AC 81333, paper submitted). The structure of PPH with its two subunits, α and β, is shown in Figure 2. The sub-units have a similar multidomain structure, consisting of an N-terminal signal peptide and a propeptide sequence followed by the actual astacin protease domain. Following the catalytic protease domain is a MAM or adhesive domain, an intervening sequence, an EGF-like domain, a transmembrane domain and a short cytosolic domain. The two subunits are over 40% identical and about 60% similar. Similarity in the C-terminal region is less prominent, the α subunit having an additional domain immediately in front of the EGF-like domain, termed I-domain, which is not present in the β subunit. The X-ray crystal structure of astacin has recently been solved to a resolution of 1.8 Å[15,16]. The MAM domain was first found in protein tyrosine phosphatase μ, A5 protein, and the α and β subunit of PPH (meprin)[17]. Recently, enteropeptidase (enterokinase), the intestinal protease responsible for the initiation of the activation cascade for pancreatic proteases, has also been shown to contain this domain[18]. The exact function of the MAM domain is not known, but the four conserved cysteine residues suggested that it may serve a common adhesive function in these proteins. For rat and mouse meprin cysteine residues within this domain have been shown to be involved in dimerization of the subunits[19,20]. Another prominent feature in

72

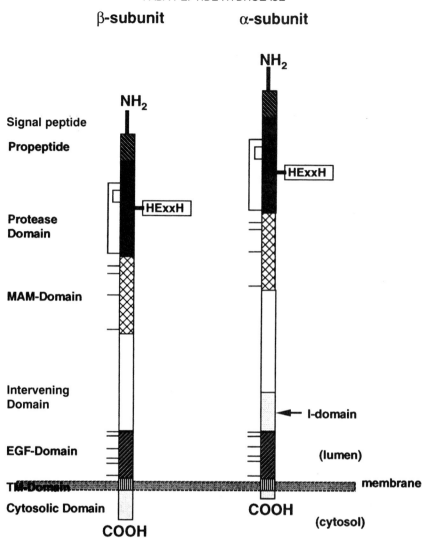

Figure 2: Domain structure of PPH α and β subunits of: signal peptide (■), propeptide (▨), astacin (protease) domain (■), MAM domain (▨), intervening sequence (☐), inserted domain (▨), EFG-like domain (▨), transmembrane domain (▥), and cytosolic domain (▨).

PPH is an EGF-like domain comprising approximately 40 amino acids and including six conserved cysteine residues[21]. EGF-like domains have been found in a number of proteins with diverse functions[22] including some proteases[23,24]. Some EGF-like domains are involved in calcium-binding while others are not[22,25]. They are all believed to be involved in regulatory mechanisms.

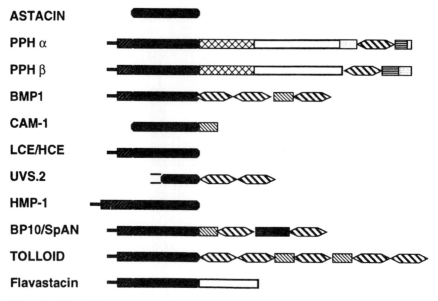

Figure 3: Schematic representation of the domain structure of the astacin family members. Signal peptide (▮), propeptide (▨), astacin (protease) domain (▬), MAM domain (⊠), intervening sequence (☐), inserted domain (▢), EFG-like domain (◥), transmembrane domain (▤), cytosolic domain (▥), CUB domain (▧) and S/T rich domain (▨). EGF, epidermal growth factor; MAM, adhesion domain; CUB, Clr/s complement-like domain; S/T, serine/threonine-rich domain

PPH IS A MEMBER OF THE ASTACIN FAMILY OF METALLOENDOPEPTIDASES

To date over 20 proteins have been identified as members of the astacin family. The astacins are grouped in family 12A which belongs to clan MB of the metallo-endopeptidases (N. Rawlings, Classification of peptidase, SWISS-PROT Protein Sequence Data Bank; http://expasy.hcuge.ch/cgi-bin/lists?peptidas.txt). X-ray crystal structure analyses of members of clan MB have revealed a strong overall topological similarity, with an extended HEXXHXXGXXH zinc-binding motif. In addition, a so-called 'Met-turn' provides the hydrophobic basis for the zinc and the three histidine residues that bind this metal ion. The family, also known as metzincins, includes adamalysins (snake venoms), serralysins (*Serratia* proteases) and matrixins in addition to astacins[26–28].

Astacin proteases are found in diverse species among eukaryotes and also prokaryotes. They include bone morphogenetic protein-1 from human, mouse, frog, sea urchin and fruit fly[29–32], CAM-1 from the Japanese quail[33], LCE and HCE from fish[34], UVS-2 from frog[35], HMP-1 from hydra[36], BP10 and SpAN from sea urchin[37,38], and tolloid from human, mouse and fruit fly[39–41]. In addition, there are members from crab-beetle and worm and the prokaryote member flavastacin[42].

The multi-domain assembly of astacins is shown in Figure 3. Most astacins are secreted from the cells. PPH and meprin α and β subunits are the only members identified so far to have transmembrane domains.

Some astacins appear to be involved in embryonic development through proteolytic modification of growth factors or tissue remodelling through interactions with the extracellular matrix. The different domains may mediate contact with cells or extracellular matrix or are involved in the regulation of these proteases.

BIOSYNTHESIS OF PPH

First insights into the biosynthesis and posttranslational processing of PPH were obtained from cultured human intestinal explants using pulse-chase labelling protocols with [^{35}S]methionine and protein analysis by SDS–polyacrylamide gel electrophoresis and fluorography after immunoprecipitation with specific antibodies[43]. Data from these experiments showed that the enzyme is secreted into the organ culture medium. After cloning, biosynthesis and processing of the two subunits was studied in heterologous expression systems. The cDNAs coding for the prepro-forms of PPH α and β were used to transfect COS-1, MDCK and 293 cells[12,44].

Synthesis and processing of human PPH α in transiently transfected COS-1 cells is shown in Figure 4. Two days after transfection, cells were pulse-labelled for 15 min with [^{35}S]methionine and chased for the times indicated at the top of Figure 4A and 4B. The α subunit is synthesized as a polypeptide of approximately 100 kDa (Figure 4A, lane 1) in an immature form (PPHα_h) that does not exit the rough endoplasmic reticulum (RER). A second species (PPHα_h*), which appears later, represents a proteolytically cleaved form of the 100 kDa form. After 2 h a mature form of PPHα_{sec} appears in the culture medium (Figure 4A, Lane 8). Secretion of the α subunit thus requires proteolytic removal of the C-terminal hydrophobic anchor peptide. This transmembrane domain may contain a signal for retention of the membrane bound α subunit in the RER. Once removed the protein is transported very rapidly to the cell surface and secreted. Co-translationally, the α subunit forms disulphide-linked homodimers which in vivo may form non-covalently linked tetramers with either α or β subunits[43].

Transfection of cells with the PPH β cDNA results in two protein species of 95 and 104 kDa (Figure 4B). The 94 kDa band (PPHβ_h) represents an immature form located in the RER (Figure 4B, lanes 1–4) whereas the 104 kDa polypeptide represents the mature form (Figure 4B, lanes 2–5). Small amounts of the latter species are secreted into the culture medium (Figure 4B, lane 9) but the protein remains predominantly inserted into the cell membrane.

Co-transfection experiments and immunoprecipitation using subunit-specific antibodies have clearly shown that both subunits are associated with the cell membrane (J. Eldering et al., manuscript submitted). Therefore the β subunit is necessary for retention of the α subunit at the cell membrane.

The difference in COOH-terminal processing of the two subunits is due to the inserted domain (I-domain) of 56 amino acids which is present only in the α subunit (Figure 2). It is located immediately NH$_2$-terminal to the EGF-like domain and contains several potential protease processing sites including dibasic residues as well as a recognition sequence for furin (RXKR). Inserting the I-domain sequence in the β subunit just in front of the EGF domain leads to the secretion

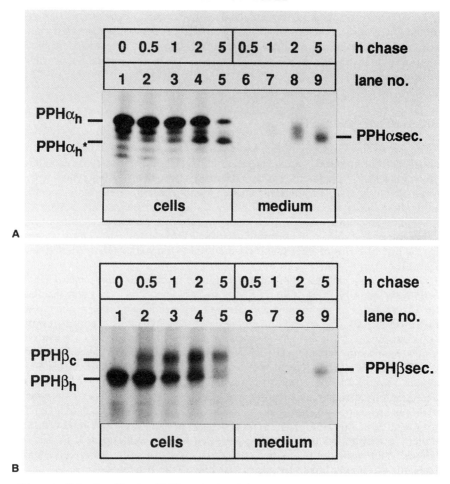

Figure 4 Pulse chase kinetics of PPH α subunit and β subunit transfected COS-1 cells. COS-1 cells transfected with the cDNA of subunit α (A) or subunit β (B) were metabolically labelled for 15 min and chased for the indicated times. The cells and the media were harvested and the proteins were immunoprecipitated with subunit specific polyclonal antibodies. The immunoprecipitates were subjected to SDS–PAGE (7.5%) under reducing conditions and the proteins were detected by fluorography

of this subunit. Deletion of the I-domain from the α subunit, on the other hand, leads to retention of this mutated subunit in the RER[45]. Thus, the I-domain is essential for proteolytic processing and the TM- and/or the C-terminal domain may contain ER retention signals[45].

PPH expressed in COS cells is synthesized as an inactive zymogen. Activation may be achieved in vitro by treatment with trypsin[44]. In vivo, both subunits of PPH are most likely activated by luminal trypsin. Activation of the kidney enzyme (α subunit) on the other hand requires a so far unidentified protease. The β subunit of meprin is present in a latent form but it is not clear how it is activated[46-48].

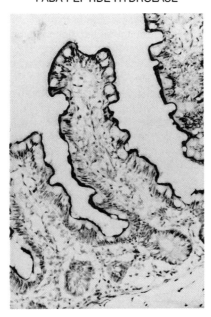

Figure 5 Immunostaining of the PPH β subunit in human small intestine. Cryostat sections were obtained from surgical specimens. The endopeptidase 24.18 β subunit was detected by immunohisto-chemistry using a subunit specific polyclonal rabbit antiserum, a biotinylated second antibody, an avidin-biotin-peroxidase complex and DAB (diaminobenzidine) as substrate. Counterstain was with Giemsa

DISTRIBUTION OF PPH IN CELLS AND TISSUES

Expression of human PPH is restricted to intestine[43] and possibly kidney[49]. In rodents, in addition to kidney expression of meprin has been demonstrated in salivary glands (mouse)[50] and craniofacial structures (rat embryo)[51]. Expression of meprin in different tissues seems confined to epithelial cells and more specifi-cally to the apical domain of polarized cells.

Using Southern blot analysis the PPH/meprin α gene has been detected in human, monkey, rat, mouse, dog, cow, rabbit and chicken, but not in yeast[52]. The gene has thus been conserved among a wide range of animals extending into non-mammalian species. In rodents meprin makes up $5-20\%$ of the total brush border protein from mouse kidney epithelial cells[53]. The enzyme is localized to the proximal tubuli in a subpopulation of nephrons in the deeper renal cortex, the so-called juxtamedullary region[53,54]. Some inbred laboratory mouse strains (C3H, CBA) secrete only low levels of meprin into the urine. These strains are deficient in the meprin α subunit but still express the β subunit (meprin B) in the kidney and intestine[8,14,53]. In contrast to mouse[52,55] the α subunit is not detectable in human kidney by RT–PCR[56]. Conversely, in one study PPH-like protein and enzymatic activity was found in human kidney[57].

Both PPH α and β subunits have been immunoprecipitated from human small intestine[3,43]. Immunocytochemistry of human small intestinal tissue sections localized PPH to the apical side of mature epithelial cells (Figure 5). A longitudinal gradient of PPH has been observed in human intestine with lowest activity in proximal duodenum and highest activity in distal ileum[3]. Recent findings have confirmed this to be the case also in mouse intestine[55]. RT–PCR has detected the α subunit in human small intestine, human colon and colon tumour tissue[57]. Recently, a variant β' subunit message larger in size than the normal mRNA (2.7 kb compared with 2.5 kb for the 'normal' β mRNA) has been detected in a human colon adenocarcinoma cell line (HT29-18C1) and in two undifferentiated mouse teratocarcinoma cells lines (F9 and Null-SSC-1)[58]. In Null-SSC-1 cells the β' message was found to be up-regulated by the differentiating agent retinoic acid. The deduced amino acid sequence of this variant differs significantly in the N-terminal portion including the signal peptide and part of the propeptide and may confer different targeting and/or activation to the β' subunit. It was suggested that different promoter usage and alternative splicing might be responsible for the generation of the β' mRNA in tumour cell lines. Gene expression may be regulated by such mechanisms depending on the differentiation/proliferative status of the cells.

FUNCTION OF PPH

The physiological substrates for PPH are not known and statements about the function of the enzyme are still speculative. In rodents, certain urinary proteins, like some MHC-molecules and so-called MUPS (major urinary proteins[59,60]), were proposed to be cleaved by meprin secreted into the urine, thereby releasing pheromones which control social behaviour, mating selection and recognition of self and non-self[61].

PPH/meprin may contribute to the catabolism of filtered or secreted biologically active peptides in the urine. Bradykinin, angiotensin I and II, substance P and insulin β-chain[3], parathyroid hormone (PTH) and parathyroid hormone-related protein (PTHrP)[62,63] are all in vitro substrates. It has been suggested that PPH/meprin is the crucial renal brush border protease degrading PTH and PTHrP, both involved in the regulation of calcium metabolism. Human PPH may inactivate or activate luminal hormones and/or growth factors and regulate epithelial cell proliferation and differentiation[9]. This may be particularly important during the fetal and postnatal periods. As the ileum is very rich in lymphatic tissue, ileal PPH may also have an immunological function such as antigen processing and presentation[3,55].

In a screen for gelatin-degrading proteases in renal cortex membrane preparations, a PPH-like endopeptidase was isolated and shown to degrade laminin, collagen type IV and fibronectin in vitro[49]. Modification of extracellular matrix compounds by such a membrane-bound protease from epithelial cells could play a role in renal cell injury and regeneration. Mouse strains with low and high meprin activity and rats have been assessed for their susceptibility to toxic or ischaemic experimental renal disease[64–66]. The results were contradictory and no clear correlation of mortality or renal injury to enzyme activity was found.

The MEP1A locus is linked to MHC loci in human and mouse, which in turn are linked to numerous diseases. A role of meprin in the pathogenesis of these diseases has been discussed[67].

Acknowledgements

This work was supported by grant no. 32-40571.94 from the Swiss National Science Foundation. Special thanks to Dagmar Hahn, Eric Dumermuth, Joyce A. Eldering, Jürgen Grünberg, Daniel Lottaz, Ursula Luginbühl, and Elizabeth Mandac, who during the last years have all contributed to the work on the human PPH.

References

1. Sterchi EE, Green JR, Lentze MJ. Non-pancreatic hydrolysis of N-benzoyl-L-tyrosyl-p-aminobenzoic acid (PABA-peptide) in the human small intestine. Clin Sci. 1982;62:557–60.
2. Sterchi EE, Green JR, Lentze MJ. Nonpancreatic hydrolysis of N-benzoyl-L-tyrosyl-p-aminobenzoic acid (PABA peptide) in the rat small intestine. J Pediatr Gastroenterol Nutr. 1983; 2:539–47.
3. Sterchi EE, Naim HY, Lentze MJ, Hauri HP, Fransen JA. N-benzoyl-L-tyrosyl-p-aminobenzoic acid hydrolase: a metalloendopeptidase of the human intestinal microvillus membrane which degrades biologically active peptides. Arch Biochem Biophys. 1988;265:105–18.
4. Kenny AJ, Fulcher IS, Ridgwell K, Ingram J. Microvillar membrane neutral endopeptidases. Acta Biol Med Ger. 1981;40:1465–71.
5. Kenny AJ, Ingram J. Proteins of the kidney microvillar membrane. Purification and properties of the phosphoramidon-insensitive endopeptidase ('endopeptidase-2') from rat kidney. Biochem J. 1987;245:515–24.
6. Beynon RJ, Shannon JD, Bond JS. Purification and characterization of a metallo-endoproteinase from mouse kidney. Biochem J. 1981;199:591–8.
7. Butler PE, McKay MJ, Bond JS. Characterization of meprin, a membrane-bound metallo-endopeptidase from mouse kidney. Biochem J. 1987;241:229–35.
8. Butler PE, Bond JS. A latent proteinase in mouse kidney membranes. Characterization and relationship to meprin. J Biol Chem. 1988;263:13419–26.
9. Dumermuth E, Sterchi EE, Jiang WP et al. The astacin family of metalloendopeptidases. J Biol Chem. 1991;266:21381–5.
10. Jiang W, Gorbea CM, Flannery AV, Beynon RJ, Grant GA, Bond JS. The alpha subunit of meprin A. Molecular cloning and sequencing, differential expression in inbred mouse strains, and evidence for divergent evolution of the alpha and beta subunits. J Biol Chem. 1992;267:9185–93.
11. Corbeil D, Gaudoux F, Wainwright S et al. Molecular cloning of the alpha-subunit of rat endo-peptidase-24.18 (endopeptidase-2) and co-localization with endopeptidase-24.11 in rat kidney by in situ hybridization. FEBS Lett. 1992;309:203–8.
12. Dumermuth E, Eldering JA, Grünberg J, Jiang W, Sterchi EE. Cloning of the PABA peptide hydrolase alpha subunit (PPH alpha) from human small intestine and its expression in COS-1 cells. FEBS Lett. 1993;335:367–75.
13. Johnson GD, Hersh LB. Cloning a rat meprin cDNA reveals the enzyme is a heterodimer. J Biol Chem. 1992;267:13505–12.
14. Gorbea CM, Marchand P, Jiang W et al. Cloning, expression, and chromosomal localization of the mouse meprin beta subunit. J Biol Chem. 1993;268:21035–43.
15. Bode W, Gomis Ruth FX, Huber R, Zwilling R, Stöcker W. Structure of astacin and implications for activation of astacins and zinc-ligation of collagenases. Nature. 1992;358:164–7.
16. Gomis Ruth FX, Stöcker W, Huber R, Zwilling R, Bode W. Refined 1.8 A X-ray crystal structure of astacin, a zinc-endopeptidase from the crayfish *Astacus astacus* L. Structure determination, refinement, molecular structure and comparison with thermolysin. J Mol Biol. 1993;229:945–68.
17. Beckman G, Bork P. An adhesive domain detected in functionally diverse receptors. Trends Biochem Sci. 1993;18:40–1.
18. Kitamoto Y, Yuan X, Wu Q, McCourt DW, Sadler JE. Enterokinase, the initiator of intestinal digestion, is a mosaic protease composed of a distinctive assortment of domains. Proc Natl Acad Sci USA. 1994;91:7588–92.
19. Chevallier S, Ahn J, Boileau G, Crine P. Identification of the cysteine residues implicated in the formation of alpha 2 and alpha/beta dimers of rat meprin. Biochem J. 1996;317:731–8.

20. Marchand P, Volkmann M, Bond J. Cysteine mutations in the MAM domain result in monomeric meprin and alter stability and activity of the protease. J Biol Chem. 1996;271:24236–47.
21. Appella E, Weber IT, Blasi F. Structure and function of epidermal growth factor-like regions in proteins. FEBS Lett. 1988;231:1–4.
22. Davis C. The many faces of epidermal growth factor repeats. New Biol. 1990;2:410–19.
23. Clarke B, Ofosu F, Sridhara S, Bona R, Rickles F, Blajchman M. The first epidermal growth factor domain of human coagulation factor VII is essential for binding with tissue factor. FEBS Lett. 1992;298:206–10.
24. Zhong D, Smith K, Birktoft J, Bajaj S. First epidermal growth factor-like domain of human blood coagulation factor IX is required for its activation by factor VIIa/tissue factor but not by factor XIa. Proc Natl Acad Sci USA. 1994;91:3574–8.
25. Campbell ID, Bork P. Epidermal growth factor-like modules. Curr Opin Struct Biol. 1993;3: 385–92.
26. Bode W, Gomisruth FX, Stöcker W. Astacins, serralysins, snake venom and matrix metalloproteinases exhibit identical zinc-binding environments (HEXXHXXGXXH and met-turn) and topologies and should be grouped into a common family, the metzincins. FEBS Lett. 1993;331: 134–40.
27. Stöcker W, Bode W. Structural features of a superfamily of zinc-endopeptidases: the metzincins. Curr Opin Struct Biol. 1995;5:383–90.
28. Stöcker W, Zwilling R. Astacin. Methods Enzymol. 1995;248:305–25.
29. Wozney JM, Rosen V, Celeste AJ et al. Novel regulators of bone formation: molecular clones and activities. Science. 1988;242:1528–34.
30. Maeno M, Xue Y, Wood TI, Ong RC, H.F. K. Cloning and expression of cDNA encoding Xenopus laevis bone morphogenetic protein-1 during early development. Gene. 1993;134:257–61.
31. Fukagawa M, Suzuki N, Hogan BL, Jones CM. Embryonic expression of mouse bone mor-phogenetic protein-1 (BMP-1), which is related to the Drosophila dorsoventral gene tolloid and encodes a putative astacin metalloendopeptidase. Dev Biol. 1994;163:175–83.
32. Hwang SP, Partin JS, Lennarz WJ. Characterization of a homolog of human bone morphogenetic protein 1 in the embryo of the sea urchin, Strongylocentrotus purpuratus. Development. 1994; 120:559–68.
33. Elaroussi MA, DeLuca HF. A new member to the astacin family of metalloendopeptidases: a novel 1,25-dihydroxyvitamin D-3-stimulated mRNA from chorioallantoic membrane of quail. Biochim Biophys Acta. 1994;1217:1–8.
34. Yasumasu S, Yamada K, Akasaka K et al. Isolation of cDNAs for LCE and HCE, two constituent proteases of the hatching enzyme of Oryzias latipes, and concurrent expression of their mRNAs during development. Dev Biol. 1992;153:250–8.
35. Sato SM, Sargent TD. Molecular approach to dorsoanterior development in Xenopus laevis. Dev Biol. 1990;137:135–41.
36. Yan L, Pollock GH, Nagase H, Sarras MPJ. A 25.7×10(3) M(r) hydra metalloproteinase (HMP1), a member of the astacin family, localizes to the extracellular matrix of Hydra vulgaris in a head-specific manner and has a developmental function. Development. 1995;121:1591–602.
37. Lepage T, Ghiglione C, Gache C. Spatial and temporal expression pattern during sea urchin embryogenesis of a gene coding for a protease homologous to the human protein BMP-1 and to the product of the Drosophila dorsal-ventral patterning gene tolloid. Development. 1992;114: 147–63.
38. Reynolds DS, Angerer LM, Palis J, Nasir A, Angerer RC. Early mRNAs, spatially restricted along the animal-vegetal axis of sea urchin embryos, include one encoding a protein related to tolloid and BMP-1. Development. 1992;114:769–86.
39. Shimell MJ, Ferguson EL, Childs SR, O CMB. The Drosophila dorsal-ventral patterning gene tolloid is related to human bone morphogenetic protein 1. Cell. 1991;67:469–81.
40. Finelli AL, Bossie CA, Xie T, Padgett RW. Mutational analysis of the Drosophila tolloid gene, a human BMP-1 homolog. Development. 1994;120:861–70.
41. Takahara K, Lyons GE, Greenspan DS. Bone morphogenetic protein-1 and a mammalian tolloid homologue (mTld) are encoded by alternatively spliced transcripts which are differently expressed in some tissues. J Biol Chem. 1994;269:32572–8.
42. Tarentino AL, Quinones G, Grimwood BG, Hauer CR, Plummer THJ. Molecular cloning and sequence analysis of flavastacin: an O-glycosylated prokaryotic zinc metalloendopeptidase. Arch Biochem Biophys. 1995;319:281–5.
43. Sterchi EE, Naim HY, Lentze MJ. Biosynthesis of N-benzoyl-L-tyrosyl-p-aminobenzoic acid hydrolase: disulfide-linked dimers are formed at the site of synthesis in the rough endoplasmic reticulum. Arch Biochem Biophys. 1988;265:119–27.

44. Grünberg J, Dumermuth E, Eldering JA, Sterchi EE. Expression of the alpha subunit of PABA peptide hydrolase (EC 3.4.24.18) in MDCK cells. Synthesis and secretion of an enzymatically inactive homodimer. FEBS Lett. 1993;335:376–9.
45. Marchand P, Tang J, Johnson G, Bond J. COOH-proteolytic processing of secreted and membrane forms of the alpha subunit of the metalloprotease Meprin A. Requirement of the I domain for processing in the endoplasmic reticulum. J Biol Chem. 1995;270:5449–56.
46. Corbeil D, Milhiet PE, Simon V et al. Rat endopeptidase-24.18 alpha subunit is secreted into the culture medium as a zymogen when expressed by COS-1 cells. FEBS Lett. 1993;335:361–6.
47. Milhiet PE, Corbeil D, Simon V, Kenny AJ, Crine P, Boileau G. Expression of rat endopeptidase-24.18 in COS-1 cells: membrane topology and activity. Biochem J. 1994;300:37–43.
48. Johnson GD, Hersh LB. Expression of meprin subunit precursors. Membrane anchoring through the beta subunit and mechanism of zymogen activation. J Biol Chem. 1994;269:7682–8.
49. Kaushal GP, Walker PD, Shah SV. An old enzyme with a new function: purification and characterization of a distinct matrix-degrading metalloproteinase in rat kidney cortex and its identification as meprin. J Cell Biol. 1994;126:1319–27.
50. Craig SS, Mader C, Bond JS. Immunohistochemical localization of the metalloproteinase meprin in salivary glands of male and female mice. J Histochem Cytochem. 1991;39:123–9.
51. Spencer-Dene B, Thorogood P, Nair S, Kenny AJ, Harris M, Henderson B. Distribution of, and putative role for, the cell-surface neutral metalloendopeptidases during mammalian craniofacial development. Development. 1994;120:3213–26.
52. Jiang W, Sadler PM, Jenkins NA, Gilbert DJ, Copeland NG, Bond JS. Tissue-specific expression and chromosomal localization of the alpha subunit of mouse meprin A. J Biol Chem. 1993;268:10380–5.
53. Craig SS, Reckelhoff JF, Bond JS. Distribution of meprin in kidneys from mice with high- and low-meprin activity. Am J Physiol. 1987;253:C535–40.
54. Yamaguchi T, Kido H, Kitazawa R, Kitazawa S, Fukase M, Katunama N. A membrane-bound metallo-endopeptidase from a rat kidney: its immunological characterization. J Biochem (Tokyo). 1993;113:299–303.
55. Bankus JM, Bond JS. Expression and distribution of meprin protease subunits in mouse intestine. Arch Biochim Biophys. 1996;331:87–94.
56. Sterchi E, Dumermuth E, Eldering J, Grünberg J. Paba-peptide hydrolase (PPH): structure and expression of a metalloendopeptidase from human small intestinal epithelial cells. In: Lentze MJ, Naim HY, Grand RJ, eds. Mammalian Brush Border Membrane Proteins II. Georg Thieme Verlag Stuttgart. New York Thieme Medical Publishers, Inc., New York, 1994.
57. Yamaguchi T, Fukase M, Sugimoto T, Kido H, Chihara K. Purification of meprin from human kidney and its role in parathyroid hormone degradation. Biol Chem Hoppe Seyler. 1994;375:821–4.
58. Dietrich J, Jiang W, Bond J. A novel meprin beta′ mRNA in mouse embryonal and human colon carcinoma cells. J Biol Chem. 1996;27:2271–8.
59. Finlayson JS, Asofsky R, Potter M, Runner CC. Major urinary protein complex of normal mice: origin. Science. 1965;149:981–2.
60. Shaw PH, Held WA, Hastie ND. The gene family for major urinary proteins: expression in several secretory tissues of the mouse. Cell. 1983;32:755–61.
61. Flannery AV, Dalzell GN, Beynon RJ. Proteolytic activity in mouse urine: relationship to the kidney metallo-endopeptidase, meprin. Biochim Biophys Acta. 1990;1041:64–70.
62. Yamaguchi T, Fukase M, Kido H, Sugimoto T, Katunuma N, Chihara K. Meprin is predominantly involved in parathyroid hormone degradation by the microvillar membranes of rat kidney. Life Sci. 1994;54:381–6.
63. Yamaguchi T, Fukase M, Sugimoto T, Chihara K. Hydrolysis of a carboxy-terminal fragment of parathyroid hormone-related protein by rat kidney: evidence for a crucial role of meprin. Horm Metab Res. 1995;27:131–6.
64. Reckelhoff JF, Craig SS, Beynon RJ, Bond JS. Meprin phenotype and cyclosporin A toxicity in mice. Adv Exp Med Biol. 1988;240:293–304.
65. Trachtman H, Valderrama E, Dietrich J, Bond J. The role of meprin A in the pathogenesis of acute renal failure. Biochem Biophys Res Commun. 1995;208:498–505.
66. Trachtman H, Greenwald R, Moak S, Tang J, Bond JS. Meprin activity in rats with experimental renal disease. Life Sci. 1993;53:1339–44.
67. Jiang W, Dewald G, Brundage E et al. Fine mapping of MEP1A, the gene encoding the alpha subunit of the metalloendopeptidase meprin, to human chromosome 6P21. Biochem Biophys Res Commun. 1995;216:630–5.

8
Paneth cells, host defence, and the crypt microenvironment

A. J. OUELLETTE, D. DARMOUL and M. E. SELSTED

Paneth cells release endogenous antimicrobial proteins and peptides into the lumen of the crypts of Lieberkühn in the small intestine. Cell-specific defensins, termed cryptdins, are among the secreted granule components of these cells, and evidence suggests that they contribute to innate immunity in the crypt microenvironment. As members of the defensin peptide family, cryptdins are cationic, 3–4 kDa, amphipathic peptides that contain six Cys residues in three, invariantly-paired disulphide bonds. Mouse cryptdins are potent antimicrobial agents, and certain microorganisms differ in their sensitivity to individual peptides; N-terminal modification and amino acid substitutions at residue positions 10 and 15 modulate antimicrobial function, and appear to be determinants of microbicidal potency. Defensin transcripts are abundant in mouse and human Paneth cells, and the known peptides are coded by separate, two-exon genes clustered on chromosome 8. Mouse Paneth cell defensin genes are expressed selectively both along the length of the small intestine and during postnatal intestinal development. In adult mice, cryptdin-4 mRNA, undetectable in duodenum, occurs at maximal levels in distal ileum, cryptdin genes are expressed in neonatal intestinal epithelium before the appearance of recognizable Paneth cells. Cryptdin-containing cells in newborn intestine are distributed throughout the newborn intestinal epithelium, with the cryptdin peptide found in apparent association with intracellular granules and also on mucosal surfaces. Thus, cryptdins appear to contribute to mucosal barrier function in both the adult and neonatal intestine. Knowledge of defensin function during epithelial differentation may improve the understanding of crypt ontogeny.

PANETH CELLS AND THE MUCOSAL BARRIER

Paneth cells release large, basophilic granules apically into the lumen of small intestinal crypts. Originating from crypt stem cells which give rise to the four intestinal epithelial lineages, these secretory granulocytes mature below the proliferative zone and have apparent half-lives of 20–25 days[1]. The appearance of

Paneth cells in rodents coincides with crypt ontogeny during the first 2–3 post-natal weeks, corresponding with events in human gestation that occur during the first trimester.

Paneth cells contribute to mucosal barrier function by synthesizing and secreting proteins associated with innate immunity and host defence into the extracellular space[2,3], including lysozyme and defensins. Release of Paneth cell granules can be stimulated by muscarinic/cholinergic agonists[4], and degranulation induced by NaF and $AlCl_3$ demonstrates the involvement of G-protein signalling mechanisms[5]. Luminal concentrations of lysozyme increase 20- to 40-fold minutes after pilocarpine administration, and cryptdins have been isolated from luminal rinses of mouse small intestine without prior administration of pharmacological agents[6]. Although Paneth cell morphology in germ-free mice and conventionally-reared animals is modestly different[7] and challenge of gnotobiotic mice and rats with an oral bolus of bacteria elicits a degranulation response[8], Paneth cell development does not require luminal bacteria or dietary factors[9,10]. Colonization and overgrowth of the epithelium by bacteria[11], a rare event, may, therefore, involve resistance to Paneth cell secretory products, including cryptdins.

Defensins are cysteine-rich, highly cationic, 3–4 kDa peptides that were originally described as antimicrobial peptide components of phagocytic leukocyte granules[12–14]. Preformed antimicrobial peptides are viewed as providing a means of responding to or inhibiting colonization of mucosal surfaces by infectious agents. Peptide antibiotics may function intracellularly, as in circulating leuko-cytes, or in a degradative external environment after release by Paneth cells and possibly other epithelia[5,16]. The primary and secondary structures of antimicrobial peptides are highly varied, yet nearly all are amphipathic, a consistent biochemical feature that is necessary for the ability to kill microbial cells by membrane dis-ruption. The six cysteines in defensins form three invariantly paired disulphide bonds[12]: Cys1 to Cys6, Cys2 to Cys4, and Cys3 to Cys5 that result in an amphipathic peptide that consists predominantly of β-sheet backbone. Neutrophil defensins mediate multimeric pore formation by mechanisms involving sequential electrostatic and hydrophobic interactions between non-covalent peptide dimers and the target membrane[17]. The diameter of pores formed by human neutrophil defensin HNP-2 has been estimated at approximately 20 Å, based on the atomic structure of HNP-3 and the size of dextran polymers released from preloaded vesicles[18]. A pore model involving the intercalation of six HNP-2 dimers in the bilayer has been reviewed recently[19].

CRYPTDINS

mRNAs coding for defensins are highly abundant in mouse[6,20] and human Paneth cells[21], and several aspects of their biological and biochemical features have been reviewed recently[22]. Six mouse Paneth cell defensins, cryptdins 1–6, have been purified from mouse small bowel, sequenced, and cryptdins 1–3 and 6 have been localized to the epithelium immunohistochemically[6]. In situ hybridization and immunodetection by light microscopy with an anti-cryptdin-1 antibody show the exclusive localization of cryptdins in Paneth cells but not in infiltrating leukocytes[6]. Ultrastructural detection experiments with immunogold conjugates have definitively localized cryptdins to Paneth cell granules and shown that the peptide(s) is present and evenly distributed in every granule examined (Ouellette et al., unpublished). Except for cryptdin-4, the amino termini of cryptdins are 5–6 residues longer than those of most phagocyte-derived defensins, yet the functional importance of the extended N-termini for action in the extracellular space following secretion has not been demonstrated. Relevant to this point, however, certain full-length and N-terminally truncated cryptdins have been purified from the mouse small intestinal lumen, and, although full-length luminal cryptdins are as active as corresponding tissue forms, the antimicrobial activity of N-terminally truncated peptides against *Escherichia coli* and *Salmonella typhimurium* is ablated or greatly diminished[23].

MOUSE CRYPTDINS ARE ANTIMICROBIAL PEPTIDES

Against *E. coli* ML35, cryptdins 1, 3, and 6 have approximately equivalent antimicrobial activities that are 3–5-fold greater than that of cryptdin-2[24]; cryptdin-4 is the most active of the peptides[24]. Of these peptides, cryptdin-4 is the most cationic and the most active enteric defensin, and it has an unusual chain-length variation between the fourth and fifth cysteine residues. In microbicidal assays performed in solution, all cryptdins except cryptdin-2 kill *E. coli* at a concentration of $10\,\mu g/ml$. Since cryptdins 2 and 3 differ only at position 10 (Thr vs. Lys, respectively), that residue position appears to be important in the bactericidal interaction of cryptdins with *E. coli*.

STRUCTURE OF ENTERIC DEFENSIN GENES

The known mouse and human Paneth cell defensin genes have a highly-conserved, two-exon structure in which the preprosegment and mature peptide coding sequences are on different exons that are separated by an approximately 550 pb intron[21,25]. In contrast, all reported neutrophil defensin genes contain an additional intron interrupting the 5′-UTS in those transcripts[26–28]; that intron distinguishes Paneth cell and myeloid defensin genes. In mice, cryptdin genes are closely linked, as evidenced by the isolation of several bacteriophage clones containing two different and complete defensin family genes[25] (Ouellette et al., unpublished data). The genes map to the proximal region of mouse chromosome 8[29] and to 8p23 in humans[30,31]. In addition to mRNAs for the six known cryptdin peptides, mouse Paneth cells express 14 additional cryptdin isoform mRNAs with extensive homology to cryptdins 1–3[24]. In contrast to the apparently expanded defensin gene family of the mouse, only two Paneth cell defensin genes have been found in the human genome[30,32]. Nucleotide substitutions affecting coding function in mouse cryptdin isoform mRNAs occur only at a few nucleotide positions: codons 38 and 52 of the prosegment and codons 68, 73, 76, 87, 87 and 89 in the peptide-coding region are the most frequently substituted positions.

DEFENSIN-RELATED MOUSE GENES

The mouse genome contains two-exon, Paneth cell-specific genes consisting of cryptdin-like first exons linked to divergent second exons that code for novel cysteine-rich sequence (CRS) peptides. As deduced from cDNA sequence analysis, the prototypic CRS gene products, CRS1C and CRS4C, are cationic, cysteine-rich peptides with 9 or 11 cysteine residues, respectively, in a series of [C]-[X]-[X] triplet repeats. The two-exon CRS genes closely resemble cryptdin genes, with highly conserved transcription start sites, intron/exon junctions, and each contains a single intron of approximately 550 bp[34]; all members of these defensin gene subfamilies map to loci on chromosome 8[33]. Thus far, mRNAs for 20 different cryptdins[24], seven CRS1C isoforms (A.J. Ouellette et al., unpublished), and eight sequence variants of CRS4C[33] are expressed by mouse Paneth cells. The extensive conservation of the prosegment in these mouse defensin family precursors suggests that it may help to target varied peptides to Paneth cell secretory granules for release into the lumen.

REGULATION OF CRYPTDIN GENES

The cryptdin-4 isoform gene is expressed with positional specificity along the longitudinal axis of the small intestine, and a subset of cryptdin genes is expressed in the immature intestinal epithelium of newborn mice prior to the appearance of recognizable Paneth cells. Assays based on reverse transcription–polymerase chain reaction (RT–PCR) do not detect cryptdin-4 mRNA in the proximal 5 cm of mouse small intestine, and the mRNA occurs at maximal levels in distal ileum[34]. In contrast, cryptdin-1 and cryptdin-5 mRNA levels are equivalent throughout the small intestine. The distribution of cryptdin-4 mRNA correlates with the greater bacterial numbers of the ileum relative to the proximal small bowel, perhaps contributing specifically to innate immunity in the distal small intestine.

Studies in transgenic mice show that a putative cryptdin-2 gene promoter can direct reporter transgene expression appropriately to Paneth cells[35]. Mice transgenic for approximately 6.5 kb upstream of the mouse cryptdin-2 gene linked to human growth hormone coding sequence (Crp2/hGH) have been established and investigated. The reporter gene was detected in proliferating and nonproliferating epithelial cells until postnatal day 5 (P5), then becoming restricted to the Paneth cell lineage during crypt ontogeny[35]. Cells positive for an anti-cryptdin-1 antibody were detected interspersed in the gut epithelium of normal mice as early as embryonic day 15 (E15). At P5, intestinal cells at the base of crypts and villus-associated goblet cells co-express hGH and cryptdin[35]. By P7, most cryptdin-positive cells have the morphological appearance of rudimentary Paneth cells[35]. RNA blot hybridization and RT–PCR analysis showed that, like cryptdin mRNA, transgene expression in a certain line was restricted to the small bowel, with distal hGH mRNA levels greater than those in proximal gut. Curiously, hGH gene expression became extinguished in adults in several pedigrees[35].

Cryptdin genes are differentially expressed during postnatal crypt ontogeny, providing an opportunity to investigate the development of this component of enteric host defence. As the Crp2/hGH transgenic mouse studies would predict[35],

RT–PCR assays readily detect cryptdin mRNAs in P1 mice[36] even though Northern blot analysis of P1 gut RNA is consistently negative[37,38]. Cells containing cryptdin peptides have been identified in newborn intestinal epithelium using a rabbit antibody to mouse cryptdin-1. Additionally, RT–PCR assays have shown that Paneth cell mRNAs for lysozyme, matrilysin, and CRS1C also are present at P1. Analysis of cryptdin-specific cDNA sequences amplified from P1 mouse intestinal RNA showed that cryptdin isoform mRNAs are present and that cryptdin-6 is the most abundant Paneth cell defensin mRNA in the P1 mouse intestine (A.J. Ouellette, unpublished).

The presence of cryptdin peptides in the developing intestinal epithelium has been confirmed immunohistochemically. In P1 mice, immunoreactive cryptdins are found in cells distributed throughout the intestinal epithelium rather than the intense, highly specific immunoreactivity of Paneth cells in adult small intestinal crypts. The peptides may be released into the lumen by these maturing small intestinal cells, since the punctate antibody staining in the neonate is consistent with localization to granules. Immunoreactive antigen was often apparent on villous luminal surfaces, suggesting an association with cell surface components. Genes characteristic of differentiated Paneth cells are, therefore, active in the newborn mouse intestinal epithelium prior to crypt formation. In humans, Paneth cell defensin mRNAs HD-5 and HD-6 have been detected by in situ hybridization in crypts at 13.5 weeks gestation[32]; the presence of HD-5 and HD-6 mRNAs at this gestational age in consistent with the appearance of Paneth cells in human intestinal development[39]. The role of cells expressing cryptdins and Paneth cell genes prior to crypt morphogenesis is unknown, but an understanding of the biology of cryptdin-positive cells during crypt morphogenesis may provide insights into cellular events in crypt development.

Since Paneth cell defensins are implicated in mucosal immunity in the adult[24,40], involvement of cryptdins in neonate enteric host defence is a possibility. The factor(s) inducing cryptdin genes are not known, but microbial antigens are unlikely activators for at least three reasons. First, cryptdins are found in late gestation[36]; second, although cryptdin gene expression has not been assessed, normal Paneth cells develop from fetal intestinal implants grown under sub-cutaneous flaps in mice[10,41]; third, cryptdin mRNA levels in adult germ-free mice are the same as in conventionally-reared mice[20]. As in adults, the Paneth cell mRNAs for lysozyme and matrilysin are co-expressed with cryptdins. However, until the primary structures of P1 mouse intestinal cryptdin peptides are known, one cannot assume that intestinal defensins in newborns are the functional equivalents of the adult Paneth cell peptides. Nevertheless, it seems reasonable to hypothesize that the release of antimicrobial cryptdins into the lumen of the newborn mouse intestine would influence the local microenvironment and con-tribute to protecting the neonatal intestine from colonization by ingested bacteria.

Acknowledgements

Supported by NIH grants DK44632, DK33506, and HD31852 (AJO), AI22931 (MES) and by the Center for the Study of Inflammatory Bowel Disease at the Massachusetts General Hospital (NIH grant DK43351).

References

1. Cheng H. Origin, differentiation and renewal of the four main epithelial cell types in the mouse small intestine. IV. Paneth cells. Am J Anat. 1974;141:521–35.
2. Geyer G. Lysozyme in Paneth cell secretions. Acta Histochem. 1973;45:126–32.
3. Harwig SSL, Tan L, Qu X-D, Cho Y, Eisenhauer PB, Lehrer RI. Bactericidal properties of murine intestinal phospholipase A₂. J Clin Invest. 1995;95:603–10.
4. Satoh Y, Ishikawa K, Oomori Y, Yamano M, Ono K. Effects of cholecystokinin and carbamyl choline on Paneth cell secretion in mice: a comparison with pancreatic acinar cells. Anat Rec. 1989;225:124–32.
5. Satoh Y, Ishikawa K, Oomori Y, Takeda S, Ono K. Bethanechol and a G-protein activator, NaF/AlC13, induce secretory response in Paneth cells of mouse intestine. Cell Tissue Res. 1992;269:213–20.
6. Selsted ME, Miller SI, Henschen AH, Ouellette AJ. Enteric defensins: antibiotic peptide components of intestinal host defense. J Cell Biol. 1992;118:929–36.
7. Satoh Y, Ishikawa K, Tanaka H, Oomori Y, Ono K. Immunohistochemical observations of lysozyme in the Paneth cells of specific-pathogen-free and germ-free mice. Acta Histochem. 1988;83:185–8.
8. Satoh Y. Effect of live and heat-killed bacteria on the secretory activity of Paneth cells in germ-free mice. Cell Tissue Res. 1988;251:87–93.
9. Rubin DC, Roth KA, Birkenmeier EH, Gordon JI. Epithelial cell differentiation in normal and transgenic mouse intestinal isografts. J Cell Biol. 1991;113:1183–92.
10. Winter HS, Hendren RB, Fox CH et al. Human intestine matures as nude mouse xenograft. Gastroenterology. 1991;100:89–98.
11. Saadia R. Trauma and bacterial translocation. Br J Surg. 1995;82:1243–4.
12. Kagan BL, Ganz T, Lehrer RI. Defensins: A family of antimicrobial and cytotoxic peptides. Toxicology. 1994;87:131–49.
13. Selsted ME, Brown DM, DeLange RJ, Lehrer RI. Primary structures of MCP-1 and MCP-2, natural peptide antibiotics of rabbit lung macrophages. J Biol Chem. 1983;258:14485–9.
14. Selsted ME, Szklarek D, Lehrer RI. Purification and antibacterial activity of antimicrobial peptides of rabbit granulocytes. Infect Immun. 1984;45:150–4.
15. Boman HG. Antibacterial peptides: key components needed in immunity. Cell. 1991;65:205–7.
16. Selsted ME, Ouellette AJ. Defensins in granules of phagocytic and non-phagocytic cells. Trends Cell Biol. 1995;5:114–19.
17. Lehrer RI, Barton A, Daher KA, Harwig SS, Ganz T, Selsted ME. Interaction of human defensins with Escherichia coli. Mechanism of bactericidal activity. J Clin Invest. 1989;84:553–61.
18. Wimley WC, Selsted ME, White SH. Interactions between human defensins and lipid bilayers: evidence for formation of multimeric pores. Protein Sci. 1994;3:1362–73.
19. White SH, Wimley WC, Selsted ME. Structure, function, and membrane integration of defensins. Curr Opin Struct Biol. 1995;5:521–7.
20. Ouellette AJ, Greco RM, James M, Frederick D, Naftilan J, Fallon JT. Developmental regulation of cryptdin, a corticostatin/defensin precursor mRNA in mouse small intestinal crypt epithelium. J Cell Biol. 1989;108:1687–95.
21. Jones DE, Bevins CL. Paneth cells of the human small intestine express an antimicrobial peptide gene. J Biol Chem. 1992;267:23216–25.
22. Ouellette AJ, Selsted ME. Paneth cell defensins: Endogenous peptide components of intestinal host defense. FASEB J. 1996;10:1280–9.
23. Ouellette AJ, Hsieh MM, Selsted ME. Structure and function of cryptdins isolated from mouse small intestinal lumen. Gastroenterology. 1996;110(Suppl.):A985.
24. Ouellette AJ, Hsieh MM, Nosek MT et al. Mouse Paneth cell defensins: primary structures and antibacterial activities of numerous cryptdin isoforms. Infect Immun. 1994;62:5040–7.
25. Huttner KM, Selsted ME, Ouellette AJ. Structure and diversity of the murine cryptdin gene family. Genomics. 1994;19:448–53.
26. Ganz T, Rayner JR, Valore EV, Tumolo A, Talmadge K, Fuller F. The structure of the rabbit macrophage defensin genes and their organ-specific expression. J Immunol. 1989;143:1358–65.
27. Linzmeier R, Michaelson D, Liu L, Ganz T. The structure of neutrophil defensin genes. FEBS Lett. 1993;321:267–73.
28. Nagaoka I, Someya A, Iwabuchi K, Yamashita T. Structure of the guinea pig neutrophil cationic peptide gene. FEBS Lett. 1992;303:31–5.

29. Ouellette AJ, Pravtcheva D, Ruddle FH, James M. Localization of the cryptdin locus on mouse chromosome 8 (published erratum appears in Genomics. 1992;12:626). Genomics. 1989;5:233–9.
30. Bevins CL, Jones DE, Dutra A, Schaffzin J, Muenke M. Human enteric defensin genes: Chromosomal map position and a model for possible evolutionary relationships. Genomics. 1996;31:95–106.
31. Sparkes RS, Kronenberg M, Heinzmann C et al. Assignment of defensin gene(s) to human chromosome 8p23. Genomics. 1989;5:240–44.
32. Mallow EB, Harris A, Salzman N et al. Human enteric defensins – gene structure and developmental expression. J Biol Chem. 1996;271:4038–45.
33. Huttner KM, Ouellette AJ. A family of defensin-like genes codes for diverse cysteine-rich peptides in mouse Paneth cells. Genomics. 1994;24:99–109.
34. Darmoul D, Ouellette AJ. Positional specificity of defensin gene expression reveals Paneth cell heterogeneity in mouse small intestine. Am J Physiol. 1996;271:G68–74.
35. Bry L, Falk P, Huttner K, Ouellette AJ, Midtvedt T, Gordon JI. Paneth cell differentiation in the developing intestine of normal and transgenic mice. Proc Natl Acad Sci USA. 1994;91:10335–9.
36. Darmoul D, Wang A, Ouellette AJ. Differential expression of cryptdin genes during crypt ontogeny and along the longitudinal axis of mouse small intestine. Gastroenterology. 1994;106(Suppl.):A603.
37. Ouellette AJ, Cordell B. Accumulation of abundant messenger ribonucleic acids during postnatal development of mouse small intestine. Gastroenterology. 1988;94:114–21.
38. Ouellette AJ, Lualdi JC. A novel mouse gene family coding for cationic, cysteine-rich peptides. Regulation in small intestine and cells of myeloid origin. J Biol Chem. 1990;265:9831–7; addition and corrections: J Biol Chem. 1994;269:18702.
39. Moxey PC, Trier JS. Specialized cell types in the human fetal small intestine. Anat Rec. 1978;191:269–86.
40. Aley SB, Zimmerman M, Hetsko M, Selsted ME, Gillin FD. Killing of *Giardia lamblia* by cryptdins and cationic neutrophil peptides. Infect Immun. 1994;62:5397–403.
41. Rubin DC, Swietlicki E, Roth KA, Gordon JI. Use of fetal intestinal isografts from normal and transgenic mice to study the programming of positional information along the duodenal-to-colonic axis. J Biol Chem. 1992;267:15122–33.

9
Gastrointestinal peptide receptors and neoplastic growth processes

J. C. REUBI

INTRODUCTION

Gastrointestinal peptides, also called regulatory peptides, are molecules with very potent biological effects which are synthesized in several types of tissues, primarily in the brain and in the gut, but also in endocrine or lymphatic tissues. They regulate key functions in the body and act through G-protein coupled receptors. They may act as neurotransmitters, hormones, gut peptides, vasoactive substances, immunoregulators or growth factors. Clinically relevant is the fact that they can be applied exogenously (subcutaneous or intravenous injection) and penetrate easily into most tissues, except for the brain which is separated from the periphery by the blood–brain barrier. They are, however, rapidly degraded by peptidases; this disadvantage can often be overcome since these compounds can be modified chemically to more stable analogues. Table 1 shows a non-exhaustive list of such regulatory peptides.

Over the last 15 years, we have tried to evaluate whether selected peptides can be used as model substances for the targeting, via specific receptors, of various human diseases, in particular tumours[1]. We first tried to identify regulatory peptide receptors in normal human tissues: most of the basic information available stems from rat or other animal studies, but not humans. I will therefore first summarize our studies performed in human tissues, in particular in the gastrointestinal tract. Second, we tried to identify pathologies characterized by over-expression of

Table 1 Selected regulatory peptides

Opioid peptides	Bradykinin
Substance P	Bombesin/gastrin-releasing peptide
Gastrin	Neuropeptide Y
Cholecystokinin	Galanin
Vasoactive intestinal peptide	Neurotensin
Pituitary adenylate cyclase activating peptide	Secretin
Angiotensin	Somatostatin
Calcitonin	Endothelin

regulatory peptide receptors that is sufficiently high to be relevant and of clinical interest as diagnostic tool or for therapy. To reach both goals, the method of in vitro receptor autoradiography has been considered the method of choice: in complex human tissue biopsies, such as those investigated in this study, it is essential to identify at the histological level the tissue expressing the respective receptors.

REGULATORY PEPTIDE RECEPTORS IN NORMAL GASTROINTESTINAL TISSUE

Somatostatin receptors

Somatostatin receptors are expressed in the mucosa of the gastrointestinal tract from the stomach to the colon[2] and in lymphoid tissue, in particular in the gut associated lymphoid tissue consisting in tonsils, appendix, Peyer patches, or solitary follicles[3]. In all these cases, the germinal centres of the lymphoid follicles preferentially express somatostatin receptors. Somatostatin receptors are also expressed in neural tissues, such as the plexus submucosus and the plexus myentericus. Somatostatin, therefore, has an extremely complex and significant role in the gut, mediated through multiple biological systems.

Substance P receptors

Substance P receptors in the gastrointestinal tract have a completely different pattern from that of somatostatin receptors. The mucosa only weakly expresses substance P receptors whereas the vessels, in particular the submucosal vessels, including both veins and arteries, are heavily labelled. Substance P is known to have a strong vasodilatory function mediated by these vascular receptors[4].

VIP receptors

Gastrointestinal VIP receptors show a pattern of expression different from that of somatostatin and substance P receptors. In colon tissue, for instance, the mucosa is labelled, with a particularly strong labelling of the superficial layer of the mucosa (Figure 1). The vessels in the submucosa are also labelled (Figure 1); most importantly, the lymphoid tissues are always labelled: Figure 1 shows a lymphoid follicle expressing VIP receptors.

CCK receptors

CCK-A and CCK-B receptors are heavily expressed in various parts of the gastrointestinal tract[5]. In the human, for instance, CCK-B receptors are found in the fundic mucosa, in particular in the midglandular part of the mucosa. CCK-A receptors are found predominantly in the basal part of the mucosa. Circular and longitudinal muscles of the stomach also express CCK receptors: CCK-B receptors

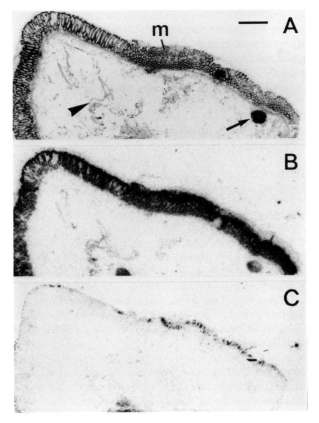

Figure 1 VIP receptors in human colon. (A) Haematoxylin–eosin-stained section showing the mucosa (m) and submucosa with vessels (arrowhead) and a lymphatic follicle (arrow). Bar = 1 mm. (B) Autoradiogram showing total binding of ^{125}I-VIP. Strong labelling is seen in the mucosa and lymphatic follicle, while moderate labelling is seen in vessels. (C) Autoradiogram showing non-specific binding (in the presence of 10^{-6} M VIP)

in the circular muscles and CCK-A receptors in the longitudinal muscles. In the antrum of the stomach a completely different picture is observed: no CCK-B receptors are found, but CCK-A receptors are present in the basal mucosa and in the muscle layers. The gall bladder expresses CCK-A receptors within the muscle layers, but no CCK-B receptors. It is possible to differentiate CCK-A and CCK-B receptors through their different affinity for CCK-A or CCK-B receptor-selective antagonists. L-364,718, a CCK-A selective antagonist, has a high affinity for CCK-A receptor in the gallbladder, while L-365,260, a CCK-B selective antagonist, has only weak affinity for these receptors. In CCK-B receptor-expressing gastric mucosa, however, L-365,260 has a higher affinity for the CCK-B receptor than has L-364,718[5]. Finally, neuronal systems express CCK receptors primarily in the colonic nerve plexus.

These results show the enormous variability and extremely broad distribution of regulatory peptide receptors in the human gastrointestinal tract. These receptors are expressed by almost all possible cell types, including various cells in the mucosa, vascular system, neuronal system, lymphoid system and muscles. These receptors are likely to represent the molecular basis for the various functional roles of these peptides in the gastrointestinal tract; this aspect is however beyond the scope of this short article. I will now discuss whether human diseases originating from these receptor-positive tissues can also express regulatory peptide receptors, whether they can over-express these receptors, and whether these receptors can be used as markers for such diseases.

REGULATORY PEPTIDE RECEPTORS IN TUMOURS

Somatostatin receptors

Somatostatin receptors are over-expressed in a large number of human tumours, including the great majority of neuroendocrine tumours and tumours of the nervous system[6]. An example of somatostatin receptor expression by an inactive pituitary adenoma is shown in Figure 2, where homogeneous distribution of this receptor in the whole tumour region is found. Combination of in vitro autoradiography with in situ hybridization provides a complementary method to identify not only the receptor protein but the receptor mRNA; Figure 2 shows abundance of the sst2 subtype mRNA in that same tumour.

Not all tumours express somatostatin receptors: colonic cancers only rarely express somatostatin receptors. However, it is intriguing to observe that around the colorectal tumours the somatostatin receptors are expressed in the peritumoral vessels, in particular in the veins[7]. We have shown a direct topographical relationship between the over-expressed somatostatin receptors and the tumour in that there was a strong correlation between the density of receptors in these vessels and their proximity to the tumour. The nearer to the tumour (0–2 cm), the higher the expression of somatostatin receptors in peritumoral veins, at 5 and 10 cm away from the tumour only low levels of vascular receptors remained, similar to the level seen in normal tissue. A similar feature was seen with substance P receptors[7]. The possible action of somatostatin through somatostatin receptors in peritumoral vessels can be described as follows. First, somatostatin may induce a vasoconstriction of these vessels, which may lead to local hypoxia and then to tumour necrosis. Second, somatostatin may induce inhibition of angiogenesis and therefore inhibit tumour growth. Finally, somatostatin may decrease the extravasation of plasma and inflammatory cells and, as such, decrease the peritumoral inflammation, which is considerable in colorectal cancers.

Somatostatin may therefore act in a dual way on tumours: first directly, as a tumour growth inhibiting factor on the somatostatin receptor-expressing tumour tissue itself, second on peritumoral vessels, as described above.

VIP receptors

Unfortunately, somatostatin receptors are not often expressed by the more common and aggressive epithelial tumours such as exocrine pancreatic cancer,

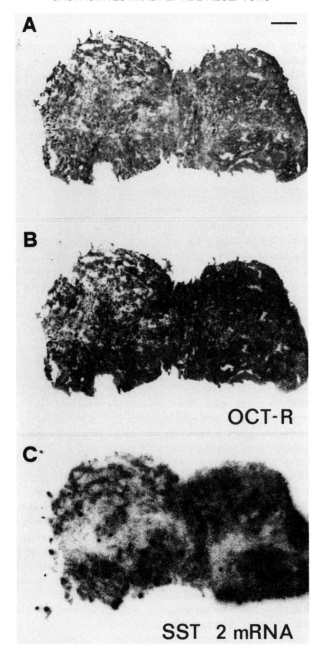

Figure 2 Somatostatin receptors and sst2 mRNA in an inactive pituitary adenoma. (A) Haema-toxylin–eosin-stained section showing the tumour. Bar = 1 mm. (B) Autoradiogram showing total binding of ^{125}I-[Tyr^3]-octreotide. The whole tumour is labelled. Non-specific binding is negligible. (C) Autoradiogram showing abundance of sst2 somatostatin receptor subtype mRNA detected by in situ hybridization in an adjacent section

bladder cancer, colon cancer, glioblastoma or non-small cell lung cancers (nSCLC). It is therefore of interest to know whether other regulatory peptide receptors may be expressed by these tumours. We observed that VIP receptors are highly expressed in the majority of human epithelial tumours, including those tumours mentioned above[8]. It is of interest to the gastroenterologist that a majority of colonic cancers and pancreatic exocrine cancers (Figure 3) express VIP receptors. It should also be mentioned that a majority of tumours preferentially express VIP_1-PACAP II receptors, a minority of tumours, mainly brain tumours, have PACAP-I receptors (with low affinity for VIP), and a significant number have a mixed PACAP-I/PACAP-II receptor distribution (Reubi, unpublished data).

Substance P receptors

Substance P receptors can also be expressed in some, but by far not all, human tumours[9]. Primarily, medullary thyroid cancers (MTC), breast tumours, neuro-blastomas and glial tumours express substance P receptors in a high incidence and density, whereas most gastrointestinal tumours appear to be negative for these receptors[9]. However, in most samples of the tumours investigated in that study we observed a high expression of substance P receptors in peritumoral vessels, whether or not the tumour expressed substance P receptors. An example of a nSCLC with SP receptors expressed by peritumoral vessels is shown in Figure 4. The receptors are present both in veins and arteries, suggesting, as mentioned previously for somatostatin receptors, the possibility of a dual action of substance P: on one hand, at the level of the tumour tissue, one the other hand, on the level of the peritumoral vessels, where substance P has a strong vaso-dilatatory action.

CCK receptors

We were unable to identify a significant amount of CCK-B/gastrin receptors in colorectal cancers, confirming recent reports by others[10]. However, we confirmed that a majority of SCLC express CCK-B/gastrin receptors whereas nSCLC do not express gastrin receptors. Unexpectedly, we also showed that almost all medullary thyroid cancers (MTC) expressed CCK-B receptors whereas differentiated thyroid cancers, including follicular and papillary thyroid cancers, did not[11]. CCK-B/gastrin receptors in MTC may be the molecular basis for the pentagastrin test, which elicits a strong stimulation of the calcitonin release in these tumours and is therefore routinely used to detect MTCs at early stages.

CCK-A receptors were rarely found in human tumours except for gastro-enteropancreatic tumours and meningiomas.

Figure 3 (Opposite) VIP receptors in an exocrine pancreatic adenocarcinoma. (A) Haema-toxylin–eosin-stained section showing the tumour. Bar = 1 mm. (B) Autoradiogram showing total binding of ^{125}I-VIP. The whole tumour is labelled. (C) Non-specific binding

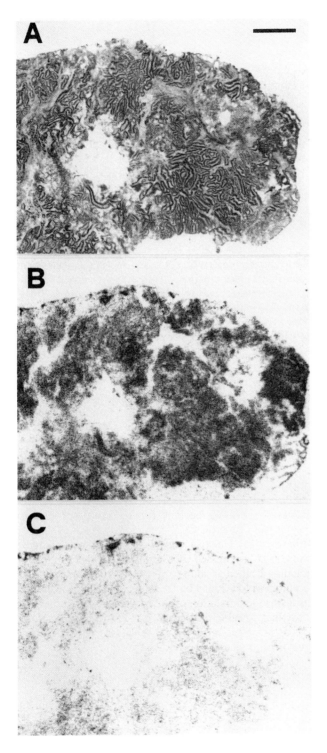

95

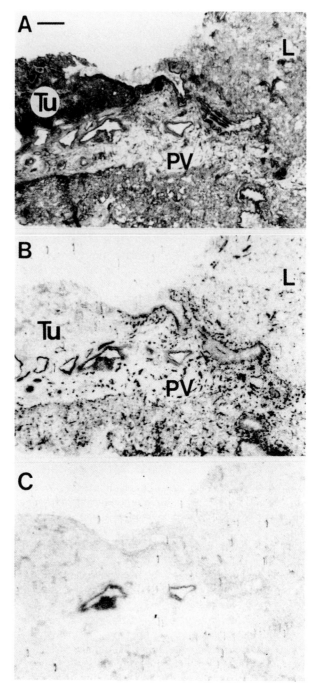

Figure 4 Substance P receptors in the surrounding vessels of a non-small cell lung cancer. (A) Haematoxylin–eosin-stained section showing the tumour (Tu), peritumoral vessels (PV), and adjacent lung (L). Bar = 1 mm. (B) Autoradiogram showing total binding of ^{125}I-SP with receptor expression primarily in the peritumoral vessels. (C) Non-specific binding

These results show that a majority of human tumours express one or several types of regulatory peptide receptors. We do not yet know much about the mechanisms and the triggers responsible for the over-expression of these receptors in neoplasms. Moreover, it seems extremely difficult to predict the receptor expression in a given tumour type based on the receptor expression in the healthy tissue from which the tumour originates. Extensive studies will have to be performed to understand these various issues.

CLINICAL IMPLICATIONS OF REGULATORY PEPTIDE RECEPTOR EXPRESSION IN TUMOURS

It is now well established that the selective pattern of high receptor expression in numerous human tumours is clinically relevant. There are two aspects of this finding: diagnostic and therapeutic.

Recent studies have shown that somatostatin receptors in tumours can be visualized by in vivo somatostatin receptor scintigraphy. An injection of radio-labelled somatostatin analogue in a patient will permit visualization of somatostatin receptor-positive tumours since the radioactive label will be enriched in the tumour due to binding to the receptors[12]. This method is particularly successful for GEP tumours and all other tumours which have a high density of somatostatin receptors. A similar development was recently reported for VIP receptor-positive tumours, for which in vivo VIP receptor scintigraphy can be performed with success[13]. However, it is likely that the development of more stable and less degradable VIP ligands will be necessary to optimize a method which may be extremely valuable for the localization of pancreatic and colonic cancers.

The regulatory peptide receptors are also a target for therapy. For instance, somatostatin receptor-positive GEP tumours are highly responsive to somatostatin analogue therapy, which mediates inhibition of hormone secretion and therefore lowers the symptoms due to the high hormone level in these patients[14]. Furthermore, a VIP receptor antagonist was able to inhibit the growth of VIP receptor-positive tumours significantly[15]. Perhaps the most attractive implication of these results will be the potential for radiotherapy of tumours expressing a very high regulatory peptide receptor density, provided that analogues linked to adequate β-emitting isotopes will be developed. Preliminary data using therapeutic doses of the [111]indium-DTPA-octreotide in GEP tumour patients appear promising[16].

A further clinical development may arise from the recent findings that tumours can express multiple regulatory peptide receptors at the same time. We have shown, for instance, that an individual MTC can express not only somatostatin receptors, but also substance P receptors and CCK-B receptors. This observation has two consequences for diagnosis and therapy. First, multiple radioligands, targeting the respective receptors, may be used simultaneously in a given tumour to increase the radioactive signal and give a much better in vivo visualization. Second, agonists or antagonists of the corresponding receptors may be used to adequately suppress growth of a given tumour type. This means that for treatment of a somatostatin-, VIP-, and gastrin-receptor-expressing tumour for instance, not only a somatostatin analogue, known to inhibit tumour growth, should be given, but that a VIP antagonist and a CCK-B receptor antagonist should be applied concomitantly to induce a more effective tumour growth inhibition.

References

1. Reubi JC. Neuropeptide receptors in health and disease: The molecular basis for in vivo imaging. J Nucl Med. 1995;36:1825–35.
2. Reubi JC, Laissue J, Waser B, Horisberger U, Schaer JC. Expression of somatostatin receptors in normal, inflamed and neoplastic human gastrointestinal tissues. In: Wiedenmann B, Kvols LK, Arnold R, Riecken EO, editors. Annals of the New York Academy of Sciences, New York: New York Academy of Sciences, 1994:122–37.
3. Reubi JC, Horisberger U, Waser B, Gebbers JO, Laissue J. Preferential location of somatostatin receptors in germinal centers of human gut lymphoid tissue. Gastroenterology. 1992;103:1207–14.
4. Pernow B. Substance P. Pharm Rev. 1983;35:85–141.
5. Reubi JC, Waser B, Läderach U et al. Localization of cholecystokinin A and cholecystokinin B/gastrin receptors in the human stomach and gallbladder. Gastroenterology. 1997;in press.
6. Reubi JC, Krenning E, Lamberts SWJ, Kvols L. In vitro detection of somatostatin receptors in human tumors. Metabolism. 1992;41:104–10.
7. Reubi JC, Mazzucchelli L, Hennig I, Laissue J. Local upregulation of neuropeptide receptors in host blood vessels around human colorectal cancers. Gastroenterology. 1996;110:1719–26.
8. Reubi JC. In vitro identification of vasoactive intestinal peptide receptors in human tumors: Implications for tumor imaging. J Nucl Med. 1995;36:1846–53.
9. Hennig IM, Laissue JA, Horisberger U, Reubi JC. Substance P receptors in human primary neoplasms: Tumoural and vascular localisation. Int J Cancer. 1995;61:786–92.
10. Imdahl A, Mantamadiotis T, Eggstein S, Farthmann EH, Baldwin GS. Expression of gastrin, gastrin/CCK-B and gastrin/CCK-C receptors in human colorectal carcinomas. J Cancer Res Clin Oncol. 1995;121:661–6.
11. Reubi JC, Waser B. Unexpected high incidence of cholecystokinin B/gastrin receptors in human medullary thyroid carcinomas. Int J Cancer. 1996;67:644–7.
12. Krenning EP, Kwekkeboom DJ, Pauwels S, Kvols LK, Reubi JC. Somatostatin receptor scintigraphy. In: Freeman LM, editor. Nuclear Medicine Annual. New York: Raven Press, 1995:1–50.
13. Virgolini I, Raderer M, Kurtaran A et al. Vasoactive intestinal peptide-receptor imaging for the localization of intestinal adenocarcinomas and endocrine tumors. N Engl J Med. 1994;331:1116–21.
14. Lamberts SWJ, Krenning EP, Reubi JC. The role of somatostatin and its analogs in the diagnosis and treatment of tumors. Endocr Rev. 1991;12:450–82.
15. Zia H, Hida T, Jakowlew S et al. Breast cancer growth is inhibited by vasoactive intestinal peptide (VIP) hybrid, a synthetic VIP receptor antagonist. Cancer Res. 1996;56:3486–9.
16. Krenning EP, Valkema R, Kooij PPM et al. Radionuclide therapy with (111-In-DTPA-D-Phe-1)-octreotide. Preliminary data of a phase 1 study. In: Continuing Education Course Manual. Reston, VA, USA: Society of Nuclear Medicine, 1996:148–56.

10
Molecular analysis of novel genes differentially expressed during gut development

G. PEROZZI, C. MURGIA, D. BARILÀ, J. CERASE, F. FELICIOLI and F. LOMBARDO

INTRODUCTION

We have chosen the small intestine as a model system to study epithelial differentiation. The morphogenetic events that lead to formation of a functional gastrointestinal tract during development occur in parallel with the acquisition of differentiated traits by the epithelial cells of the mucosal layer. This process continues in adult animals, where continuous cell renewal occurs throughout life with precise temporal and spatial patterns: commitment to differentiation and loss of proliferation capacity occur at very early stages of cell migration along the crypt–villus axis, before the epithelial cells reach the crypt–villus junction[1]. Both during development and in the adult, epithelial differentiation is accompanied by increasing expression of specific proteins necessary to perform the absorptive functions of the mature epithelium. In the enterocytes, which represent the most abundant villus cell type, the major classes of proteins whose expression is turned on during differentiation are digestive enzymes, transport proteins and structural components of the microvillar cytoskeleton. The coordinate expression of such functions results from transcriptional activation of the corresponding genes, and it is regulated by common mechanisms involving promoter elements and transcription factors that are still largely unknown. Several studies have been conducted in recent years to identify the key factors involved in transcriptional activation of differentiation-specific intestinal genes. Molecular analysis of the promoters of cloned intestinal genes has shown that each one contains distinct combinations of binding sites for different transcription factors, and a clear picture has not yet emerged of the general mechanisms underlying the regulation of transcription in this tissue[2,3]. One aspect that can be further pursued to provide information on common mechanisms is the isolation of novel genes that are up-regulated during development and differentiation in the small intestine. For this reason we have undertaken in the past few years a search for novel genes differen-

99

tially expressed during development and differentiation of intestinal epithelial cells. Using subtractive hybridization for the construction of a sensitive cDNA probe, we have isolated from an intestinal cDNA library, enriched in epithelial-specific transcripts, several clones that are expressed in a stage-specific manner during development[4]. The isolated *Dri* clones (differentially expressed in rat intestine) correspond to genes expressed in the mature villus epithelium of 21-day-old rats, but either absent or barely expressed in the fetal undifferentiated gut at 15 days of gestation. The DNA sequences of two of these clones (*Dri 27* and *Dri 42*) are novel. Molecular analysis of these two clones has been the focus of our research, to uncover the function of their gene products in the enterocyte, as well as to contribute to the identification of the regulatory mechanisms responsible for transcriptional regulation during intestinal development and epithelial differentiation.

MATERIALS AND METHODS

Tissue preparation and RNA extraction

The portion of small intestine between the pylorus and the ileocaecal valve was dissected from Sprague–Dawley rats, anaesthetized with Farmotal (20 mg/100 g, i.p.; Farmitalia-Carlo Erba, Milano, Italy). The dissected tissue was quickly rinsed in cold Hank's buffered saline (Flow Laboratories, Irvine, UK) and immediately frozen in liquid nitrogen. Total RNA was extracted from frozen pulverized tissues or cell lysates as described by Chirgwin et al.[5]. Total RNA from the myogenic cell line C2[6] was a kind gift from Dr A. Felsani (Istituto di Ricerca Regina Elena, Roma, Italy).

cDNA library

The rat intestinal cDNA library, synthesized in our laboratory, has been described previously[7]. The rat brain cDNA library was purchased from Stratagene, La Jolla, CA. Both libraries were cloned into the *Eco*RI site of the phage vector λZAP II. Library screening and in vivo excision of insert-containing pBluescript SK– from plaque-purified, recombinant λ phages were performed according to standard procedures[8].

DNA sequence

The DNA sequence was determined on double stranded templates using the Sanger's method of dideoxy chain termination, as modified by the use of Sequenase (USB Corporation, Cleveland, OH) and ³⁵S-labelled dATP[9]. Comparative sequence analysis was performed on the GenEMBL nucleotide sequence database using the FastA package for Apple-Macintosh[10].

Cell cultures and transfections

The cell line FRIC B (fetal rat intestinal cells) was isolated in our laboratory from fetal rat intestine and displays a relatively undifferentiated phenotype[11]. The

Caco 2 cell line[12] was a kind gift of Professor A. Zweibaum (INSERM, Villejuif, France) and was used between passages 80 and 100. Both cell lines were grown as described previously[11]. Transfections were carried out with Lipofectamine (Gibco BRL-Life Technologies Italia, Milan, Italy) as described by the manufacturer. Neomycin-resistant, stably transfected clones were selected in complete medium containing $400\,\mu g/ml$ G 418 (Geneticin, Sigma). Transfected Caco 2 cells for toxicity studies were seeded on 96-well tissue culture plates and grown for 15 days after reaching confluency. The metal ion to be assayed was added as either chloride or sulphate salt in complete medium. Cell survival was determined with the method of neutral red absorption[13].

RESULTS AND DISCUSSION

Molecular isolation of *Dri 27* and *Dri 42* cDNA clones

The two novel cDNA clones *Dri 27* and *Dri 42* were isolated following a subtraction screening of an intestinal cDNA library on the basis of their up-regulation during development. We have previously reported the results of Northern and in situ hybridization experiments showing that the expression of both genes in rat small intestine is up-regulated, not only during development but also in adult animals, along both the horizontal (duodenum to ileum) and the vertical (crypt to villus) axes of the intestinal epithelium[4]. As for their tissue distri-bution, detectable levels of *Dri 27* mRNA are found in a restricted number of tissues, namely the small intestine, testis and brain, while transcription of *Dri 42* is ubiquitous.

Since both clones were initially isolated as partial fragments that did not contain a complete open reading frame (ORF), we have used them as probes for the isolation of full-length clones. Screening of a rat intestinal cDNA library, synthesized in our laboratory from RNA extracted from villus epithelium, led us to isolate two overlapping *Dri 42* clones, both of which contained a complete ORF of 930 bp, but differed in the lengths of their 5' and 3' untranslated regions (UTR). The encoded protein of 312 amino acids has a calculated molecular mass of 35.3 kDa[7]. Screening of the same library with the *Dri 27* probe yielded several clones at increasing distances (up to 3 kb) from the polyadenylation site, but their DNA sequence did not contain the ORF. A full-length *Dri 27* cDNA of 5.4 kb could be isolated only from a rat brain cDNA library. The DNA sequence of this clone has shown that the *Dri 27* ORF is located in the 5' portion of the mRNA, almost 4 kb upstream of the polyadenylation site. The significance of such a long 3' UTR is still unclear. The primary sequence of the Dri 27 protein is 339 amino acids long, with a predicted molecular mass of 37.7 kDa (Murgia et al., manuscript in preparation). The most prominent feature of both Dri 27 and Dri 42 protein sequences is a high degree of hydrophobicity. The hydropathy profile of the two sequences, calculated according to Kyte and Doolittle[14], is shown in Figure 1. The presence of alternating hydrophobic and hydrophilic domains is indicative of membrane bound proteins.

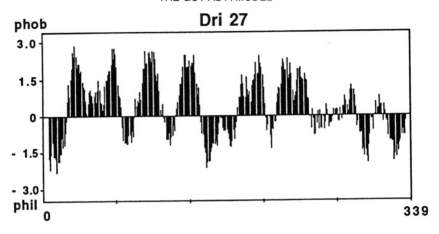

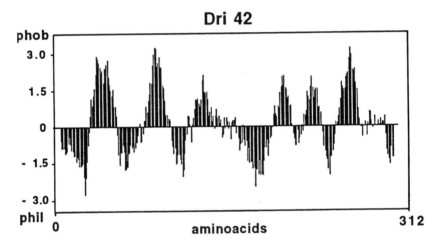

Figure 1 Hydropathy profile of the Dri 27 and Dri 42 proteins. Phob and Phil indicate hydro-phobicity and hydrophilicity, respectively. Numbers in the bottom refer to amino acid residues from the amino-terminus

Molecular analysis of Dri 42

By a combination of in vitro translation experiments in the presence of micro-somal membranes, and confocal fluorescence microscopy, we have recently demonstrated that Dri 42 is a glycoprotein, that all six of its hydrophobic domains are membrane spanning and that this protein is localized in the endoplasmic reticulum (ER) membrane[7]. The primary sequence of Dri 42 shares no homology with previously isolated proteins of known function. The only significant homology that was found in the EMBL and GenBank sequence databases is with a recently isolated protein of yet unknown function (HIC-53), which is induced transcriptionally by hydrogen peroxide treatment of *ras*-transformed mouse

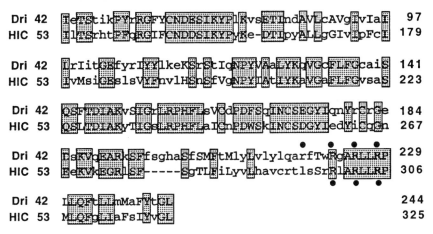

Figure 2 Alignment of the primary sequences of Dri 42 and HIC-53. Capital letters indicate either identity or conservative amino acid substitutions. Identical residues in the two sequences are boxed. Closed circles are positioned above the arginine residues in the conserved (R-X-X) repeat. The HIC-53 protein sequence was retrieved from the GenEMBL Databases using the on-line internet resources for sequence comparisons offered by the European Bioinformatics Institute (http://www.ebi.ac.uk). The alignment was obtained locally, using the MACAW software for Apple Macintosh

osteoblasts[15]. Comparison of the primary sequences of the two proteins is shown in Figure 2. Although the cloned portion of HIC-53 is incomplete at the amino-terminus, the two proteins share 48% homology over a stretch of 211 amino acid residues (33–244 in the Dri 42 sequence), encompassing the first five hydrophobic segments of Dri 42 (Figure 1). Within the homologous stretch both proteins contain a repeat of the motif (R-X-X), preceded and followed by a series of conserved leucine residues that could be responsible for protein–protein interactions. This structural motif is frequently found in the sequence of voltage-gated ion channel proteins[16], suggesting a possible function for both Dri 42 and HIC-53. Although very little information is available at present on HIC-53, we believe that a more detailed study of the expression profile of these two proteins is necessary to determine whether they exert their function in a cooperative fashion. Using Northern hybridization we have determined that Dri 42 expression is not induced by treatment of intestinal cell lines with hydrogen peroxide (data not shown). However, differentiation-dependent regulation of the expression of *Dri 42* appears to be specific for epithelial tissues.

Dri 42 gene expression is up-regulated during developmental maturation not only in the small intestine, but also in other rat epithelia (liver, kidney, lung). We compared *Dri 42* expression in the human adenocarcinoma cell line Caco 2, which is able to undergo spontaneous epithelial differentiation after 2 weeks of confluency[12], and in the non-epithelial cell line C2, which undergoes myogenic differentiation under specific culture conditions[6]. The steady-state levels of *Dri 42* mRNA in these cells, analysed by Northern hybridization, are presented in Figure 3. *Dri 42* mRNA levels increased almost three-fold during in vitro differentiation of Caco 2 cells, while no quantitative difference was observed during

A

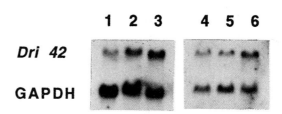

B

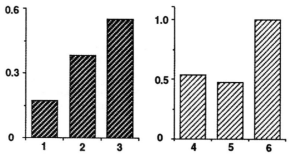

Figure 3 *Dri 42* expression in differentiating epithelial and non-epithelial cell lines. (A) Northern hybridizations of the radioactively labelled *Dri 42* cDNA probe to total RNA (20 μg/lane) extracted from: undifferentiated (lane 1) and differentiated (lane 2) Caco 2 cells; FRIC B cells (lane 3); undifferentiated myoblasts (lane 4), and differentiated myotubes (lane 5) of the C2 cell line; rat skeletal muscle dissected from an adult animal (lane 6). (B) Quantitative analysis of the relative mRNA levels, obtained by laser densitometry of the autoradiographs in (A). The plotted values are normalized for the amount of GAPDH mRNA in each lane

myoblast to myotube conversion. On the basis of sequence homology and of their expression patterns, we suggest that Dri 52 and HIC-53 may represent a novel class of channel proteins, whose members could share a common substrate, yet to be identified, but they probably act in distinct cellular compartments and/or in response to different external stimuli. Further studies on the role of Dri 42 in intestinal epithelial differentiation, its putative function as a channel protein and its possible interaction with itself or with HIC-53 are currently in progress in our laboratory.

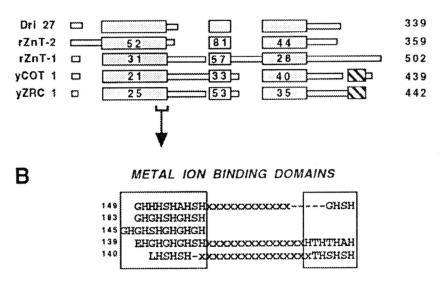

Figure 4 Protein sequence comparison among Dri 27 and different metal ion transporters. (A) Schematic alignment in which the blocks of highest similarity among the five proteins are depicted as filled boxes. The numbers within each box represent the percentage similarity with the corresponding Dri 27 sequence. This value is expressed in terms of chemical identity and includes conservative amino-acid substitutions. The numbers on the right indicate the number of residues in each sequence. Computer analysis was performed using the programs described in the legend to Figure 2. (B) Enlargement of the region defined by the arrow, which contains the alternating histidine domain. Numbers indicate the position of the first amino acid residue of the histidine motif within the corresponding sequences

Molecular analysis of Dri 27

Comparison of the Dri 27 primary sequence with those in the GenEMBL data-base has shown that it belongs to a family of highly related proteins, previously isolated from yeast and mammals. A characteristic feature of the protein family is the presence of a conserved stretch of alternating histidine residues, which confers the ability to transiently bind metal ions. A schematic alignment of the Dri 27 sequence with those of rat ZnT-1[17], rat ZnT-2[18], yeast Cot 1[19] and yeast Zrc 1[20] is shown in Figure 4A. The highest level of overall homology with the Dri 27 sequence (47%) is observed with ZnT-2, a protein responsible for vesicular sequestration of excess cytoplasmic zinc ions[18]. However, alignment of all five protein sequences identifies three blocks of significant similarity. Although these five proteins differ in their overall length (varying between 339 and 502 amino acids) their histidine-rich domains are found at very similar positions, between 132 and 184 amino acids from the amino-terminus. This conservation is even more striking when the hydropathy profiles of the five proteins are com-pared. The extremely conserved amino acid sequence of the histidine-rich domains is shown in Figure 4B. Of the four homologous proteins, ZnT-1, ZnT-2 and Zrc

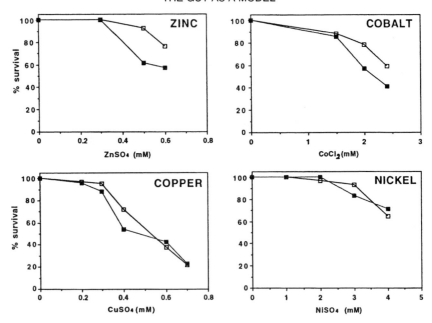

Figure 5 Survival of Dri 27-over-expressing subclones of Caco 2 cells in the presence of increasing concentrations of different metal ions. Each value represents the mean of two different determinations on two independent subclones of Dri 27 over-expressors (closed squares) and vector-transfected subclones (open squares)

1 are involved in zinc transport, while Cot 1 confers specific resistance to cobalt ions in yeast cells. Therefore, the presence of a conserved histidine motif is not sufficient in itself to identify the substrate specificity of Dri 27, although the overall structure of this protein and the presence of such conserved features strongly suggest that it functions as a metal ion transporter.

To identify the specific substrate that binds with high affinity to the Dri 27 histidine motif, we fused it to the bacterial reporter protein glutathione-S-transferase (GST) and overproduced it in *Escherichia coli*. Both GST alone and the Dri 27–GST fusion protein were assayed for their ability to bind different transition metal ions (Zn, Cu, Ni, Co) immobilized on a Sepharose matrix. Step elution with increasing imidazole concentrations has shown that GST alone is not retained on the column, while GST-Dri 27 is stably bound, up to 250 mM imidazole, but no difference is observed, among the metal ions tested, in the imidazole concentration required to displace binding in vitro (data not shown). We concluded that the entire sequence of the protein, within its specific cellular environment, is probably a prerequisite for proper functioning. The *Dri 27* ORF region was, therefore, cloned in the mammalian expression vector pCB6 and transfected into Caco 2 cells. Stably transfected, Dri 27-expressing clones were selected and subcloned. Preliminary results on two independent Dri 27-expressors and vector-transfected controls indicate that over-expression of Dri 27 increases the sensitivity of differentiated Caco 2 cells to the presence of zinc salts, and to a lesser extent to cobalt salts, added to the culture medium for 24 h (Figure 5). On the contrary, no difference in cell survival is observed when copper or nickel salts are added to the medium. To compare the kinetics of uptake and transport of these two candidate substrates, we are presently using atomic absorption spectroscopy to measure the kinetics of uptake and transport of zinc and cobalt by Caco 2 cells, grown as monolayers on filter supports.

Regulation of *Dri 27* gene expression

To determine whether transcription of the *Dri 27* gene is subject to metal-dependent regulation, Northern hybridization experiments were performed in the intestinal cell line FRIC B[11]. The results of this analysis, shown in Figure 6, indicate that when FRIC B cells are grown in the presence of 200 μM $ZnSO_4$, the steady-state levels of *Dri 27* mRNA decrease by three-fold after 24 h. The same effect is seen when cells are treated in the presence or in the absence of serum (data not shown). This decrease in *Dri 27* mRNA levels appears to be a specific response to zinc, as it is not seen in the presence of 300 μM $CuSO_4$, at which concentration normal induction of the metallothionein gene occurs (Figure 6). Negative regulation of gene expression by zinc has never been described. Therefore experiments are in progress to determine whether lower steady-state levels of *Dri 27* mRNA in response to zinc treatment are due to post-transcriptional regulation.

Having determined that Dri 27 is a tissue-restricted, differentiation-induced protein involved in metal ion transport we sought to determine which promoter elements and *trans*-acting factors are involved in regulating the tissue- and stage-specificity of expression of the corresponding gene. We have cloned the genomic region containing the promoter of the *Dri 27* gene from a mouse C126 genomic library. The DNA sequence of 3 kb upstream of the transcriptional start site contains several consensus sequences that could potentially bind known transcription factors. To determine which of these sites are involved in transcriptional regulation of this gene, we are presently testing the ability of different *Dri 27* promoter constructs to drive expression of the bacterial reporter gene luciferase in cell lines derived from several tissues. The results of this analysis will help to elucidate which elements and factors are responsible for the regulation of *Dri 27* tran-scription in different tissues and developmental stages.

Acknowledgements

This work was supported in part by the National Research Council of Italy, special project RAISA, subproject 4, paper no. 2671. D.B. was the recipient of a CNR-RAISA fellowship.

References

1. Gordon JI. Intestinal epithelial differentiation: new insights from chimeric and transgenic mice. J Cell Biol. 1989;108:1187–94.
2. Crabtree GR, Schibler U, Scott MP. Transcriptional regulatory mechanisms in liver and midgut

A

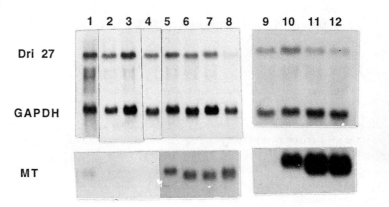

B

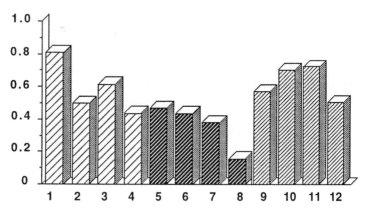

Figure 6 *Dri 27* expression in FRIC B cells treated with zinc and copper salts. (A) Northern hybridizations of radioactively labelled probes to total RNA (20 μg/lane) extracted from: adult rat small intestine (lane 1); FRIC B cells grown in the presence (lane 2) and in the absence (lane 3) of serum for 24 h; FRIC B cells grown in the presence of 200 μM $ZnSO_4$ for 0, 2, 6, 8 and 24 h (lanes 4–8); FRIC B cells grown in the presence of 300 μM $CuSO_4$ for 0, 2, 6, and 24 h (lanes 9–12). GAPDH, glyceraldehyde-3-phosphate dehydrogenase; MT, metallothionein. (B) Quantitative analysis of the relative mRNA levels, obtained by laser densitometry of the autoradiographs in (A). The plotted values are normalized for the amount of GAPDH mRNA in each lane

morphogenesis of vertebrates and invertebrates. In: McKnight SL, Yamamoto KR, editors. Transcriptional regulation. Plainview, NY: Cold Spring Harbor Laboratory Press. 1992:1063–102.

3. Traber PG, Silberg DG. Intestine-specific gene transcription. Annu Rev Physiol. 1996;58:275–97.
4. Barilà D, Murgia C, Nobili F, Gaetani S, Perozzi G. Subtractive hybridization cloning of novel genes differentially expressed during rat intestinal development. Eur J Biochem. 1994;223:701–9.
5. Chirgwin JM, Przybyla AE, MacDonald RJ, Rutter WJ. Isolation of biologically active ribonucleic acid from sources enriched in ribonuclease. Biochemistry. 1979;18:5294–9.

6. Yaffe D, Sxel O. Serial passaging and differentiation of myogenic cells isolated from dystrophic mouse muscle. Nature. 1977;270:725–7.

7. Barilà D, Plateroti M, Nobili F *et al.* The *Dri 42* gene, whose expression is upregulated during epithelial differentiation, encodes a novel er resident transmembrane protein. J Biol Chem. 1996; in press.

8. Sambrook J, Fritsch EF, Maniatis T, editors. Molecular cloning, a laboratory manual, second edition. 1989, Cold Spring Harbor, NY: Cold Spring Harbor Laboratory Press.

9. Tabor S, Richardson CC. DNA sequence analysis with a modified bacteriophage T7 DNA polymerase. Proc Natl Acad Sci USA. 1987;84:4767–71.

10. Pearson WR, Lipman DJ. Improved tools for biological sequence comparison. Proc Natl Acad Sci USA. 1988;82:2444–8.

11. Plateroti M, Sambuy Y, Nobili F, Bises G, Perozzi G. Expression of epithelial markers and retinoid binding proteins in retinol or retinoic acid treated intestinal cells in vitro. Exp Cell Res. 1993;208: 137–47.

12. Neutra M, Louvard D. Differentiation of intestinal cells in vitro. In: Matlin KS, Valentich JD, editors. Functional epithelial cells in culture. New York: Alan R. Liss. 1989:363–98.

13. Borenfreund E, Puerner JA. Toxicity determined in vitro by morphological alterations and neutral red absorption. Toxicol Lett. 1985;24:119–24.

14. Kyte J, Doolittle RF. A simple method for displaying the hydropathic character of a protein. J Mol Biol. 1982;157:105–32.

15. Egawa K, Yoshiwara M, Shibanuma M, Nose K. Isolation of a novel *ras*-recision gene that is induced by hydrogen peroxide from a mouse osteoblastic cell line, MC3T3-E1. FEBS Lett. 1995; 372:74–7.

16. Pongs O. Molecular biology of voltage-dependent potassium channels. Physiol Rev. 1992;72: S69–87.

17. Palmiter RD, Findley SD. Cloning and functional characterization of a mammalian zinc transporter that confers resistance to zinc. EMBO J. 1995;14:639–49.

18. Palmiter RD, Cole TB, Findley SD. ZnT-2, a mammalian protein that confers resistance to zinc by facilitating vesicular sequestration. EMBO J. 1996;15:1784–91.

19. Conklin DS, McMaster JA, Culbertson MR, Kung C. *COT-1*, a gene involved in cobalt accumulation in *Saccharomyces cerevisiae*. Mol Cell Biol. 1992;2:3678–88.

20. Kamizono A, Nishizawa M, Teranishi Y, Murata K, Kimura A. Identification of a gene conferring resistance to zinc and cadmium ions in the yeast *Saccharomyces cerevisiae*. Mol Gen Genet. 1989;219:161–7.

11
Intestinal proliferation and infection in childhood

T. C. SAVIDGE, A. N. SHMAKOV, J. A. WALKER-SMITH and
A. D. PHILLIPS

EPITHELIAL CELL PROLIFERATION IN THE SMALL INTESTINAL MUCOSA

The rapid and continuous renewal of epithelial cells within the small intestinal mucosa is an essential process for the digestion and absorption of nutrients, as well as for the maintenance of the integrity of the gut against infection by pathogenic organisms[1]. Although epithelial cell production rates vary greatly amongst species, the continuous cell division process is essential as it replaces epithelial cells which are extruded from the villus[2]. This replacement process is achieved by long-lived pluripotent epithelial stem cells which populate the specialized proliferative units known as the crypts of Lieberkühn[3]. These are flask shaped multicellular structures situated within the connective-tissue lamina propria which provides a microenvironment relatively devoid of luminal substances. The small intestine has evolved sophisticated mechanisms which regulate spatio-temporal control of epithelial cell proliferation and differentiation within the crypt[4]. This process is also influenced by cellular interactions with the pericryptal myofibroblast layer which embraces the crypt[5,6]. This intricate cellular cross-talk is likely to involve numerous signalling pathways mediated via integrins, extracellular matrix components, growth factors and cytokines. The small intestinal mucosa therefore constitutes an ideal tissue system for studying factors which regulate sequential cellular events, such as asymmetrical stem cell division, substem cell proliferation, lineage commitment, epithelial cytodifferentiation and cell death.

Investigation of mechanisms which regulate mucosal proliferation is important since a number of human gastrointestinal diseases, including infection, inflammatory bowel disease and colorectal cancer, are associated with altered patterns in crypt cell proliferation[2,7]. Appropriate regulation of cell division therefore plays an important role in controlling the steady-state balance between cell birth and loss in the gut, and dysregulation may have profound consequences resulting, for example, in inappropriate regeneration of damaged tissues following infection of the gastrointestinal tract.

EPITHELIAL CELL PROLIFERATION IN CHILDHOOD INFECTIVE ENTERITIS

Children suffering from enteric infection commonly display severe villous atrophy, resulting from an imbalance between epithelial cell loss and replacement within the small bowel[8]. Although the extent of mucosal damage may vary depending upon the nature of the infection, an increased crypt cell proliferation rate is a common finding in these patients. This has been demonstrated recently by measuring mitotic activity within crypt sections and correlating this with immuno-reactivity with the cell cycle associated antigen Ki67[9]. This short-lived nuclear antigen (identified using the MIB-1 monoclonal antibody) is expressed during all phases of the cell cycle (late G_1, S, G_2 and M) and may, therefore, be used to define the crypt growth fraction, i.e. the percentage of actively cycling cells within the crypt[10]. Thus, this antibody is a useful marker to measure epithelial cell pro-liferation in childhood infective enteritis to examine whether common disease-related responses exist.

Epithelial MIB-1 immunoreactivity (i.e. the crypt growth fraction) from proximal small intestinal biopsies from children with giardiasis, cryptosporidiosis and enteropathogenic *Escherichia coli* enteritis is shown in Figure 1. For the respective clinical groups, *Giardia lamblia*, *Cryptosporidium* and enteropathogenic *E. coli* were identified either in the duodenal juice or in the small intestinal mucosa using light and electron microscopy. As described previously[9], patients were divided into the following clinical groups: (a) Controls: 11 children (six female, five male; median age 22.8 ± 3.7 months ($\pm$ SEM), range 4–43 months) with a histologically normal mucosa in whom no gastrointestinal cause could be found for their symptoms. (b) Giardiasis: eight children (two female, six male), median age 20.6 ± 4.0 (range 11–46) months. (c) Cryptosporidiosis: eight children (four female, four male), median age 11.4 ± 2.3 (range 3–22) months. (d) Enteropatho-genic *E. coli* [EPEC]: five children (three female, two male), median age 8.8 ± 1.5 (range 5–14) months.

As shown in Figure 1, a hyperplastic crypt response was recorded in all of the infective enteropathies when compared with histologically normal mucosa. This included a significant increase in both the total crypt cell population and the total number of cycling cells recorded per crypt. Analysis of the spatial distribution of MIB-1$^+$ cells within the crypts demonstrated that peak MIB-1 labelling indices (I_{MIB-1}) were detected in the lower to middle portion of the crypt in all samples examined (Figure 2a). However, in the disease groups MIB-1 labelled cells were recorded in higher cell positions within the crypts. In the case of giardiasis and cryptosporidiosis this upward shift in proliferation was primarily due to the marked crypt elongation measured in these disorders as there was little evidence of an altered I_{MIB-1} distribution curve when these were plotted on a standardized crypt axis (Figure 2b). The notable exception was the EPEC group, in which a raised I_{MIB-1} was recorded throughout the crypt. The increased cellular proliferation recorded in giardiasis and cryptosporidiosis may, therefore, be accounted for by

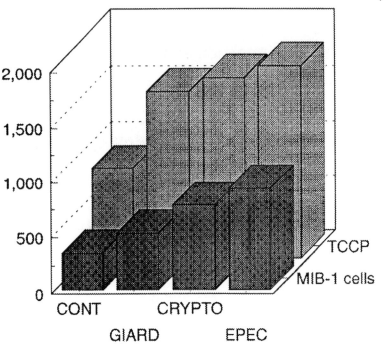

Figure 1 Total crypt cell population (TCCP) and cycling (MIB-1) cells in children suffering from giardiasis (GIARD), cryptosporidiosis (CRYPTO), and enteropathogenic *E. coli* (EPEC) enteritis

a crypt expansion alone, whereas the significantly raised I_{MIB-1} recorded in mucosal infection with EPEC indicates a substantially enlarged crypt growth fraction and a possible shortening of the cell cycle duration in this disorder. The high levels of proliferation measured in EPEC without recording a comparable increase in crypt size suggests that distinct regulatory mechanisms may operate in this type of enteropathy.

USE OF HUMAN INTESTINAL XENOGRAFTS TO STUDY EPITHELIAL CELL PROLIFERATION

Epithelial cell proliferation in human small and large bowel has now been characterized in fixed and cultured biopsy material[2]. However, a major problem remains to perturb such tissues under in vivo conditions. Short-term culture currently provides the only viable option for manipulating human intestine experimentally, but this technique is complicated since isolation procedures used to harvest intestinal tissues often constitutively activate many genes which are normally expressed at low levels in the gut epithelium, for example the proinflammatory cytokines IL-6 and IL-8[11]. Consequently, rodents are routinely used as models for human gastrointestinal disease as this remains the best

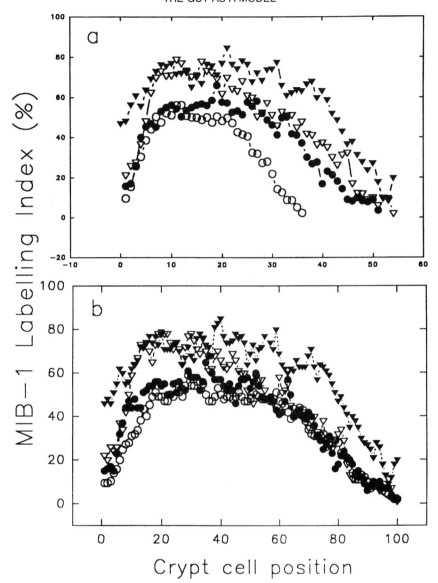

Figure 2 Longitudinal distribution of MIB-1+ epithelial cells in control and disease patients. Crypts have been adjusted to (a) mean group lengths and (b) a standardized axis where the crypt base and crypt–villus junction represent 0% and 100%, respectively (open circles, controls; filled circles, giardiasis; open triangles, cryptosporidiosis; filled triangles, EPEC enteritis)

practical option for perturbating normal steady-state kinetics. In addition, with recent advances in trans-genic technology, murine models have the advantage in that over-expression or deletion of a defined gene product may be investigated in vivo within the context of intestinal proliferation and function[4,12]. However,

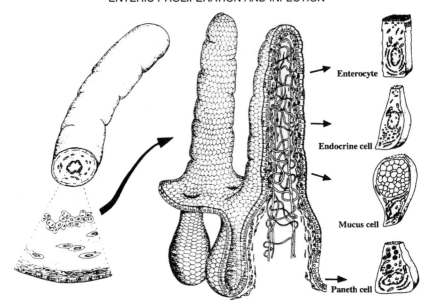

Figure 3 Schematic representation of xenograft development following transplantation of human fetal small intestine into *scid* mice

caution still needs to be exercised when extrapolating such data back to humans as fundamental species differences in genetics, intestinal structure and kinetics are common[2].

Xenotransplantation of human intestinal tissues into immunocompromised mice represents one possible approach to overcome such limitations since it is possible to measure human epithelial cell kinetics in this type of tissue under in vivo conditions[13–15]. The model system which we have adopted in our laboratory involves xenotransplanting human fetal intestinal segments subcutaneously into C.B-17 severe-combined immunodeficient (*scid*) mice[15]. In this site the tissue vascularizes and regenerates to form a mucosa displaying region-specific differentiation pathways, with well developed crypts (Figure 3). We have examined intestinal proliferation within these crypts to assess how closely this reflects measurements made in healthy paediatric gut[16,17]. In addition, by infecting intestinal xenografts with *Salmonella* species we have been able to investigate altered patterns of epithelial cell proliferation in an experimentally induced enteritis, and have compared this with infective enteropathies seen in children.

Epithelial MIB-1 immunoreactivity was very similar in xenograft and paediatric small intestinal crypts. The frequency distribution of MIB-1+ cycling cells along the longitudinal crypt axis is illustrated in Figure 4, where crypts have been adjusted to the mean crypt group length and a standard crypt length of 100%, respectively. These frequency distributions clearly demonstrate that proliferation is appropriately confined to the lower portion of the crypt in xenografted intestine, although peak labelling indices were recorded in a lower crypt cell position when compared with paediatric mucosa. However, as demonstrated previously for the

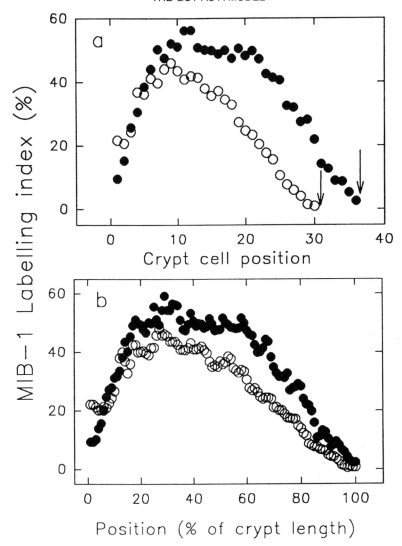

Figure 4 Longitudinal crypt distribution of MIB-1⁺ epithelial cells in xenograft (open circles) and paediatric (filled circles) small intestine. Crypts have been adjusted (a) to mean group lengths (arrows) and (b) a standard length of 100%

infective enteropathies, the MIB-1⁺ cells recorded in higher crypt cell positions in paediatric bowel is primarily due to the longer crypts as this difference is less pronounced after the crypt lengths have been standardized (Figure 4b).

Intestinal epithelial cell division often shows a high degree of synchrony as groups or 'runs' of proliferating cells are often recorded in adjacent crypt cell positions[18]. We investigated the ability of epithelial cells in xenograft crypts to form similar runs of proliferating cells by defining these as an uninterrupted series of MIB-1⁺ cells in consecutive crypt cell positions. Comparisons of the frequency of run lengths and the number of runs per crypt in xenograft and paediatric intestine are shown in Figure 5. Although this demonstrates that both types of tissue possess similar MIB-1⁺ run lengths, significantly more runs were recorded per crypt in paediatric bowel. However, this difference may be attributed to the fact that paediatric crypts were significantly larger than xenograft crypts, and the former possessed significantly more cycling cells.

SALMONELLA ENTERITIS IN HUMAN INTESTINAL XENOGRAFTS

We next explored whether rates of epithelial cell proliferation could be elevated to levels measured in the childhood infective enteropathies by inoculating an enteric pathogen into the lumen of the intestinal xenografts[19]. For these investigations we acutely infected fully differentiated xenografts with 5×10^7 invasive *Salmonella typhimurium* BRD847 for 8 and 24 h. Inspection of haematoxylin and eosin-stained sections demonstrated marked villous atrophy and evidence of crypt damage within 24 h of infection. The tissue characteristically possessed a heavy murine-derived leukocytic infiltrate, predominantly neutrophils. These regularly infiltrated the epithelium, which often formed crypt abscesses. The resultant effect of the infection was a temporal increase in the crypt MIB-1 labelling index, reaching a maximum 24 h after infection (Figure 6).

DISCUSSION

The present chapter describes how the pattern of epithelial cell proliferation changes in the small intestinal mucosa from children infected with either *G. lamblia, Cryptosporidium* or enteropathogenic *E. coli*. In addition, the chapter has detailed an experimental human intestinal xenograft model which may now be used to investigate putative disease factors that regulate epithelial cell proliferation in intestinal mucosa infected with human-specific pathogens.

Studies of epithelial MIB-1 immunoreactivity in crypts from non-infected xenograft tissues demonstrated many similarities with healthy small intestine from children. These included closely matched MIB-1 crypt labelling indices and frequency distribution curves, as well as an ability for cell division to show synchronized behaviour in xenografted bowel. These findings reflect common kinetic parameters in both types of tissue, for example growth fractions, cell cycle durations, epithelial migration rates and the number of transit divisions before cells decycle and exit the crypts. This indicates that there are basic regulatory mechanisms in ectopically transplanted xenograft intestine which are sufficient to initiate and maintain the spatial arrangement of cellular proliferation in a way which is very similar to the in vivo situation. Thus, human fetal small intestine possesses predetermined genetic information, provided by the epithelial stem cell population and/or the juxtaposed mesenchyme, which permits tissue development and differentiation in the absence of conventional luminal stimuli, such as dietary factors, indigenous flora, pancreatic and biliary secretions[6,15,20].

Luminal factors do not, therefore, appear to play an essential role in the spatio-

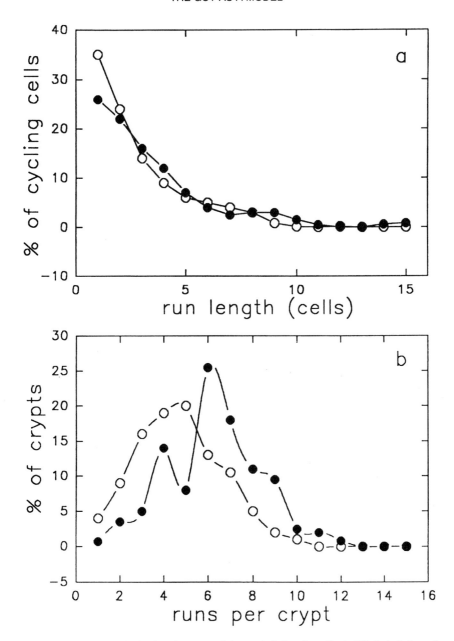

Figure 5 MIB-1⁺ run distributions in xenograft (open circles) and paediatric (filled circles) small intestinal crypts. The graphs illustrate (a) the percentage of the total MIB-1⁺ population recorded in runs (i.e. show synchronized cell proliferation) and (b) the number of runs per crypt (i.e. run frequency distribution) in the different tissues

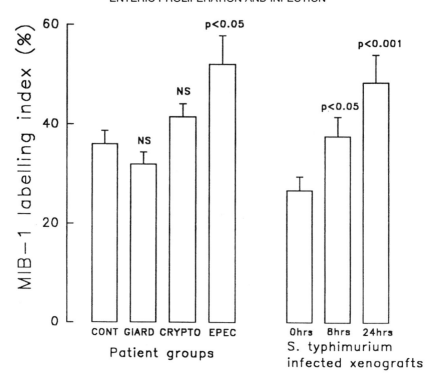

Figure 6 Crypt MIB-1 labelling indices for the different patient and xenograft groups (NS, no significant difference as assessed by the Mann–Whitney U-test for ranks)

temporal regulation of crypt cell proliferation. However, these factors may play a 'fine tuning role' as subtle differences were noted in the pattern of proliferation in xenograft and paediatric bowel. First, the intestinal crypts were significantly shorter in the former. Second, minor differences were apparent in the MIB-1 labelling pattern in xenograft intestine, which included lower crypt labelling indices and a shift in MIB-1+ immunostaining towards the base of the crypt. The absence of conventional luminal stimuli in xenografted tissues, especially bacterial flora, is the most likely explanation for these differences[21–23]. This has been clearly demonstrated in germ-free mice reconstituted with an indigenous bacterial flora, where crypt cell proliferation recovered to conventional levels[24]. We have demonstrated a similar elevation in crypt cell proliferation following luminal infection of intestinal xenografts with *Salmonella typhimurium*. The nature of this proliferative response showed similarities to enteropathogenic *E. coli* infections in children, in that the crypt growth fraction was significantly elevated in both enteropathies. However, it remains to be established whether chronic infection in the xenograft model, as is evident in the childhood infective enteropathies, maintains similarly high proliferation rates. We are currently using this model system to investigate potential disease factors which mediate this rapid up-regulation in crypt cell proliferation. Preliminary evidence utilizing quantitative reverse-transcription polymerase chain reaction has demonstrated a several hundred-fold up-regulation of mucosal-derived human IL-6 and IL-8 mRNA species in *Salmonella*-infected xenografts (unpublished findings). This pattern of up-regulation has been described in a number of gut-related diseases, including infection and inflammatory bowel disease[25,26], which suggests that we are observing an appropriate 'mucosal disease response' in our experimental enteritis. We are now actively investigating the role of these cytokines in regulating intestinal proliferation, particularly in view of the fact that at present there is no murine structural homologue for IL-8.

Acknowledgements

The authors thank Drs D. Brown (The Babraham Institute), S. Roberts and Professor C. Potten (Paterson Institute for Cancer Research, Christie Hospital, Manchester, UK) for helpful comments, and Dr L. Wong (The MRC Tissue Bank) for his assistance. This work was funded by the Biotechnology and Biological Sciences Research Council.

References

1. Cheng H, Leblond CP. Origin, differentiation and renewal of the four main epithelial cell types in the mouse small intestine. V. Unitarian theory of the origin of the four epithelial cell types. Am J Anat. 1974;141:537–62.
2. Wright NA, Alison MR. The Biology of Epithelial Cell Populations (Volumes I and II). Oxford: Clarendon Press, 1984.
3. Potten CS, Loeffler M. Stem cells: attributes, spirals, pitfalls and uncertainties. Lessons for and from the crypt. Development. 1990;110:101–20.
4. Gordon JI, Hermiston ML. Differentiation and self-renewal in the mouse gastrointestinal epithelium. Curr Opin Cell Biol. 1994;6:795–803.
5. Haffen K, Kedinger M, Simon-Assmann P. Cell contact dependent regulation of enterocyte differentiation. In: Lebenthal E, editor. Human Gastrointestinal Development. New York: Raven Press. 1989:19–39.
6. Duluc I, Freund J, Leberqueier C, Kedinger M. Fetal endoderm primarily holds the temporal and positional information required for mammalian intestinal development. J Cell Biol. 1994;126: 211–21.
7. Lipkin M. Proliferation and differentiation of normal and diseased gastrointestinal cells. In: Johnson LR, editor. Physiology of the Gastrointestinal Tract. New York: Raven Press. 1989: 255–84.
8. Thomas A, Phillips AD, Walker-Smith JA. The value of proximal small intestinal biopsy in the differential diagnosis of chronic diarrhoea. Arch Dis Childh. 1992;67:741–4.
9. Savidge TC, Shmakov AN, Walker-Smith JA, Phillips AD. Epithelial cell proliferation in childhood enteropathies. Gut. 1996;39:185–93.
10. Schluter C, Duchrow, Wohlenberg C et al. The cell proliferation-associated antigen of antibody Ki-67: A very large, ubiquitous nuclear protein with numerous repeated elements, representing a new kind of cell cycle-maintaining proteins. J Cell Biol. 1993;123:513–22.
11. Jung HC, Eckmann L, Yang SK et al. A distinct array of proinflammatory cytokines is expressed in human colon epithelial cells in response to bacterial invasion. J Clin Invest. 1995;95:55–65.
12. Hauft SM, Kim SH, Schmidt GH et al. Expression of SV-40 T antigen in the small intestinal epithelium of transgenic mice results in proliferative changes in the crypt and reentry of villus-associated enterocytes into the cell cycle but has no apparent effect on cellular differentiation programs and does not cause neoplastic transformation. J Cell Biol. 1992;117:825–39.

13. Verstijnen CPHJ, Kate JT, Arends JW, Schutte B, Bosman FT. Xenografting of normal colonic mucosa in athymic mice. J Pathol. 1988;155:77–85.
14. Winter HS, Hendren RB, Fox CH *et al.* Human intestine matures as nude mouse xenograft. Gastroenterology. 1991;100:89–98.
15. Savidge TC, Morey AL, Ferguson DJP, Fleming KA, Shmakov AN, Phillips AD. Human intestinal development in a severe-combined immunodeficient xenograft model. Differentiation. 1995;58: 361–71.
16. Shmakov AN, Morey AL, Ferguson DJP, Fleming KA, O'Brien JA, Savidge TC. Conventional pattern of human intestinal proliferation in a severe-combined immunodeficient xenograft model. Differentiation. 1995;59:321–30.
17. Shmakov AN, Savidge TC. Cellular proliferation in the crypt epithelium of human small intestinal xenografts. Epithel Cell Biol. 1995;4:104–12.
18. Potten CS, Chwalinski S, Swindell R, Palmer M. The spatial organization of the hierarchical proliferative cells of the crypts into clusters of 'synchronised' cells. Cell Tissue Kinet. 1982;15: 351–70.
19. Huang GTJ, Eckmann L, Savidge TC, Kagnoff MF. Infection of human intestinal epithelial cells with invasive bacteria upregulates apical intercellular adhesion molecule-1 (ICAM-1) expression and neutrophil adhesion. J Clin Invest. 1996;98:572–83.
20. Rubin DC, Swietlicki E, Roth KA, Gordon JI. Use of fetal intestinal isografts from normal and transgenic mice to study the programming of positional information along the duodenal-to-colonic axis. J Biol Chem. 1992;267:15122–33.
21. Rossi TM, Lee PC, Young C, Tjota A. Small intestinal mucosa changes, including epithelial cell proliferative activity of children receiving total parenteral nutrition (TPN). Dig Dis Sci. 1993; 38:1608–13.
22. Philpott DJ, Kirk DR, Butzner JD. Luminal factors stimulate intestinal repair during the refeeding of malnourished infant rabbits. Can J Physiol Pharmacol. 1993;71:650–6.
23. Sharma R, Schumacher U, Ronaasen V, Coates M. Rat intestinal mucosal responses to a microbial flora and different diets. Gut. 1995;36:209–14.
24. Abrams GD, Bauer H, Sprinz H. Influence of the normal flora on mucosal morphology and cellular renewal in the ileum. A comparison of germ-free and conventional mice. Lab Invest. 1963;12:355–64.
25. Przemioslo RT, Ciclitira PJ. Cytokines and gastrointestinal disease mechanisms. Bailliere's Clin Gastroenterol. 1996;10:17–31.
26. Krueger J, Ray A, Tamm I, Sehgal PB. Expression and function of interleukin-6 in epithelial cells. J Cell Biochem. 1991;45:327–34.

12
Perspectives on stem cells and gut growth: Tales of a Crypt – From the Walrus to Wittgenstein

I. M. MODLIN, M. KIDD and A. SANDOR

INTRODUCTION

For years, questions of gut ontogeny and phylogeny have perplexed clinicians and biologists alike. More recently, however, it has become evident that the elucidation of the origin of the cells and the molecular regulation of both their phenotype and function are critical issues. This recognition reflects a need to further understand both the molecular physiology of the system and also to identify key elements and events related to malfunction. In this respect it is crucial to delineate the biology of the disease processes culminating in either loss of gut function or neoplasia.

The two opening sessions of this symposium were devoted to the subject of stem cells and gut growth and development. It was soon apparent that an understanding of the issues within the areas defined for discussion often resembled attempts of an inhabitant of a distant archipelago to solve the New York Times crossword puzzle. Potential hopes of further solution of the issues by discussion were often dissolved by a recognition of the paucity of data available, the epistemological nature of the questions and the lack of an obvious framework for interpolation of facts. Indeed, the discussion between the participants sometimes resembled Lewis Carroll's recounting of the colloquy between Tweedledee and Alice:

> 'The time has come', the walrus said,
> 'To talk of many things:
> 'Of shoes – and ships – and sealing wax –
> Of cabbages – and kings –
> And why the sea is boiling hot –
> And whether pigs have wings.'

Discourse regarding crypts, niches, molecular regulation, growth factors and cryptdins eerily echoed the sagacity of the walrus but in much the same way was quite difficult to resolve. Sapient members of the assembled cognoscenti claimed that the mere thought of crypts evoked Nietzchean if not Freudian fantasies of mystical progenitors.

On the surface, it appeared that there was a meaningful basis within which the nature of stem cells and the regulation of their division could be accommodated to embrace a framework of growth regulation and lineage transformation. On closer inspection, however, it was apparent that diverse and diffuse components of information were simply being pinned to a board which could be broadly recognized as an important intellectual backdrop against which an unknown area was being explored. After hours of most informative presentation, one was left with the impression of having surveyed a seventeenth century Hondian concep-tualization of the world. There were recognizable continents, definable seas, yet strange denizens were apparent and vast areas of the chart were simply blank (Figure 1). Such comments should not be interpreted as nigratory, since both speakers and subjects were of the highest calibre. Rather they reflect a recognition of our woeful ignorance of this vital area.

This overview seeks not to specifically critique any particular area and indeed all the presentations were of an extraordinarily high level. It rather aspires to define the lack of cohesion and the major areas of nescience that currently exist in a most critical area of gut biology. What is desperately needed is a framework from which to define a series of questions and goals which should be resolved in an attempt to generate a cohesive understanding of the area. Certainly, without the gut and its ability to function appropriately, all other systems are impotent. Indeed, if one views the historical perspective, our current concepts of gut growth and development and the molecular regulation of cell type and its function closely approximate Galenic concepts of human anatomy. Thereafter, Vesalius defined and made their geographic relationship to each other apparent and delineated the potential function of the system as a whole. Yet, as mirrored in the medical musings and drawings of da Vinci, we have minimal knowledge of origin, interrelation-ship, regulation of function and know even less of malfunction. What is needed is the Morgagni of the new millennium.

The origin of the stem cells and the regulation of their proliferation is an area of considerable importance and is the subject of both molecular and mathematical debates. Clonality presentations generated the impression of ritual tribal musings and the concept of a stem cell niche, whilst Abraxian in its elegance, left one with shimmering visions of Atlantis. Coleridge in his deepest of opiate reveries would have been proud of the sophistry which allowed the interweaving of Wittgenstinian mathematical modelling with cell proliferation, the niche theory and clonal expansion. Nevertheless, information provided on each of these subjects was dramatic in its relevance and lucid in its presentation. Somewhat lacking were explanations of the biological mechanics by which these diverse but heuristic propositions could be reconciled.

Dare a meeting take place where genes and gene therapy are not evoked as either the new holy grail or the star in the sky over the Judean desert. The relevance of the somatic mutations of the *APC* gene were further adumbrated upon and the relevance to intestinal pathology once again drawn in a stark and apposite fashion. The dreaded spectre of cystic fibrosis as a lurgy capable of management by gene therapy was raised with hopeful fervor by the Scottish group. Who can

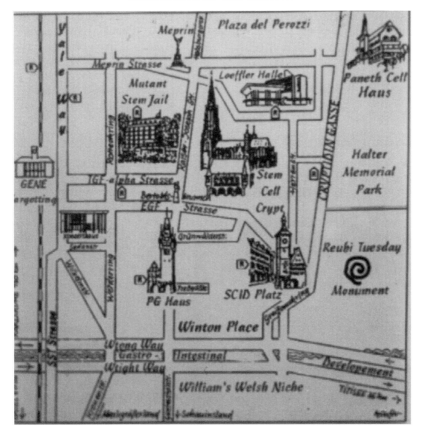

Figure 1 Freiberg (aka) Stem Cell City after the Falk Gut Biology Meeting of 1996. Blank areas represent lack of knowledge. Where any of the streets leads to is unknown. The names of certain buildings may be incorrect after 1996

deny the allure of the skirl of pipes and the drumming of the fife as the molecular therapists sally forth. ('Lest we scoff, ye of little faith', remember the comments in regard to James Watt when he initially proposed steam as a motive force.) Nevertheless, flaws in the vector remain to be resolved as do complex and unresolved issues of appropriate nuclear activation.

While an understanding of 'the jeans' (Levi-Strauss) is still lacking, the further expansion of Montalcini Levi's work in the area of growth factors shed some pleasant light on the regulation of cell proliferation. The role of transforming growth factor-α (TGF-α) appears to be resolving with caffeine-like intensity as its effect on basolateral membrane receptors, prostaglandin synthesis and COX-2 became apparent. Nevertheless, how all this interfaces with meprin, a brush border enzyme of crayfish derivation and debatable function, is utterly unknown. A second comet-like series of observations regarding the Dri-42 and Dri-26 proteins, which appear to be the gemelli (Romulus/Remus) of intestinal cell metal transporters, flashed through the heavens of our comprehension. Fortunately, a panegyric on the Paneth cell restored some balance to the recognition that there were cell types which actually produced specific substances – defensins or cryptdins which had a definable function. This reassuring concept of a group of molecular policemen in the gut with a defined role of protecting the barrier provided a sense of order in the hitherto disparate constellation of information placed before the Cognoscenti.

The subject of the nature and function of the myriads of receptors present on cells was painted in a Rubenesque fashion. A utopian vision was floated that potential diagnostic and therapeutic strategies could be implemented using appropriate probes. In a chiaroscuro commentary on the congeners available for such receptors, the ephemeral outline of the possibility (dare one allude to it) of the regulation of neoplastic proliferation was dimly illuminated. The last presentation chosen with Dickensian skill as if to outline the glissade-like nature of its chimeric phenotype dealt with the unique murine xenograft model, the *scid* mouse. Its unique possibilities in the exploration of gut biology supported the concept of a scenario within which a unifying hypothesis might be developed.

Since no current scientific explanations exist to synthesize the superb individual pieces of information presented in these sessions, it is probably most appropriate to summate using poetic reflection and licence. The information, like a star, was globulating, scintillating, and viviscent in its appeal. Yet like the evening star, it was distant and as yet difficult to place in the galactic immensity of this unexplored biological space.

Nevertheless, some explanations should be attempted and in this respect, I feel much like Humpty Dumpty in responding to Alice's request to explain the 'Jabberwocky', which is probably the earliest attempt by a mathematician (Dodgson) to embrace the concept of crypt cell activity,

> 'T'was brillig, and the slithy toves
> Did gyre and gimble in the wabe~:
> All mimsy were the borogroves,
> And the mome raths outgrabe'

Humpty explained that brillig meant it was 4:00 pm at the time when one began to broil things for dinner and meeting sessions wound down. Slithy meant lithe and slimy which is active so that the word is actually like a portmanteau and has two meanings packed up in one word. Presumably this would also reflect gut cell motogenicity and mitogenicity. Toves, on the other hand, are more difficult to understand because they are in between lizards and are something like corkscrews. Possibly they represent cells of dubious lineage or even bacteria which have mated with gut cells. In addition, it is proposed that toves live under sun dials where they also survive by eating cheese. This surely is a comment on the role of luminal nutrients in cell activation. The nature of their cellular motion is like a gyroscope, hence the word gyre, and their other function is to gimble which is how a gimlet makes its hole. Of course, such holes and membrane pores are obviously allusions to ion channels and tight junctions. The wabe, of course, is a grass plot around the sun dial and is the milieu within which the toves function.

Clearly an early description of the unstirred layer concept and crypt matrix. Mimsy means to be flimsy and miserable and is another portmanteau word which presumably reflects the desperate feeling of investigators lost in the immensity of this field, whereas borogrove is a shabby bird with feathers sticking all around it, something much like an ambient mop and as early a description of a cell membrane receptor site as one can find. Hardest of all to understand is the mome raths since rath is a type of green pig and mome means lost or away from home. Whether this is an allusion to the derivations of persons involved in this field is unlikely but may be resolved at a future meeting. Of particular interest is the derivation of outgrabe which is a sound similar to something between bellowing and whistling with a sneeze in the middle. The final concept of outgrabe is the collective sound made by the audience at the recognition of the extraordinary value of the information provided at this novel meeting.

This brief whimsical view of the information presented is extended in a series of synoptic paragraphs which comprise the remainder of this article.

STEM CELLS

Stem cells were defined by Steel in 1977 as 'cells which have the capacity to produce a large family of descendants within their own natural environment'[1]. These are considered the most unspecialized or primitive of cells and are thought to engender numerous cells which may differentiate or produce new stem cells. Stem cells are located at specific positions at the bottom of the intestinal crypt, where they are self-maintaining and regenerate after perturbation. It seems likely that, in steady state, the number of active stem cells in a crypt can fluctuate and the life cycle of macroscopic crypts can be linked to stem cell dynamics. The progeny of a single stem cell can replace other stem cells thus culminating in monoclonality. Since the entire process appears to be age dependent, the organization and control of stem cells has assumed the role of a key issue in epithelial biology. Given the critical nature of stem cells in gut neoplasia the intestinal epithelium provides a fine model in which to study these issues, particularly as they relate to epithelial cell transformation and malignancy.

Clonal studies

The objective of clonality studies is to infer the properties and organization of stem cells by following the fate of the marked clones of cells which arise following mutagenesis affecting a marker locus (e.g. G6PD, Dlb-1)[2]. Unequivocal observations indicate that after a latent period, marked clones occupy a crypt unit, thus over time several (4–6?) stem cells are replaced by the progeny of one resulting in a monoclonal crypt. The mechanisms by which this occurs are the subject of debate but include the following: ancestral stem cells, stochastic competition, environmental factors, crypt cell fission and combinatorial.

The precise role of each has been difficult to delineate in experimental conditions induced by measuring the effects of different mutagens[3]. Although high doses of mutagen result in an increased number of induced clones, the toxicity may also affect growth rate and the extent of crypt fission. Alternatively, the effects of low doses of mutagen may be overshadowed by the occurrence of spontaneously arising clones. This effect may be compounded in young mice (6 weeks of age), where gut development may not be complete, and a low background mutation rate is evident. It is also likely that different mechanisms may provide similar predictions for the fate of induced clones. Probably the most satisfactory strategy would be to determine how clonal growth and susceptibility to mutations alters with pathological status. In order to determine the precise lineage relationships between stem and proliferative cells these cells should be examined under different conditions irrespective of their mechanism of renewal.

Stem cell niche theory

The stem cell niche concept predicts that intestinal crypts are maintained by a group of cells which only retain stem cell properties while they remain within the confines of a niche (nested, sequestered environment)[4]. Such properties are lost as they pass out of the niche. It is proposed that the niche is maintained by interaction between the stem cells and a specialized group of pericryptal fibroblasts. This hypothesis proposes that the asymmetry of division inherent in any stem cell is not intrinsic, but extrinsic and dependent on movement of the stem cell out of the niche.

Evidence for stem cell niche has been provided by Potten[26] using uptake of tritiated thymidine. He concluded that 16 long-lived 'stem' cells were present in the small intestine, while only three were present in the large intestine. Alternatively, using mutagen administration, and different mouse models, Williams[4,5], and Ponder and Winton[6], have reported that the scattered individual crypts become entirely replaced by the mutant phenotype cells, suggesting only one progenitor (stem) cell. In addition these studies indicated that the time taken for mixed phenotype crypts to disappear was longer in the small than in the large intestine. The 'gestalt' of such is consistent with the existence of a stem cell niche, with external control of asymmetry of stem cell division and random or partial loss of cells from the niche. The alternative hypothesis of a single stem cell model which predicts that crypts are maintained either by a single stem cell or a group of stem cells which are dependent on an intrinsic control of symmetry is inconsistent with current experimental observations.

Carcinogenesis is a multistep phenomenon, but it seems likely that retention of somatic mutations in stem cells must play a critical role in this process. It is well established that the carcinogen dimethylhydrazine (DMH) causes both mutations and crypt neogenesis in the murine colon. In contrast, ethylnitrosourea (ENU) acts as a pure mutagen. Under experimental conditions the effect of administering both these agents together appears to be additive. However, studies indicate that application of ENU 2–3 days after DMH results in a 40% increase in the frequency of mutations. This would suggest that stem cells may be more susceptible to somatic mutations when exposed to a mutagen during regeneration. This in turn might be due to either increased stem cell mitotic activity during crypt fission or to the retention of a mutation which would otherwise have been lost. A similar pattern of phenotypic changes following mutagen exposure has been identified in the human colon, except that the time course is far longer. This could be due to either more stem cells/niche or to other changes in crypt cell kinetics[5].

Mathematical modelling

Crypts contain active stem cells with equal growth potential which are subject to local autoregulatory control. A stochastic model of stem cell growth can therefore be derived[6]. Thus at cell division each stem cell may be assumed to produce either 2, 1 or none (0) daughter cells with probabilities of p, q and r respectively. If the population of the crypts exceeds a certain threshold S_f it is assumed that the crypt divides into 2, segregating its stem cells at random. The original model which assumed constant values for p, q and r could explain the majority of data on crypt extinction rates, crypt size distribution and the times to monoclonality conversion after mutagenic events in adult mice. However, the acquisition of more recent data on crypt fission rates and the occurrence of patches of adjacent monoclonal crypts, have led to a reassessment of this model. It is now proposed that a modification of this model should involve the introduction of a state dependent generalization which includes differing values for p, q and r. This formulation has more recently been used to reanalyse the in vivo data of Park and Wright[27]. In contrast to these authors' conclusion that crypt fission per se plays a large role in the monoclonality conversion of crypts, the model modification asserts that stochastic behaviour of stem cells may be of more importance. Modelling analysis of the dynamics of crypt fission and monoclonality in juvenile mice has also been undertaken and has been found to be consistent with the experimental evidence. At this time it would therefore appear that a model of co-existing stochastically growing stem cells with autoregulatory features (fluctuating self-regulated stem cell population), is able to comprehensively describe the small intestine crypt situation in both juvenile and adult mice.

Adenomatous polyposis coli (APC)

Somatic mutation of the *APC* gene in intestinal epithelial cells may be one of the first, if not the first step in intestinal carcinogenesis and clones derived from such mutant cells gradually expand into adenomas. This clonal expansion of the population of mutant cells is of biological significance since it increases the numbers of cells at risk for mutations of other genes (e.g. K-*ras*, *DCC*, *p53*) leading to carcinoma. Little is however known about the process of clonal expansion[7]. In normal intestinal epithelium, growth results primarily from a process of crypt replication which is thought to be driven by expansion of the stem cell population. Although some information is available regarding this process, these studies have for the most part utilized markers with no known impact on function. In contrast, mutation of the *APC* gene has a significant impact on cell behaviour but still allows for classical analysis of these clinically significant cell populations. In adenomas derived from familial adenomatous polyposis patients with an *APC* mutation, the number of aberrant crypt foci (ACF; a measure of crypt proliferation rates) is > 11 times normal. By contrast, in hyperplastic mucosa with K-*ras* mutations, ACF is < 11 times normal. Thus a threshold limit, in terms of crypt proliferation (ACF), appears to exist for carcinogenesis.

In a separate set of experiments the progeny of mice which are heterozygous for the APC mutation (+/– crossed with mice with a homozygous defect in the DNA mismatch repair enzyme MSH2 (–/–) have > 100 times the normal ACF[8]. These animals have reduced survival, secondary to a greater number of and more rapidly developing adenomas. These observations in concert with that of patient data suggest that somatic *APC* mutations are responsible for the formation of the additional tumours and that contrary to expectation ACF are postnatal events.

Gene therapy

Gene therapy is touted as an increasingly viable alternative for a number of acquired hereditary diseases. To date, major work has been undertaken in the treatment of cystic fibrosis (CF) which has become the paradigm for the genetic therapeutic treatment of a disease. Current experimental protocols require the need to introduce extrachromosomal copies of the *cftr* gene under the control of a ubiquitously expressed promoter[9]. This approach is somewhat limited by the inefficiency of gene delivery, immunological reaction to the vector, and incorrect temporal and spatial gene expression. In addition, the requirement for repeated delivery exists since the cell targets of such therapy are differentiated, cannot therefore divide and will be replaced over time. This problem is amplified in the small intestine, where cell turnover is extraordinarily high. It is therefore necessary to develop alternative strategies. A promising possibility is the method of ex vivo homologous recombination to precisely correct the mutation in the endogenous gene. The results of this technique should allow for the correct temporal expression of *cftr* under the control of the endogenous promoter in the relevant epithelial cells.

A series of *cftr* mutant mice (–/–) generated by intercrossing various mutant alleles created by gene targeting in embryonal stem cells have been developed[10]. These mice display the characteristic CF chloride channel defect and have varying degrees of intestinal abnormality with gross mucus accumulation leading to intestinal blockage. These transgenic animals provide good experimental models to determine what proportion of intestinal cells must be derived from wild type or 'corrected cells' to achieve a non-CF phenotype. Preliminary data from these *cftr* mice demonstrate the alterations in electrical potential difference across the intestinal mucosa observed normally in patients with CF. An alternative strategy to achieve ex vivo uptake of genetic products involves a cultured murine stem cell system, since the standard method of gene incorporation utilizing liposome complex delivery is neither effective nor efficient. However, the preliminary results even under such constraints have been encouraging. For survival, *cftr* (–/–) animals require only 30% restoration of chloride conductance which is the equivalent of only 5% of normal mRNA levels. In order to increase efficiency of gene transfer an alternative method of nuclear microinjection is currently under investigation. Once the basic methodologies have become established, such techniques may become useful in the treatment of other genetic disorders afflicting the intestine.

GROWTH AND DEVELOPMENT

The control of growth in the gut is mediated by a number of pathways. One of these comprises negative feedback mechanisms which operate after mucosal damage. The origin of this control lies in the villus cells rather than in the crypt cells. A second consists of a chemical regulator of intestinal cell proliferation responsible for mucosal hyperplasia, which probably acts both systematically and locally. It is also possible that luminal ingesta exert an influence via a local humoral mechanism. Overall it appears that stem cells are the most important cellular target for these controlling agents, but effects on transit cells of the crypts cannot yet be excluded.

Functional redundancy or auxiliary mechanisms in gut development

Intestinal development can be broadly classified into two major phases: a perinatal phase in which proteins important in the suckling period begin to be expressed and a weanling phase in which the suckling phenotype is replaced by the mature phenotype. The major motif which is continuously reiterated in the developing intestine is an apparent 'functional redundancy'. An alternative, more attractive view is that the intestine has developed a number of auxiliary mechanisms.

The small intestine is replete with examples of auxiliary mechanisms. Experimental grafting of fetal tissue reveals that essentially normal development can occur in the absence of luminal factors and ontogenetically programmed hormonal surges. Exogenous glucocorticoids can precociously elicit the mature phenotype, as does in vivo manipulation which elevates endogenous glucocorticoids[11]. Although glucocorticoids appear to be necessary for early maturation, it is not known which cell type is activated. Two alternatives include either the last dividing cell rather than stem cells themselves or an effect on mesenchymal cells.

c/EBP-α is a transcription factor whose expression is associated with cessation of proliferation and the onset of differentiation. Observations in knockout mice which are homozygous negative for this gene reveal the counterintuitive observation that they have approximately normal intestines. Of particular interest is the role of TGF-α epidermal growth factor (EGF) in postnatal intestinal growth. Surprisingly, however, EGF receptor knockout mice survive with a normal intestine suggesting that TGF-α/EGF may bind to other members of the EGF receptor superfamily: erb B2,3,4 receptors. Other factors which may have a modulatory effect on intestinal development include bacterial infection. Yet in germ free mice intestinal development appears to be normal.

The conclusion arrived at from these observations is a general hypothesis, that gut maturation, like other critical aspects of mammalian development, has evolved a multiplicity of regulatory mechanisms during evolutionary development to enable mammals to survive various selective pressures.

EGF receptor and TGF-α

The EGF superfamily comprises an ever-expanding number of membrane-anchored growth factors which display high affinity binding to different members of the EGF tyrosine kinase receptor family[12,13]. Recent work has focused on the trafficking of human TGF-α and EGF in polarized MDCK cells and indicates that TGF-α is targeted preferentially to the basolateral surface, the compartment where the EGF receptor resides. EGF is not targeted but accumulates at the apical surface due to rapid proteolytic cleavage at the basolateral surface. Amphiregulin and heparin binding EGF-like growth factor are also targeted to this surface.

A model of polarized cells (HCA-7) grown on Transwell membrane filters has been developed to evaluate the effects of EGF-like growth factors on cell proliferation and cyclo-oxygenase activation. Basolateral administration of TGF-α leads to an induction of COX-2, increased nuclear COX-2 immunostaining, and the exclusive basolateral release of prostaglandins. EGF receptor blockade decreases levels of COX-2 and prostaglandins and also reduces mitogenesis. A specific COX-2 inhibitor, SC-58125, attenuates TGF-α-induced mitogenesis and inhibits both in vitro and in vivo growth of these cells.

These results have been corroborated in a second series of experiments, utilizing the TGF-α over-expressing mutant cell line, RIE-1,which autoregulates growth via activation of the EGF receptor and stimulation of COX-2 activity and PG2 release. These studies further confirm the role of TGF-α in epithelial cell growth and activity.

Meprin: an interesting brush border enzyme

The metabolism and expression of brush border enzymes are highly regulated in the mucosal cells of the gastrointestinal tract and this is correlated with growth and differentiation. PABA-peptide hydrolase, or human meprin, is a zinc metalloendopeptidase initially isolated from the brush border membrane of epithelial cells from the human small intestine[14,15]. The prototype of this family is the crayfish enzyme, astacin, which was the first to be isolated and characterized although more than 20 family members have now been identified in species as diverse as hydra and human. The proposed functions of this enigmatic enzyme include degradation of polypeptides, activation of growth factors, and processing of extracellular matrix proteins both in mature and developing systems.

Meprin is a unique protease since it possesses a multidomain structure and is composed of a protein complex with two glycosylated disulphide-linked subunits, α and β. It exhibits the structural characteristics of receptors with a transmembrane, an epidermal growth factor-like, and an adhesion domain. The α and β subunits are differentially expressed and processed to yield latent and active proteases in membrane-bound as well as in secreted forms. There are indications that the two subunits may be expressed differently in intestinal tissue. Expression of meprin in humans is highest in the small intestine with an increasing activity gradient from the proximal duodenum to the distal ileum. Some expression is also found in the colon. It is possible that the spatial and structural differences of meprin make it a potentially important enzyme in the regulation of growth and development of the intestinal epithelium. Little evidence exists, however, to support this proposal.

Paneth cells

Paneth cells are epithelial granulocytes located at the base of the crypts of Lieberkühn in the small intestine of many mammalian species. They generally occupy the first few cell positions in the crypt column and are interspersed with other cells with a distinct inverse gradient of Paneth cell density with distance from the crypt base in both mouse and rat. It is of note that these cells exhibit distinct ultrastructural features which have been interpreted as characteristic of stem cells. Their function has long been a mystery but two theories exist. A high protein-producing activity coupled to the production of lysozyme and zinc has suggested a role in the control of local bacterial flora. Indeed, apical release of granules by Paneth cells appears to contribute to the mucosal barrier function in the crypt microenvironment, since these granules contain an array of endogenous antimicrobial proteins and peptides. The alternative, and possibly complementary, hypothesis is that these cells have a managerial role in the control of cell pro-liferation[16,17].

Paneth cells produce defensins, known as cryptdins (crypt defensins), which are also expressed in the bone marrow. Six defensins have been characterized at the peptide level, and each is encoded by a separate two-exon gene on chromosome 8[18]. A minimum of 19 mouse cryptdin isoforms are predicted from the peptide and cDNA sequencing data. The Paneth cell cryptdins are similar to typical defensins, and are cationic, 3–4 kDa proteins with six cystine residues that form three disulphide bonds to create an amphipathic peptide. Antimicrobial assays utilizing cryptdins isolated from intact small bowel and from the intestinal lumen, suggest that the N-terminus and residues in positions 10, and particularly 15 (arginine) are potential determinants of antimicrobial activity[19]. However, target microbes (S. typhimurium, E. coli) differ in their sensitivity to individual cryptdins, although type 4 appears to be most consistently potent. It is noteworthy that peptides with apparently minor structural differences exhibit variable activities particularly against the trophozoites of Giardia lamblia.

Cryptdins are early markers of crypt ontogeny, and individual genes are differ-entially expressed in the undifferentiated epithelium of newborn mice and along the length of the proximal to distal gut axis in humans. Cryptdin genes, however, are active in the intestinal epithelium prior to Paneth cell differentiation and using PCR, cryptdin gene activity can be identified as early as 24 h after birth in the intestinal mucosa of mice. Using immunocytochemical localization it is apparent that cryptdin-containing cells are localized throughout the newborn intestinal epithelium; cryptdin itself is found within the intracellular granules. After birth, cryptdin mRNAs accumulate to high levels in differentiating Paneth cells during crypt ontogeny particularly in the second and third weeks after birth. Cryptdin-6 appears to be the most abundant cryptdin in the newborn intestine. In adult mice, cryptdin-4 is expressed with positional specificity along the longitudinal intestinal axis (undetectable in the duodenum, maximal in distal ileum), but is not evident in the stomach or the duodenum.

Overall it would appear that cryptdins probably mediate innate immunity in the hostile environment of the intestinal lumen. It would thus be of considerable interest to define the particular biochemical and biophysical attributes that enable these peptides to exert a barrier function at mucosal surfaces. In addition, the temporal and spatial asymmetries of these genes as well as their number confer upon them the possible utility of specific markers in the developing intestine. A potential role in the control of cell proliferation remains to be firmly established.

Gastrointestinal receptors

Receptors for gastrointestinal peptides such as somatostatin (SST), vasoactive intestinal polypeptide (VIP), substance P, cholecystokinin (CCK) and gastrin can be identified in targets as diverse as the gut mucosa, smooth muscle, vessels, gut-associated lymphoid tissue and neural plexus. Under certain pathological conditions, such as neoplasia, these peptides may be either abnormally expressed (present on cells which usually do not exhibit them) or even over-expressed. SST receptors are expressed in most neuroendocrine tumours, although it is not uncommon to identify SST receptor-positive vessels in SST receptor-negative tumours (e.g. colonic tumours). Most epithelial tumours express VIP receptors (75%). Substance P receptors are mostly expressed in breast cancers, medullary thyroid cancers and astrocytomas, and it is of potential therapeutic interest that levels of these receptors are also increased in the intra- and peritumoral vessels of such neoplasms. CCK-B receptors are identifiable in small cell lung cancer and the vast majority of medullary thyroid cancers. It may be of both biological and therapeutic relevance that CCK-B receptors have not been identified in colon cancer. CCK-A receptors are only occasionally present in gastroenteropancreatic tumours and meningiomas. While some lesions are occasionally positive for only one of these receptors, tumours are often composed of a combination of the above. It is of clinical and biological relevance that in a large proportion of tumours the receptors are functional and may thus mediate growth by stimulation or inhibition[20].

At this time a number of relevant diagnostic and therapeutic applications have been developed on the basis of in vitro human studies. First, intravenous injection of labelled SST or VIP to localize receptor-bearing tumours and metastases in vivo has been most successful in lesions expressing the SST subtype 2 receptor and are probed using [111]Indium-labelled octreotide[21]. VIP receptor imaging has not been particularly successful to date, mainly because of the high background levels consequent upon degradation of the probe. Second, synthetic polypeptide agonists or antagonists have been utilized for treatment of receptor-positive tumours. This has proved most useful in the instance of somatostatin congener therapy indirectly targeting tumour growth and metastases by induction of either vasoconstriction, inhibition of angiogenesis, direct tumour and anti-trophic effect or indirect inhibition of growth factors from adjacent cells[22].

Novel developmental genes

Subtractive hybridization is a powerful tool which has been used to isolate novel genes which are selectively expressed under certain conditions. Utilizing intestinal development as a model, two novel clones which are transcriptionally up-regulated during development in rat small intestine have been isolated[23]. The expression of these two genes appears to be regulated both during development and during cell differentiation, along both the duodenum–ileum and crypt–villus axes.

The first clone, identified as Dri27, consists of 341 amino acids, and is predicted to be a hydrophobic protein. Immunocytochemical studies indicate that this protein is inserted into the basolateral plasma membrane domain of the rat enterocyte but that it is also expressed in the brain. The function of this novel protein has been evaluated in a series of fusion protein studies. Segments of the protein were linked to the bacterial reporter GST protein and it was noted that a histidine-rich domain bound to different transition metal ions, including Zn, Cu, Ni, Co. When Dri27 was overproduced in Caco-2 cells, transport of these metal ions was up-regulated but no metal specificity could be identified. However, since the primary sequence of the transporter shares significant homology with two recently isolated Zn transporters, it seems likely that this protein may transport Zn in vivo.

The second clone, identified as Dri42, is expressed ubiquitously throughout the body, but has only been demonstrated to be up-regulated in the epithelium of the small intestine. It is a 6-transmembrane spanning domain protein with a weak homology to a variety of potassium gated proteins. Using laser confocal microscopy, this protein, when over-expressed in the MDCK cell line, can be detected in the endoplasmic reticulum (ER), suggesting that it is an ER-resident transmembrane protein. Pulse-chase labelling experiments further confirm that it does not accumulate in the Golgi apparatus even after 4 h. Membrane insertion of the protein is achieved co-translationally by the action of alternating insertion signals and halt transfer signals, resulting in the exposure of both termini of the protein to the cytosolic side. Although no ionic channel data are currently available for this ER protein, a putative role for these two proteins in the regulation of small intestinal development has been proposed.

Ex vivo SCID xenograft

The severe-combined immunodeficient (SCID) murine xenograft model has been utilized to resolve some fundamental questions regarding human gastrointestinal ontogenesis. The model was initially used to evaluate whether human fetal gut when transplanted subcutaneously into such mice underwent region specific morphogenesis and epithelial cytodifferentiation[24]. However the model is also of utility in the investigation of human gastrointestinal drug targeting[25], and the biology of childhood and adult enteropathy. In particular the potential role of non-epithelial cells in the regulation of epithelial differentiation can also be addressed.

Ten weeks after grafting with human material, characteristic small intestine mucosa develops which resembles the stratified type of epithelium present during early fetal gastrointestinal development. However, idiosyncratic epithelial differentiation pathways can thereafter be identified during xenograft regeneration. These specifically reflect both an absence of Paneth cells and an abundance of enteroendocrine cells. It is possible that such differences are as a result of the loss of conventional luminal and hormonal stimuli normally present during pregnancy. In situ hybridization shows that the intestinal xenograft epithelium, muscularis mucosa and externa are of exclusively human origin. It is of interest that although the submucosa and lamina propria were comprised of a chimeric mix, murine cells were rarely detected in contact with the epithelium. Human myofibroblasts and intraepithelial lymphocytes were most commonly seen in contact with the xenograft epithelium. The lack of murine:human cell contact suggests that species-specific interactions are maintained in this model via a selection process. These differences appear to be important for regulating epithelial cell differentiation.

References

1. Steel GG. Growth kinetics of tumors. Oxford: Oxford University Press, 1977.
2. Brooks RA, Gooderham NJ, Zhao K *et al.* 2-Amino-1-methyl-6-phenylimidazo[4,5-b]pyridine is a potent mutagen in the mouse small intestine. Cancer Res. 1994;54:1665–71.
3. Potten CS, Li YQ, O'Connor PJ, Winton DJ. A possible explanation for the differential cancer incidence in the intestine, based on distribution of the cytotoxic effects of carcinogens in the murine large bowel. Carcinogenesis. 1992;13:2305–12.
4. Williams ED, Lowes AP, Williams D, Williams GT. A stem cell niche theory of intestinal crypt maintenance based on a study of somatic mutation in colonic mucosa. Am J Pathol. 1992;141: 773–6.
5. Campbell F, Fuller CE, Williams GT, Williams ED. Human colonic stem cell mutation frequency with and without irradiation. J Pathol. 1994;174:175–82.
6. Loeffler M, Birke A, Winton D, Potten C. Somatic mutation, monoclonality and stochastic models of stem cell organization in the intestinal crypt. J Theor Biol. 1993;160:471–91.
7. Bjerknes M. Simple stochastic theory of stem cell differentiation is not simultaneously consistent with crypt extinction probability and the expansion of mutated clones. J Theor Biol. 1994;168: 349–65.
8. Reitmair AH, Cai JC, Bjerknes M *et al.* MSH2 deficiency contributes to accelerated APC-mediated intestinal tumorigenesis. Cancer Res. 1996;56:2922–6.
9. Dorin JR. Development of mouse models for cystic fibrosis. J Inher Metab Dis. 1995;18:495–500.
10. Dorin JR, Dickinson P, Emslie E *et al.* Successful targeting of the mouse cystic fibrosis trans-membrane conductance regulator gene in embryonal stem cells. Transgenic Res. 1992;1:101–5.
11. Nanthakumar NN, Henning SJ. Distinguishing normal and glucocorticoid-induced maturation of intestine using promodeoxyuridine. Am J Physiol. 1995;268:G139–G145.
12. Coffey RJ, Gangarosa LM, Damstrup L, Dempsey PJ. Basic actions of transforming growth factor-alpha and related peptides. Eur J Gastroenterol Hepatol. 1995;7:923–7.
13. Barnard JA, Graves-Deal R, Pittelkow MR *et al.* Auto- and cross-induction within the mammalian epidermal growth factor-related peptide family. J Biol Chem. 1994;269:22817–22.
14. Dumermuth E, Eldering JA, Grunberg J, Jiang W, Sterchi EE. Cloning of the PABA peptide hydrolase alpha subunit (PPH alpha) from human small intestine and its expression in COS-1 cells. FEBS Lett. 1993;335:367–75.
15. Hall JL, Sterchi EE, Bond JS. Biosynthesis and degradation of meprins, kidney brush border proteinases. Arch Biochem Biophys. 1993;307:73–7.
16. Creamer B. The turnover of the epithelium of the small intestine. Br Med Bull. 1967;231:226–30.
17. Cairnie AB. Homeostasis in the small intestine. In: Cairnie AB, Lala PK, Osmond DG, editors. Stem cells of renewing cell populations. New York: Academic Press, 1976:67–78.
18. Huttner KM, Ouellette AJ. A family of defensin-like genes codes from diverse cysteine-rich peptides in mouse Paneth cells. Genomics. 1994;24:99–109.
19. Ouellette AJ, Hsieh MM, Nosek MT *et al.* Mouse Paneth cell defensins: primary structures and antibacterial activities of numerous cryptdin isoforms. Infect Immun. 1994;62:5040–7.
20. Reubi JC. Neuropeptide receptors in health and disease: the molecular basis for in vivo imaging. J Nucl Med. 1995;36:1825–35.
21. Krenning EP, Kwekkeboom DJ, Oei HY *et al.* Somatostatin receptor scintigraphy in carcinoids, gastrinomas and Cushing's syndrome. Digestion. Suppl. 3: 1994:54–9.
22. Reubi JC, Horisberger U, Laissue J. High density of somatostatin receptors in veins surrounding human cancer tissue: role in tumor-host interaction? Int J Cancer. 1994;56:681–8.
23. Barila D, Murgia C, Nobili F, Gaetani S, Perozzi G. Subtractive hybridization cloning of novel genes differentially expressed during intestinal development. Eur J Biochem. 1994;223:701–9.
24. Savidge TC, Morey AL, Ferguson DJ, Fleming KA, Shmakov AN, Phillips AD. Human intestinal development in a severe-combined immunodeficient xenograft model. Differentiation. 1995; 58:361–71.
25. Savidge TC, Schmakova A. Human gastrointestinal drug delivery; an experimental chimeric approach. J Drug Targeting. 1995;3:71–4.
26. Potten CS, Klimashevski K, Gushchin VA. Study of the kinetics of epithelial cell populations in normal tissues of the rats intestines and in carcinogenesis. I. A comparison of enterocyte population kinetics in different segments of the intestine and colon. Exp Pathol Jena. 1980;18:387–406.
27. Park HS, Goodlad RA, Wright NA. Crypt fission in the small intestine and colon: A mechanism for the emergence of G6PD locus-mutated crypts after treatment with mutagens. Am J Pathol. 1995;147:1416–27.

Section III
Epithelial mesenchymal interactions

13
Cellular and molecular mechanisms regulating intestinal development

M. KEDINGER, M. PLATEROTI, V. ORIAN-ROUSSEAU, O. LORENTZ,
C. FRITSCH, A. DE ARCANGELIS, G. EVANS, I. DULUC,
J. N. FREUND and P. SIMON-ASSMANN

INTRODUCTION

During intestinal development the steps of morphogenesis and differentiation, as well as the maintenance of the morphological and functional steady-state in the mature organ, result partly from cross-talk between epithelial and mesenchyme-derived cells. Due to its developmental and spatial pecularities, the intestinal tissue is of special interest as a model for more general aspects of developmental and cell biology. This chapter will focus on one hand on some characteristics of the mesenchymal cell compartment and on the other hand on the role of basement membrane (BM) molecules, such as laminins (LNs) located at the epithelial–mesenchymal interface, in this cross-talk.

FROM THE FETAL TO THE ADULT GUT

The intestinal tube derives from the association of the embryonic endoderm and the splanchnic mesoderm. In humans, the intestinal endoderm appears around the eighth day of gestation and rapidly forms the epithelial border of the digestive tract. It is surrounded at 15 days by the splanchnic mesoderm that will give rise to the connective tissue, muscle and serosal layers. Three distinct gut anlagen, the fore-, mid- and posterior gut, develop respectively into the duodenum, the major part of the small intestine and colon, and the distal colon. The same development events occur in rodents.

At 8 weeks in human and 14 days in rat fetuses, the intestinal tube is composed of an inner stratified endoderm comprising undifferentiated cells. At the tiny lumen border, intercellular junctional complexes as well as rare irregular apical microvilli become obvious. From that stage onwards, a high cellular proliferative activity and active tissue remodelling lead to the outgrowth of villi and later on to the formation of crypts by an epithelial down-growth into the mesenchyme. Crypt formation is associated to a progressive restriction of the proliferative cells in the inter-villus regions which is achieved once villus formation is complete, around 12 weeks of gestation in humans and around birth in rodents. In parallel to the conversion of the stratified into a simple epithelium, various cell types emerge from the immature primitive cells that will differentiate: absorptive, goblet, entero-endocrine and Paneth cells. Concomitant with the morphogenetic steps, the mesenchyme differentiates first into the outer muscle layers and later into cellular elements of the submucosal and mucosal connective tissue. Among the latter are subepithelial elongated myofibroblasts, muscle fibres and fibroblasts.

The mature gut is compartmentalized: the crypts comprise dividing cells which derive from a resident pluripotent stem cell population and differentiate while migrating along a vertical crypt to villus axis. Cell differentiation is bidirectional: while most phenotypes arise from cell migration and differentiation towards the apex of the villi, Paneth cells differentiate in the bottom of the crypts (for reviews see Refs. 1, 2). Differentiated absorptive cells are highly polarized; they are charac-terized by their apical brush border domain which constitutes the functional organelle subserving terminal digestion and absorption of the products of ingested food, owing to digestive enzymes and transporters.

The onset of morphological and enzymatic differentiation occurs proximo-distally and the adult gut is characterized by an antero-posterior gradient of mor-phological features and of cytodifferentiation. Contrasting with the crypt-villus structure of the small intestine, the mature colon is characterized by deep glands and a flat surface epithelium composed of hexagonal cuffs of epithelial cells that surround the orifice of each gland. However, during development, the colon exhibits a transient villus phase. These villi are covered by polarized cells carrying regular brush borders and which express small intestinal-type enzymes such as sucrase-isomaltase in the human fetal colon and lactase in the postnatal rat colon. Of particular interest, linked to this transient small intestinal-type expression in the developing colon is the finding that human colon carcinomas and established human colonic cancer cell lines express typical enterocytic differentiation markers such as sucrase-isomaltase and lactase[3]. During the last decade, these cell lines have been extensively used as models of investigation of the morphological and functional enterocytic differentiation.

THE INTESTINAL BASEMENT MEMBRANE (BM)

In the early fetal intestine, the deepest epithelial cell layer is delineated by a regular BM; the underlying mesenchymal cells are elongated and parallel to the basement membrane. In the mature organ, the subepithelial elongated myofibro-blasts are also separated from the epithelium by the BM. Because of its strategic location at the endodermal/epithelial–mesenchymal interface, the BM may play a crucial role in regulating the communication between these two cell compart-ments.

BMs are specialized sheet-like extracellular matrix (ECM), that can be visualized as a linear electron-dense material which separates the parenchymal cells from the connective tissue in most tissues. ECM molecules are considered as dynamic effectors in morphogenesis and in generation or maintenance of epithelial cell

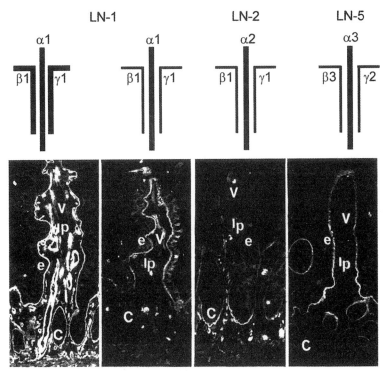

Figure 1 Differential expression of laminin isoforms in human adult intestine. The molecule or individual chains, detected with the corresponding antibodies, are indicated in bold on top of the micrographs. (e) epithelial cells, (lp) lamina propria, (V) villus, (C) crypt. Taken from Ref. 41, with permission

polarity. Each ECM molecule is composed of many domains and has multiple binding sites for other matrix molecules, for a variety of other molecules such as growth factors and, most importantly, for cells. Their association forms a complex three-dimensional network[4]. This exoskeleton interacts with cell surface receptors such as integrins, which transduce information from the cell environment to the intracellular compartment.

The subepithelial intestinal BM comprises the ubiquitous BM molecules, LN, type IV collagen, nidogen and perlecan. The tissue- and age-dependent specificity of the BMs is ensured by the expression of various isoforms of laminin and collagen IV. As an example, at least 11 isoforms of the laminin family (trimeric cross-shaped molecules) are presently known[4] (Champliaud and Burgeson, personal communication). At least three of these, LN-1, LN-2 and LN-5, are expressed in the gut subepithelial BM, with age- and location-specific patterns, and thus participate to the establishment of its functional micro-heterogeneity (Figure 1). LN-1 (α1, β1, γ1 chains) is expressed early at the intestinal epithelial–mesenchymal interface (11/12 days in the mouse/rat embryos, 7 weeks in human fetuses). In contrast, the first expression of LN-2 (α2, β1, γ1 chains) is delayed (around birth in rodents, at 15 weeks in human) and immediately confined to the crypts.

In the human mature organ, LN-1 and LN-2 have a complementary localization, with LN-1 underlying the villus and upper crypt epithelial cells and LN-2 the lower two-thirds crypt cells[5,6]. Finally, LN-5 (α3, β3, γ2 chains) which, like LN-1 is found at the level of the villus cells, is characterized in the mouse intestine by a dissociation in chain expression due to a late appearance of α3 chains[7]. Such a distinct distribution of each LN isoform together with their binding to various integrins strongly suggest their specific participation in different cellular behaviours, such as proliferation, migration and differentiation. Similar variations are seen for type IV collagen α(IV) constituent chains during human gut development[8]. There are species-specific variations in the composition of a given BM, as exemplified for LN-1 and LN-2[5]. An additional level of microheterogeneity in the composition of the BM at a given developmental stage results from the relative proportions of the different BM molecules and of qualitative changes in the constituent chains of a given molecule. As an example, the biosynthesis of LN-1 α1 chain vs. β1/γ1 chains is the highest during intestinal morphogenesis and onset of differentiation[9].

EPITHELIAL–MESENCHYMAL CELL INTERACTIONS IN THE DEVELOPING AND ADULT GUT

The requirement of epithelial–mesenchymal contact for gut morphogenesis and differentiation is supported by the above mentioned observations and by the following experimental arguments: first, isolated intestinal endoderm or mesenchyme fail to develop when grafted in the coelomic cavity of chick embryos; second, primary cultures or cell lines of fetal epithelial cells or postnatal crypt cells poorly differentiate in the absence of mesenchymal support.

During the past two decades, numerous embryonic recombination experiments have emphasized that morphogenesis and cytodifferentiation of the gastrointestinal tract are dependent on reciprocal interactions between epithelium and mesenchyme. More insight into such processes has been gained using various types of interspecies or heterotopic embryonic tissue associations. The main conclusions of such experiments have been reviewed in Haffen et al.[10] and Yasugi[11]; as far as they are related to the gut, they can be summarized as follows.

First, each of the intestinal endodermal and mesenchymal tissue component exerts permissive effects on the development of its associated counterpart. Experimentally, interspecies chick–rodent epithelial–mesenchymal associations develop as intracoelomic grafts, leading to chimeric intestines in which the morphogenetic pattern is dictated by the mesenchyme, while the epithelial functional cytodifferentiation is an intrinsic property of the endoderm[12]. Xenografts of tissue recombinants composed of endodermal and mesodermal anlagen originating from various proximo-distal segments of rat fetal small intestines lead to chimeric intestines, in which the endoderm develops its own functional cytodifferentiation characteristics[13].

Second, endodermal–mesenchymal contacts are required to allow the expression of their reciprocal permissive interactions. Indeed, epithelial or mesenchymal anlagen are unable to differentiate in vitro or in vivo unless heterologous cellular contacts are achieved[14,15]. In parallel, co-cultures and interspecies recombination experiments stress the importance of heterologous cell interactions for the elaboration of an adequate extracellular molecular organization, necessary to direct cell proliferation and differentiation. Although each cell compartment cultured independently is able to synthesize some BM molecules, no authentic BM, visualized with specific antibodies or as an electron-dense material, can be elaborated unless heterologous co-cultures are employed. In this case, LN-1, type IV collagen, nidogen and perlecan are deposited at the epithelial–mesenchymal interface[16].

The absolute requirement of close cell contacts for BM formation can be explained by the data obtained from the analysis of chick–rodent epithelial–mesenchymal hybrid associations developed as grafts in chick embryos or in nude mice. In such hybrid intestines, the deposition of BM components can be traced with species-specific antibodies. From these observations we conclude that the subepithelial BM is composed of molecules deposited either by the epithelial or mesenchymal compartment alone, or by both compartments for some BM constituents. In addition, variations in the cellular origin can be observed as a function of the morphogenetic and differentiation state of the hybrids. The detailed conclusions drawn from this study are summarized in Simon-Assmann et al.[17] These data stress the importance not only of the heterologous cell contacts but also of the maturation state of each tissue compartment. This also underlies the reciprocal, permissive or instructive cell interactions that lead to the elaboration of the appropriate exoskeleton.

Third, the morphological integrity of the endoderm or mesenchyme is not required to allow morphogenesis and/or differentiation. This is examplified in vitro by the ability of layered mesenchymal and endodermal co-cultures to express, respectively, smooth-muscle α-actin (a myofibroblastic marker) and apically located digestive enzymes. The development as intracoelomic grafts of endoderms associated with cultured mesenchymal cells, or conversely of cultured endodermal cells with intact mesenchymes, leads to well organized and functionally active intestinal structures[18,19].

Fourth, instructive interactions have been observed in various types of tissue associations developed after transplantation. These include the ability of the jejunal or ileal mesenchyme to induce fetal rat colonic endoderm to switch on small intestinal-type enzymatic differentiation[13,20]. This observation is of particular importance in the light of the peculiar expression of small intestinal-like phenotypes in colonic cancer cells. Gut mesenchyme also exerts an inductive action on avian gizzard endoderm which changes its morphological and cytodifferentiation pattern[10]. In addition, there is an instructive potency of the intestinal endoderm to the surrounding mesenchymally derived cell layer, demonstrated by its ability to induce skin fibroblastic cells to form subnormal peripheral muscle and inner lamina propria-like layers[19].

Finally, functional epithelial–mesenchymal cell interactions are maintained in the mature gut. Indeed postnatal primary crypt cell cultures and to a lesser extent crypt cell lines (IEC cells[21]) can be induced by fetal mesenchyme to achieve villus morphogenesis and complete cytodifferentiation with the emergence of various epithelial cell phenotypes[18]. Additionally, cell cultures established from postnatal intestinal lamina propria are able, like the fetal mesenchyme, to direct intestinalization of the avian gizzard endoderm[22].

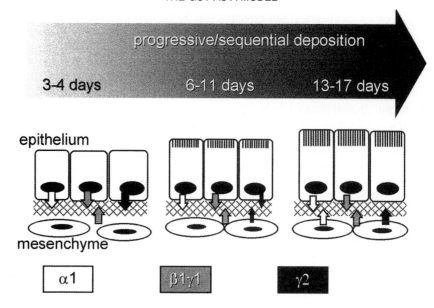

Figure 2 Cellular origin of laminin-1 α1, β1/γ1 and of laminin-5 γ2 constituent chains. Hybrid intestines were constructed by the association of chick mesenchyme and mouse endoderm and vice versa, which were grafted in the coelom of chick embryos for 3–17 days. Immunocytochemical detections of the different chains were performed on transverse cryosections, with species-specific antibodies[7,24]

FOCUS ON THE MESENCHYMAL CELL COMPARTMENT

The morphological and experimental observations described above stress the importance of both epithelial and mesenchymal cell compartments. However little is known about the mesenchyme-derived cells in the gut. Because of their localization at the epithelial–lamina propria interface, the subepithelial (myo)fibroblastic cells may be involved in signal transmission between these compartments. The current knowledge about the subepithelial mesenchymal cells has been summarized in a recent review[23].

Using the interspecies recombination experiments designed to analyse the cellular origin of the BM molecules (see above), we showed that type IV collagen and nidogen, two molecules involved in the association of laminin and perlecan, were produced by the mesenchymal cells (see Ref. 17). In addition, these experiments demonstrated that, together with the maturation of the mesenchymal cells, the expression of the α1 and γ2 chains of LN-1 and LN-5, respectively, was turned on in these cells[7,24] (Figure 2). Thus BM molecules may represent signals given by the mesenchyme and received by the epithelium, allowing morphogenesis, differentiation or growth. Other putative effectors described in various tissues, including the gut, may also be involved in the mesenchyme to epithelium cross-talk. This is exemplified by molecules such as epimorphin[25], midkine (a heparin binding component)[26] and hepatocyte growth factor/scatter factor (a secreted glycoprotein, HGF/SF)[27] whose transcripts have been located in mesenchymal cells surrounding the gut endoderm or epithelium. Interestingly, HGF/SF receptors are expressed in the intestinal epithelial cells[27,28]. In addition, epithelial differentiation agents such as retinoids and/or glucocorticoids are known to induce or enhance the expression of BM molecules, integrins or metalloproteases involved in matrix remodelling[29,30], of midkine[26] and of transforming growth factor-β (TGF-β)[31], which is known to induce the differentiation of various mesenchymal cell types into myofibroblasts[32].

Altogether these observations indicate that undifferentiated mesenchymal cells may be the target of various agents, including the cytokines produced by the immunocompetent cells present in the lamina propria. Possibly in response to such stimulation, these cells will enter different phenotypic pathways and thus modulate the epithelial–mesenchymal unit.

Recent data support this concept. Indeed, two morphologically distinct mes-enchymal cell clones derived from postnatal rat intestinal lamina propria display several interesting differences in their response to cytokines and in their ability to promote specific morphogenesis. Firstly, the proliferation of one cell line, F1G9, is inhibited by TGF-β1, that of the A1F1 cell line by interleukin-2 (IL2). In addition, TGF-β1 induces a large proportion of F1G9 cells (but not of A1F1 cells) to differentiate into myofibroblasts. Secondly, when F1G9 cells are associated with intestinal endoderms, either in vitro (co-cultures) or in vivo (grafts), they are able to induce differentiation of the epithelial cells and to support normal morphogenesis. In contrast, A1F1 cells only form deep glands devoid of epithelial expression of digestive enzymes[33] (Figure 3). One can therefore hypothesize that a change in the relative proportions of various phenotypically different mesen-chymal cells, resulting from an impaired balance in cytokines, may be responsible for morphological and functional alterations of the gut in pathological situations.

The major role of the mesenchyme in the regulation of intestinal epithelial differentiation is also strengthened by the effects of retinoic acid (RA), which is a morphogen and differentiating agent for various organs. RA treatment of undiffer-entiated fetal intestine in vitro (organ cultures) and in vivo (xenografts in nude mice), induces morphogenesis and differentiation. These effects are assessed by the outgrowth of villi, enlargement of the crypt compartment, thickening of the muscular layers and precocious expression of lactase. Interestingly, subepithelial mesenchymal clonal cell lines derived from 8-day old postnatal rat lamina propria respond to exogenous RA by increasing the expression of specific cytoplasmic and nuclear retinoid binding proteins (RBPs) and of laminin and collagen IV. When co-cultured with intestinal endodermal cells, these clones are able to enhance epithelial cell polarization and differentiation upon RA treatment; in these latter conditions, RA increased BM molecules expression and deposition[30] (Figure 4).

ROLE OF LAMININS IN CELL INTERACTION-DEPENDENT DIFFERENTIATION

Experimental evidence supporting a role for BM molecules in cell differentiation is given by the chronological steps in cell–cell contacts, the formation of the BM, and the expression of epithelial cell differentiation markers which occur in co-

THE GUT AS A MODEL

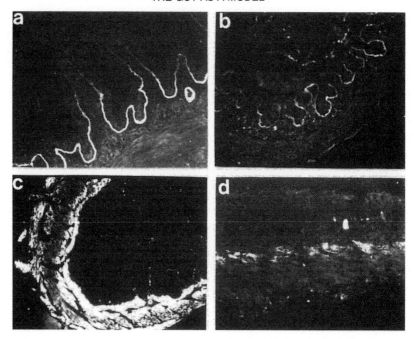

Figure 3 Differential morphogenesis induced by two mesenchymal cell clones (F1G9: a, c and A1F1: b, d) associated with 14-day intestinal endoderms and grafted for 13 days in the chick embryo. Immunocytochemical detection of laminin (a, b) and of smooth muscle α-actin (c, d). Note that the grafts composed of F1G9 cells form villi and small crypts and well developed outer muscle layers; those composed of A1F1 form glands and the muscle coat is poorly differentiated

cultures of embryonic intestinal endodermal cells and mesenchymal cells. Furthermore, in this model, the expression of apical hydrolases can be blocked by anti-laminin antibodies added in the co-culture medium[29].

An interesting correlation between the amount of laminin synthesized by two human colonic cancer cell lines (undifferentiated HT29 and differentiated Caco-2 cells) and their interactions with mesenchymal cells also stressed the potential importance of this BM molecule. Indeed, in contrast to Caco-2 cells, HT29 cells did not form close contacts with underlying mesenchyme-derived cells, nor a BM at the intercellular interface, and HT29 cells only produced low amounts of LN-1 and did not express the α1 chain[34,35]. To try to correlate LN-1 α1 chain production to the degree of cell differentiation, its expression has been inhibited in Caco-2 cells by stably transfecting the cells with an antisense cDNA. This leads to particularly interesting and informative data on the role of this molecule[36]. Inhibition of α1 chain expression in the transfected clones alters the secretion of the complementary β1/γ1 chains of LN-1. As a consequence, no BM is formed in co-cultures despite the fact that type IV collagen and nidogen are produced by the mesenchymal cell compartment. Finally, the polarization and some differentiation characteristics of the cells are significantly disturbed. These experiments clearly demonstrate the requirement of LN-1 for epithelial cell differentiation, which is also suggested by the villus localization of this laminin isoform in human

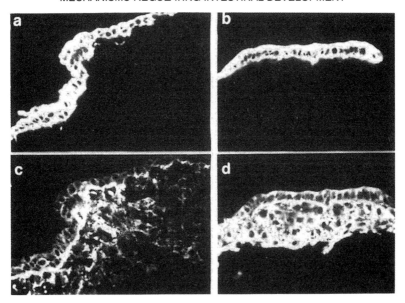

Figure 4 Epithelial polarization and differentiation is enhanced by retinoic acid in co-culture conditions of 14-day endodermal cells with cloned subepithelial myofibroblastic cells. (a, c): 3-day control co-cultures; (b, d): co-cultures in the presence of 10^{-8}M all-*trans* RA from day 2. Immunocytochemical detection of cytokeratin (a, b) and of laminin (c, d) on cryosections of the co-cultures. Note that RA treatment leads to a polarization of the epithelial cells and an accumulation of laminin in the mesenchymal cells

intestine. A correlation between the amount of laminin produced and the state of Caco-2 cell differentiation has also been reported by Vachon and Beaulieu[37].

Among the differentiation parameters of Caco-2 cells altered by the inhibition of the $\alpha 1$ chain was a drastic inhibition of sucrase-isomaltase (SI)[36]. It is worth noting that in parallel to these changes, a decrease in the expression of *cdx* 2 occurred. *cdx* 2 is an intestinal-specific homeobox gene which has been demonstrated to act as a transcription factor for several intestinal-specific differentiation genes, among which SI (for review see Ref. 38), and whose expression is correlated with the fate of the epithelium in heterotopic hybrid intestinal xenografts[39]. In the $\alpha 1$-deficient clones as well as in the clones which showed a phenotypic reversion (loss of $\alpha 1$ chain inhibition by a decrease in selection pressure), there is a clear parallel between *cdx* 2 and laminin $\alpha 1$ mRNA. A similar correlation can be made in a series of Caco-2 clones exhibiting various rates of inhibition of laminin $\alpha 1$ chain synthesis by the antisense RNA. Additionally, the culture of non-manipulated Caco-2 cells on laminin coatings led to enhanced SI and *cdx* 2 transcripts. Thus, laminin may control the expression of *cdx* 2, which subsequently regulates the expression of intestinal differentiation markers[40]. These experiments strongly suggest that, in the intestinal tissue, the effect of laminin, synthesized by both epithelial and mesenchymal cells and deposited at the cellular interface, on epithelial differentiation may be mediated by key regulatory genes such as *cdx* 2.

In conclusion, these data demonstrate the importance of epithelial–mesenchymal cell interactions in the developing and mature intestine. They indicate that specific mesenchymal cell populations can direct intestinal development and differentiation; furthermore their nature and properties can be influenced by various agents like retinoids or cytokines produced by the epithelium or the immunocompetent cells present in the lamina propria. BM molecules, including laminins, may play a crucial role in the cross-talk between the epithelial and mesenchymal cells. Dysfunction of signal transmission emanating from either cell compartment may be a crucial determinant in the pathogenesis of intestinal disease.

Acknowledgements

We would like to thank C. Arnold and C. Leberquier for their expert technical help in the work reported herein. The work was supported by funds from the Institut National de la Santé et de la Recherche Médicale, and grants from the Association pour la Recherche contre le Cancer and the Fondation Aupetit.

References

1. Potten CS, Loeffler M. Stem cells. Attributes, cycles, spirals, pitfalls and uncertainties. Lessons for and from the crypt. Development. 1990;110:1001–20.
2. Hermiston MI, Simon TC, Crossman MW, Gordon JI. Model systems for studying cell fate specification and differentiation in the gut epithelium. From worms to flies to mice. In: Johnson LR, editor, Physiology of the Gastrointestinal Tract. 3rd edn., New York: Raven Press. 1994:521–68.
3. Zweibaum A, Laburthe M, Grasset E, Louvard D. The use of cultured cell lines in studies of intestinal cell differentiation and function. In: Frizell R, Fields H, editors, Handbook of physiology: The gastro-intestinal system IV. New York: Alan Liss, 1991;7:223–55.
4. Timpl R, Brown JC. Supramolecular assembly of basement membranes. Bioessays. 1996;18: 123–32.
5. Simon-Assmann P, Duclos B, Orian-Rousseau V et al. Differential expression of laminin isoforms and $\alpha6$-$\beta4$ integrin subunits in the developing human and mouse intestine. Dev Dynam. 1994;201:71–85.
6. Beaulieu JF, Vachon PH. Reciprocal expression of laminin A-chain isoforms along the crypt-villus axis in the human small intestine. Gastroenterology. 1994;106:829–39.
7. Orian-Rousseau V, Aberdam D, Fontao L et al. Developmental expression of laminin-5 and HD1 in the intestine. Epithelial to mesenchymal shift for the laminin $\gamma2$ chain subunit deposition. Dev Dynam. 1996;206:12–23.
8. Beaulieu JF, Vachon PH, Herring-Gillam FE et al. Expression of the $\alpha5$ (IV) collagen chain in the fetal human small intestine. Gastroenterology. 1994;107:957–67.
9. Simo P, Simon-Assmann P, Bouziges F et al. Changes in the expression of laminin during intestinal development. Development. 1991;112:477–87.
10. Haffen K, Kedinger M, Simon-Assmann P. Cell contact dependent regulation of enterocytic differentiation. In: Lebenthal E, editor, Human Gastrointestinal Development. New York: Raven Press. 1989:19–39.
11. Yasugi S. Role of epithelial-mesenchymal interactions in differentiation of epithelium of vertebrate digestive organs. Dev Growth Diff. 1993;35:1–9.
12. Kedinger M, Simon PM, Grenier JF, Haffen K. Role of epithelial–mesenchymal interactions in the ontogenesis of intestinal brush border enzymes. Dev Biol. 1981;86:339–47.
13. Duluc I, Freund JN, Leberquier C, Kedinger M. Fetal endoderm primarily holds the temporal and positional information required for mammalian intestinal development. J Cell Biol. 1994;126: 211–21.
14. Kedinger M, Simon-Assmann P, Alexandre E, Haffen K. Importance of a fibroblastic support for in vitro differentiation of intestinal endodermal cells and for their response to glucocorticoids. Cell Diff. 1987;20:171–82.

15. Takiguchi-Hayashi K, Yasugi S. Transfilter analysis of the inductive influence of proventricular mesenchyme on stomach epithelial differentiation of chick embryos. Roux Arch Dev Biol. 1990; 198:460–6.

16. Simon-Assmann P, Bouziges F, Arnold C, Haffen K, Kedinger M. Epithelial–mesenchymal interactions in the production of basement membrane components in the gut. Development. 1988; 102:339–47.

17. Simon-Assmann PM, Kedinger M, De Arcangelis A, Orian-Rousseau V, Simo P. Extracellular matrix components in intestinal development. Experientia. 1995;51:883–900.

18. Kedinger M, Simon-Assmann PM, Lacroix B, Marxer A, Hauri HP, Haffen K. Fetal gut mesenchyme induces differentiation of cultured intestinal endoderm and crypt cells. Dev Biol. 1986; 113:474–83.

19. Kedinger M, Simon-Assmann P, Bouziges F, Arnold C, Alexandre E, Haffen K. Smooth muscle actin expression during rat gut development and induction in fetal skin fibroblastic cells associated with intestinal embryonic epithelium. Differentiation. 1990;43:87–97.

20. Foltzer-Jourdainne C, Kedinger M, Raul F. Perinatal expression of brush border hydrolases in rat colon: hormonal and tissue regulations. Am J Physiol. 1989;257:G496–503.

21. Quaroni A, Wands J, Trelstad RL, Isselbacher KJ. Epithelioid cell cultures from rat small intestine characterization by morphologic and immunologic criteria. J Cell Biol. 1979;80:248–65.

22. Haffen K, Kedinger M, Simon-Assmann P. Mesenchyme-dependent differentiation of epithelial progenitor cells in the gut. J Pediatr Gastroenterol Nutr. 1987;6:14–23.

23. Valentich JD, Powell DW. Intestinal subepithelial myofibroblasts and mucosal immunophysiology. Curr Opin Gastroenterol. 1994;10:645–51.

24. Simo P, Bouziges F, Lissitzky JC, Sorokin L, Kedinger M, Simon-Assmann P. Dual and asynchronous deposition of laminin chains at the epithelial-mesenchymal interface in the gut. Gastroenterology. 1992;102:1835–45.

25. Goyal A, Grapperhaus KJ, Swietlicki E, Rubin DC. Characterization of rat intestinal epimorphin expression suggests a role in crypt-villus morphogenesis. Gastroenterology. 1995;108(suppl):A727.

26. Mitsiadis TA, Salmivirta M, Muramatsu T et al. Expression of the heparan-binding cytokines, midkine (MK) and HB-GAM (pleiotrophin) is associated with epithelial–mesenchymal interactions during fetal development and organogenesis. Development. 1995;121:37–51.

27. Sonnenberg E, Meyer D, Weidner KM, Birchmeier C. Scatter factor/hepatocyte growth factor and its receptor, the c-met tyrosine kinase, can mediate a signal exchange between mesenchyme and epithelia during mouse development. J Cell Biol. 1993;123:223–35.

28. Crepaldi T, Pollack AL, Prat M, Zborek A, Mostov K, Comoglio PM. Targeting of the SF/HGF receptor to the basolateral domain of polarized epithelial cells. J Cell Biol. 1994;125:313–20.

29. Simo P, Simon-Assmann P, Arnold C, Kedinger M. Mesenchyme-mediated effect of dexamethasone on laminin in co-cultures of embryonic gut epithelial cells and mesenchyme-derived cells. J Cell Sci. 1992;101:161–71.

30. Plateroti M, Freund J-N, Leberquier C, Kedinger M. Mesenchyme-mediated effects of retinoic acid during rat intestinal development. J Cell Sci. 1997;110:in press.

31. Danielpour D. Induction of transforming growth factor-beta autocrine activity by all-transretinoic acid and 1 alpha,25-dihydroxyvitamin D3 in NRP-152 rat prostatic epithelial cells. J Cell Physiol. 1996;166:231–9.

32. Desmoulière A. Factors influencing myofibroblast differentiation during wound healing and fibrosis. Cell Biol Int. 1995;19:471–6.

33. Fritsch C, Simon-Assmann P, Kedinger M, Evans GS. Cytokines modulate fibroblast phenotype and epithelial-stroma interactions in rat intestine. Gastroenterology. 1997;112:826–838.

34. Bouziges F, Simo P, Simon-Assmann P, Haffen K, Kedinger M. Altered deposition of basement-membrane molecules in co-cultures of colonic cancer cells and fibroblasts. Int J Cancer. 1991;48: 101–8.

35. De Arcangelis A, Simo P, Lesuffleur T, Kedinger M. L'expression de la laminine est corréleé à la différenciation des cellules cancéreuses coliques humaines. Gastroenterol Clin Biol. 1994;18: 630–7.

36. De Arcangelis A, Neuville P, Boukamel R, Lefebvre O, Kedinger M, Simon-Assmann P. Inhibition of laminin α1 chain expression leads to alteration of basement membrane assembly and cell differentiation. J Cell Biol. 1996;133:417–30.

37. Vachon PH, Beaulieu JF. Extracellular heterotrimeric laminin promotes differentiation in human enterocytes. Am J Physiol. 1995;268:G857–67.

38. Traber PG, Silberg DG. Intestine-specific gene transcription. Annu Rev Physiol. 1996;58: 275–97.
39. Duluc I, Lorentz O, Leberquier C, Kedinger M, Freund J-N. Homeogene expression during intestinal development and in a model of epithelial cell heterodifferentiation. J Cell Sci. 1997;in press.
40. Lorentz O, Duluc I, De Arcangelis A, Simon-Assmann P, Kedinger M, Freund J-N. Key role of the *Cdx2* homeobox gene in the extracellular matrix-mediated intestinal cell differentation. J Cell Biol. 1997;in revision.
41. Kedinger M, Fritsch C, Evans GS *et al*. Role of stromal-epithelial cell interactions and of basement membrane molecules in the onset and maintenance of epithelial integrity. In: Kagnoff MF, Kiyono H, editors, Essentials of Mucosal Immunology. London: Academic Press, 1996: 111–23.

14
The role of the non-integrin 67 kDa laminin receptor in enterocyte proliferation, adhesion and motility

M. M. WEISER, D. E. SYKES, J. J. PISCATELLI and M. RAO

INTRODUCTION

The intestine is characterized by rapid proliferation and differentiation of its epithelial cell, the enterocyte, as it moves on a relatively stable basement membrane[1,2] to its apoptotic end at the villus tip. There is much evidence, particularly from tissue culture studies, that the components of the basement membrane, particularly laminin[3–5], serve as growth factors in addition to any scaffolding function[6–9]. In normal morphogenesis and epithelial cell differentiation during development, data have shown that mesenchymal derived cells similar to myofibroblasts are responsible for most basement membrane synthesis, but the stimulus for synthesis is induced by the presence of endodermally derived epithelial cells[10,11]. Postnatally, myofibroblasts beneath the intestinal basement membrane, and not epithelial cells, were shown to be the principal cells synthesizing collagen IV and laminin[2,12], presumably to maintain basement membrane structure and to extend the basement membrane as needed physiologically. Thus, in the post-development state the growth factor and differentiation-stimulating properties of the intestinal basement membrane relate more to dynamic cell surface interactions with an existing stable basement than to any structural changes or resynthesis of basement membrane components themselves. Crypt-villus differences have been reported in the structure of laminin[13,14], a complex protein (M_r 800000) made up of three genetically distinct polypeptide chains. In the intestine two different types of laminin have been described, one dominant in the crypts and the other under villus cells[13], but the turnover of intestinal laminin is in terms of weeks[15] in contrast to the 48–72 h lifespan of enterocytes. Sensing an appropriately structured basement membrane to which it may adhere and move, may be the major signal for the enterocyte to proceed with its genetically programmed rate of proliferation and distinct pathway of differentiation. It is true that laminin possesses epidermal growth factor (EGF)-like repeats and other necessary peptide signal sites to induce mitogenesis[16–18] but separation of these growth-stimulating amino acid sequences from cell adhesive sites has been difficult. Since epithelial cell mitogenesis, proliferation and differentiation are most assuredly intertwined with cell adhesion and cell motility, complete molecular characterization of the latter processes may not be possible without concomitantly studying how they interrelate with each other and cell growth.

The process of cell movement must, therefore, also entail cell adhesion, and both may be due to multiple plasma membrane constituents. Although these may include glycolipids[19] and the underlying cytoskeleton[20], the specificity and dynamics of the processes probably reside in plasma membrane proteins[21]. The cell that may be a model for studying the complicated properties and requirements in integrating cell movement with cell adhesion within a fixed tissue framework is the enterocyte. The enterocyte is a highly polarized cell characterized by three specialized domains of its plasma membrane, an environmentally exposed microvillus membrane, a lateral domain characterized by tight junctions, gap junctions and desmosomes[22,23] and a basal domain, defined as the zone of adherence to basement membrane. Since the enterocyte must move almost continuously during its short life and still maintain adherence to basement membrane, the basal domain must be dynamic, either in its formation (like a moving belt), or in its protein turnover. Ultramicroscopic observations of the enterocyte have revealed a clustering of the cytoskeleton actin at the basal domain of its plasma membrane[24,25], a finding more suggestive of cytoskeletal-mediated protein movement (and turnover) to account for cell movement.

If we assume, as evidence would indicate, that enterocyte adherence and motility involve binding to laminin, then two classes of laminin-binding proteins have been identified in the plasma membrane of enterocytes, integrins and non-integrins, one of the latter being the 67 kDa laminin receptor (LR)[26–28]. Originally, integrins were seen as fibronectin receptors[29], although the original observation described laminin binding[30]. At least 16 different integrins have been identified[31,32], each made up of one α and one β subunit from among 11 α and six β varieties of subunits. Integrins bind laminin partly through the RGD (arg-gly-asp) cell recognition site, but multiple sites have been invoked. Much recent work has concluded that integrin–laminin binding is a major molecular mechanism establishing cell adhesion to basement membrane. Beaulieu[33] has studied this interaction in the intestine and found differences in the amount and type of integrins along the crypt-villus axis of the human intestine. He discusses these findings in this symposium. Integrins have also been shown to effect cell movement in mouse fibroblasts when they bind fibronectin. This ligand-binding initiated integrin attachment to the retrograde moving cytoskeleton[34]. Thus, integrins are clearly important in cell motility as well as cell adhesion. However, there are non-integrin laminin-binding cell surface membrane proteins that also appear to effect cell adhesion and cell motility, perhaps in a relationship with integrins. The main subject of this chapter concerns the role of the non-integrin 67 kDa laminin-binding cell surface receptor in intestinal cell adhesion and mobility.

INTESTINAL 67 kDA LR

Malinoff and Wicha[27] used laminin affinity chromatography to isolate a high affinity ($Kd = 2 \times 10^{-9}$ M) laminin receptor of ~69 kDa from the cell surface of

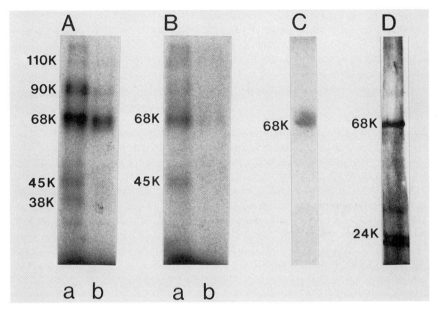

Figure 1 Identification of intestinal laminin-binding proteins. (A,B) Cell surface membrane proteins capable of binding to laminin affinity columns. The cell surface of intact isolated villus (A) and crypt cells (B) were subjected to lactoperoxidase-catalysed radioiodination. Crude plasma membrane fractions isolated by differential centrifugation were then put through laminin–Sepharose affinity columns and eluted proteins separated by SDS–PAGE. After transfer to nitrocellulose, the proteins purified by laminin affinity chromatography were detected by autoradiography. (a) [125I]-labelled proteins eluted with 0.05 M NaCl, followed by (b) with 1.0 M NaCl. (C) Villus cell membrane proteins that bind [125I]laminin. Cell membrane proteins were separated by SDS–PAGE, transferred to nitrocellulose, incubated with [125I]laminin and proteins binding laminin detected by autoradiography. (D) Membrane proteins purified by CDPGYIGSR (a laminin peptide) affinity chromatography. The eluted proteins were separated by SDS-PAGE and detected by silver stain. See Ref. 26 for detailed methods

murine fibrosarcoma cells. A similar protein was isolated from human carcinoma cells[28,35], rat Sertoli cells[36], inflammatory macrophages[37] and neural cells[38]. Earlier studies suggested that the peptide YIGSR on the β-1 chain of laminin was the binding site for LR: peptides containing this amino acid sequence could inhibit cell adhesion to laminin[39,40] and affinity columns of this peptide could be used to purify LR[26,41]. Earlier work from our laboratory used laminin affinity chromatography to isolate laminin-binding proteins from the plasma membrane of rat enterocytes (Figure 1)[26]. Laminin binding proteins ranged from 38 to 110 kDa (Figure 1A,B) in both villus and crypt cell plasma membranes, the higher molecular weight compounds being compatible with integrins. However, the most abundant laminin binding protein was at 67 kDa and this was particularly seen when plasma membrane proteins were first separated by SDS–PAGE, transferred to nitrocellulose and probed with [125I]laminin (Figure 1C).

Furthermore, the 67 kDa protein was the major protein eluted from a YIGSR-affinity column (Figure 1D). Similar findings were observed for human intestine by Stallmach and Riecken[42]. Antibodies to the rat 67 kDa LR showed relative

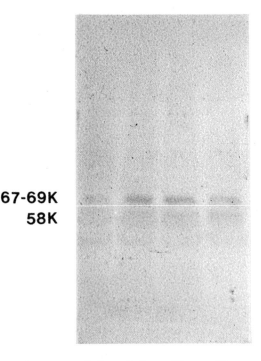

67-69K
58K

Vᴜ Vʟ Cᴜ Cʟ

Figure 2 Immunoblot detection of the 67kDa LR in villus and crypt cell membrane fractions. Detergent extracts of rat intestinal fractions (100 μg/lane) were separated by SDS–PAGE, blotted onto nitrocellulose and antigens identified using a rabbit antibody made to the antigen identified in Figure 1D. Lanes contained membrane proteins from cells of the upper villus (V_U), lower villus (V_L), upper crypt (C_U), and lower crypt (C_L)

abundance of the LR in upper crypt and over the lower half of the villus (Figure 2). Although the LR was originally reported as being localized immunohisto-chemically to rat intestine crypt basal membrane[26], we had great difficulty repeating these data. In human intestines, Stallmach and Rieken[42] found sparse immuno-fluorescence in the crypt and almost none in the villus cells; intestine from a patient with coeliac disease showed abundant immunofluorescence in 'hyper-regenerative' areas. These immunohistochemical findings seemed contradictory to the abundance of this protein found in the plasma membrane of crypt and villus cells, as illustrated in Figures 1 and 2. Our next approach was to determine whether its rate of synthesis would help explain these findings.

Having developed a rat intestinal crypt cell library to isolate crypt-specific genes[43], we used this library to clone the rat LR using a 27-mer oligonucleotide homologous to reported sequences of human, rat and mouse LR[44]. Sequence

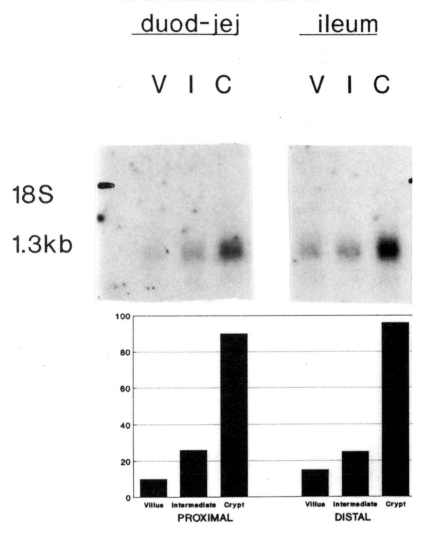

Figure 3 Detection of the 33/67 kDa LR mRNA in rat enterocytes. The cDNA probe for the LR was prepared from a crypt cell library[45]. Each lane contains 10 μg of total RNA extracted from isolated cells obtained as fractions representative of the gradient from crypt to villus of a rat intestine. Equal loading was monitored by hybridization with a cDNA to 28S RNA. The graph below represents densitometry determinations as an estimate of the relative abundance. For more detailed methods see Ref. 45

analysis of the isolated probe showed 96% identity with rat and 87% with mouse and human[45]. Steady-state content of the mRNA detected by this probe showed a 10-fold greater abundance in total RNA extracted from crypt cells than from villus cells (Figure 3). This was confirmed by in situ hybridization. Abundant levels of LR-mRNA were also seen in F9 teratocarcinoma cells, rat fetal liver and intestine[45]. In IEC6 cells, a cell line derived from normal adult rat crypt

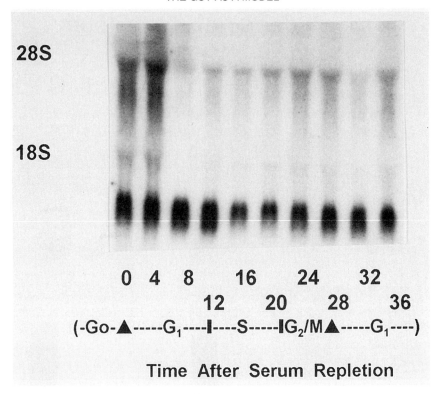

28S

18S

0　4　8　　16　　24　　32

12　　20　　28　　36

(-Go-▲-----G₁----I----S-----IG₂/M▲-----G₁----)

Time After Serum Repletion

Figure 4 Detection of the 33/67 kDa LR mRNA in IEC cells. The LR mRNA was detected at abundant levels in IEC-6 cells, a rat intestinal cell line derived from normal rat crypt cells. Shown are IEC-6 cells which have had their cell cycle synchronized by serum starvation. For details of the methods, see Ref. 83. A decrease in message levels was seen during S-phase where DNA replication is the primary function, and higher levels seemed best maintained during G_1, the phase of the cell cycle when protein synthesis is increased in preparation for DNA replication. This finding would be compatible with the need for new ribosomal proteins like the 32–40 kDa protein precursor of 67 kDa LR

cells[46], the mRNA was abundant but tended to decrease in the S-phase of the cell cycle (Figure 4). These findings would appear to support the reported immuno-histochemical findings for the protein's location in crypt or proliferative cells. The problem, however, was that the size of the transcript, 1–1.3 kb, was too small to produce a protein of 67 kDa. This had been a persistent contradiction in work on the 67 kDa LR. The human[47,48] and mouse[44] cDNAs detected mRNAs of, at most, 1400 bases long, more compatible with proteins of 33–40 kDa size. Even more confusing was the reported homology with a 33–40 kDa cytoplasmic protein(s) thought to be involved in translation and associated with tumour development[49,50].

The 67 kDa LR IN CANCER AND METASTASIS

Interest in the 67 kDa laminin receptor had been initially heightened by reports that this protein was over-expressed in cancer and associated with the metastatic

1.2-1.4kb

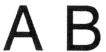

A B

Figure 5 Increased levels of the 33/67 kDa LR mRNA in cells with increased metastatic potential. The animal model used for studies on metastasis was a murine colon cancer cell line (MCA-38) that is capable of metastasizing to the liver from peripheral injection sites, including the caecal wall[56]. When metastatic MCA-38 cells were subsequently cultured on plastic (A), they lost their ability to metastasize. Those cells capable of metastasis (B) showed higher levels of LR mRNA

process. A monoclonal antibody to this LR showed the protein to be present in normal epithelial cell types but increased in human mammary and colon cancers[51]. The receptor was shown to be localized to the cell surface of metastatic carcinoma cells[52]. A parallel between the level of the 67 kDa LR in human colorectal cancer (1.5–5-fold higher than normal cells) and the level of its mRNA, as judged from in situ hybridization studies, was also shown. Blot hybridization studies of human colon cancer showed mRNA levels to correlate statistically with Dukes' classification[53]. In work from Kleinman's laboratory, a human colon cancer cell line which forms subcutaneous tumours in nude mice at the site of injection was divided into laminin-adherent and laminin non-adherent stable subpopulations after subculturing through 26 passages. The laminin-adherent cell type formed tumours that were less differentiated, as judged histologically[54]. Earlier work from the same laboratory had used laminin peptides to select B16-F10 melanoma cells and found that cells grown on YIGSR formed twice as many lung metastases[55]. It was suggested that LR binding to the YIGSR site on laminin was important to malignant potential. We have studied a murine colon cancer cell line that can metastasize to the liver from injection sites in the caecum[56]. If these cells are sub-cultured on plastic they lose their ability to metastasize. Those cells capable of metastasis show significantly higher levels of LR mRNA (Figure 5). YIGSR-containing peptides have been shown to inhibit angiogenesis by inhibiting endothelial cell migration[18]. When injected in vivo, a YIGSR peptide inhibited growth of Lewis lung cancer cells[18]. This was interpreted as an indirect effect on tumour growth secondary to inhibition of endothelial cell migration leading to decreased angiogenesis which is required for the growth of a metastatic nodule. The 67 kDa LR also appears to be important in tumour adhesion to endothelial matrix[57], where it may promote collagenolytic activity and cell migration thereby directly facilitating the metastatic process[58].

Studies highlighting the effects of the 67 kDa LR in tumour cell migration and metastasis strongly suggest that the 67 kDa LR may function normally in tissues where cell movement is required, as in the intestine. Cell movement requires cell adhesion to basement membrane components, spreading and formation of a migrating front as migration is initiated. In a study of endothelial cells, the 67 kDa LR was shown to be important in spreading and migration[59]. It was shown that in these processes the 67 kDa LR co-localizes with actin filaments[59]. A similar finding was recently shown for $\beta 1$ integrins, which are important in regulating cell movement[34]. Massia et al.[60] have further shown that immobilized YIGSR-containing peptides are required to demonstrate cell spreading and that the 67 kDa LR co-localized with cellular α-actin and vinculin. They conclude that while other plasma membrane laminin binding proteins are involved in the process of cell spreading, 'The major receptor necessary for mediating cell spreading via YIGSR is the 67-kDa protein, since it appears to be solely involved in clustering and cytoskeletal association.' More recent evidence also implicates integrins in this process in other cells[34]. Thus, evidence from experiments with normal cells, cancer cells and metastasis seemed to show that the 68 kDa LR is an important contributor to adhesion and mobility on a basement membrane. However, confusing and discordant findings need to be resolved before these observations can be given molecular relevance.

STRUCTURE AND SYNTHESIS OF THE 67 kDA LR

The 67 kDa LR has been an elusive protein with two major contradictory findings. First was the fact that an mRNA of a size capable of directing the synthesis of a 67 kDa protein has never been found. The LR mRNA appeared to be capable of synthesizing proteins of only 33–40 kDa. What was known of the amino acid structure of the 67 kDa protein was surmised from the nucleotide sequence of the cDNA. However, antibodies made to different peptides had revealed the presence of the 67 kDa LR as a plasma membrane-spanning protein[61], although there were no striking hydrophobic peptide sequences that could be characterized as membrane spanning. Second was the finding that 33–40 kDa proteins entirely homologous with the 67 kDa plasma membrane protein were identified as cytoplasmic[62], ribosomal-associated proteins similar to yeast mitochondrial ribosomal protein MRP4, and bacterial/chloroplast ribosomal S2 proteins[63]. The small 33–40 kDa proteins now appear to be represented in all cells, including plants[64]. They seem to be essential components of the 40S ribosomal subunit and form a family of ribosomal proteins that are acidic and appear to be critical to the control of translation. They are reported to be in two states, one free in the cytoplasm and the other bound to the polysome. They appear to hop on and off the ribosome, binding being required for translation to proceed[64–66]. In this regard they are similar to the acidic ribosomal phosphoproteins P0, P1, and P2 which form pentameric complexes with each other $(2P1 + P0 + 2P2)$ and then bind to the ribosome allowing translation to proceed. This process requires phosphorylation and dephosphorylation of the acidic ribosomal phosphoproteins[67]. Binding of the phosphorylated complex is to the GTPase domain of the 28S rRNA in the 60S subunit: this appears to effect elongation[67,68]. In contrast to the acidic ribosomal phosphoproteins P0, P1 and P2, the 33–40 kDa LR ribosomal protein is associated with the 40S subunit and in yeast appears to effect initiation rather than elongation[65]. It is of interest that we found the messages for the acidic ribosomal phosphoproteins P0, P1, and P2 to be highly expressed in crypt cells, similar to our findings with the LR mRNA[69].

A precursor–product relationship between the 33–40 kDa ribosomal-associated protein and the 67 kDa laminin receptor had been suggested originally by Rao et al.[44] in studies characterizing its mRNA. In an in vitro rabbit reticulo-cyte cell-free translation system using total RNA from a human pancreatic cancer cell line, the only product immunoprecipitated was a 37 kDa protein. In a similar system using mRNA specifically eluted from immobilized LRcDNA, a protein of only 37 kDa was synthesized. They concluded that the 37 kDa protein was a precursor of the 67 kDa LR, although they never showed any synthesis of a 67 kDa protein. Furthermore, Costronovo et al.[70], in pulse–chase experiments showed that the 37 kDa protein appeared first, well before any 67 kDa protein was detected. In transfection experiments with the 'full length' 37 kDa LRcDNA, only the 37 kDa protein was made. The appearance of both 37 and 67 kDa proteins required protein synthesis[71]. These data led to the suggestion that the 67 kDa protein resulted from a post-translational modification of the 37 kDa precursor which did not involve the addition of dramatically different amino acid sequences. Data recently reported suggest that the 67 kDa protein was a homodimer of the 33 kDa precursor[66]: that is, two precursor proteins are covalently linked, pre-sumably by a transpeptidation reaction, to form a homodimer. In addition, the 67 kDa protein has been shown to contain fatty acids (palmitate, stearate and oleate were extracted and isolated) acylated at four sites to the protein, making it more hydrophobic[66] and, therefore, more likely to be associated with membranes rather than cytoplasm. Figure 6 is a cartoon representation of this structure. The enzyme(s) responsible for the formation of the homodimer, the enzyme's specificity or the factors that would initiate the formation of the homodimer have not been defined. Since growth on laminin-containing matrices stimulates the formation of the 67 kDa protein and its appearance in the plasma membrane[71], it seems reasonable to assume that laminin, in some cells, is an inducer of 67 kDa synthesis. However, that induction may require internal monitoring related to the cell's state of differentiation and motility requirements.

The precise binding sites of the 33 or 67 kDa proteins to laminin have been debated. A 20 amino acid peptide, peptide G, was shown to have a high affinity for laminin[61] and peptide G-treated B16BL6 melanoma cells 'resulted in a two- to 10-fold significant increase in the number of...lung metastases.'[57] Others attributed the binding of peptide G to its high affinity for heparin, known to be bound to the globular portion of laminin A[72], and therefore non-specific. That is, LR binding to basement membrane may be related to non-specific associations to glycosaminoglycans in the basement membrane or to heparin intimately associated with the globular end of the A-chain of laminin. Heparin bound to laminin has been proposed to modulate the complex assembly of laminins and/or to alter the affinities of laminin to various laminin binding proteins[73,75]. Demianova et al.[65] have suggested that part of the binding of LR to laminin is to the heparin

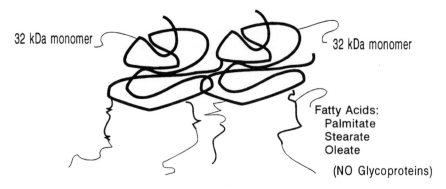

32 kDa monomer

32 kDa monomer

Fatty Acids:
Palmitate
Stearate
Oleate

(NO Glycoproteins)

32 kDa + 32 kDa + Fatty Acids = 67 kD HOMODIMER

Figure 6 Cartoon representation of the 67 kDa LR protein. This illustration is based on data reported by Landowski *et al.*[66]. They transfected hamster CHO cells with a hamster cDNA to LR and with methotrexate amplification, the transfected cells produced ample LR protein for structural analysis. The protein was purified by laminin affinity chromatography. SDS-PAGE showed only a 67 kDa protein. By mass spectra analysis the molecular weight was $66.7 \pm 0.2\%$ kDa. No disulphide binding was found and the amino acid composition was very close to that previously determined for the 32 kDa protein. Three types of fatty acids were found covalently attached: palmitate, stearate and oleate. They proposed that the 67 kDa LR was a homodimer of the 32 kDa protein monomer. The nature of the bond uniting the monomers is unknown but thought to be a peptide bond formed post-translationally. It was shown that high affinity binding of the 67 kDa LR to laminin required the presence of a detergent-soluble membrane factor

– laminin complex at the globular end of laminin A chain through a nucleic acid binding site suspected to be intrinsic to the function of the 33–40 kDa monomeric ribosomal protein. When purified laminin and 67 kDa LR were mixed, images of the mixture, viewed by rotary shadowing, showed the vast majority of LR to be bound to laminin at the intersection where the B2 chain curves to join the A-chain (see Figure 7)[76], an area on the A-chain far from the globular end. Since this study used purified laminin in which heparin would have been removed, it does not exclude the heparin–laminin site for LR binding. The importance of the high affinity binding to the YIGSR site on the B1 chain is also not excluded since LR, on purification by laminin or YIGSR affinity chromatography, loses its high affinity for laminin. In a pivotal study on LR structure, Landowski et al.[66] showed that the ability of purified LR to bind to laminin could be restored by the addition of two of the original wash fractions representing detergent extracts of cell membrane. They postulate that the high-affinity binding of LR to laminin may require or be 'modulated by an, as yet, unidentified factor…' If LR is more involved with cell movement, then a factor(s) lost when LR becomes bound to laminin (or lost when LR is released from laminin) may be critical to the mechanism of cell movement. One may postulate that the loss of this factor from the LR bound to laminin decreases the binding affinity of the LR to laminin and renders LR at the old site of attachment impotent to re-bind laminin. This would allow newly constituted LRs at the forward moving site to bind to laminin, enhancing cell spreading and forming a dynamic migrating front. Changes in LR binding to laminin may

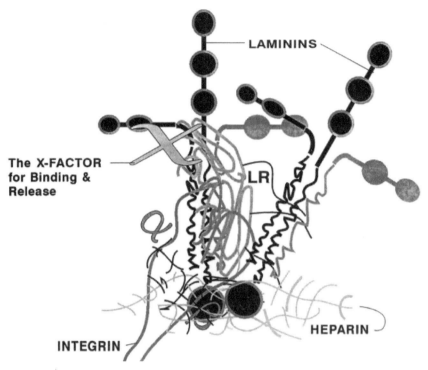

Figure 7 Cartoon illustrating possible binding relationships of LR to laminin. It is proposed that the LR, in conjunction with integrin, binds to a number of sites on laminin. The affinity of LR for laminin is dependent on a detergent-soluble, plasma membrane associated factor. It was this property, whereby binding affinities may be altered, that suggested to Landowski *et al.*[66], that the 67 kDa protein may be particularly suitable for cell mobility. Part of the integrin chains, particularly the β1 chain, spans the plasma membrane and can bind actin in the cytoskeleton[34]. The inter-relationships among the proteins that bind laminin to effect each other's affinity to laminin plus specific enzymes (protein kinases, proteases, etc.) would allow for controlled cell motility

also affect integrin affinities to laminin or to integrin binding to actin of the cytoskeleton[34]. The other laminin binding sites that have been demonstrated, including those with integrins[34,77,78], may all contribute to the flexibility required of proteins constantly altering their interactions with the cytoskeleton and the basement membrane to produce controlled and vectorially directed cell movement as required for the enterocyte.

PROPOSAL

A fundamental question in cell biology is to define the inter-related molecular mechanisms of cell movement and cell adherence as required for optimum function of a particular cell type. A related question concerns the mechanisms by which a cell perceives the need to move in a particular direction and how this information is directed to achieve the desired result, efficiently. Different tissues have different requirements for cell mobility. At one extreme is the renal tubular cell or hepato-cyte where there is little to no mobility and cell–basement membrane adherence is of relative permanence. At the other extreme is the lymphocyte or neutrophil where cell mobility is almost a constant characteristic. Lymphocytes are required to initiate a vast array of recognition/adherence proteins related to specific functions and environment and to move in different tissues and on different matrix com-positions; tissue organization is not required and cell adherence is impermanent. In between is the intestinal enterocyte whose rapid cell proliferation in the crypts and constant differentiation is coupled to cell movement along a crypt to villus vectorial axis to enterocyte death at the villus tip. The enterocyte must have properties of cell–cell and cell–matrix adherence that are of relative imperma-nence, without loss of attachment since tissue organization must be maintained. This would require cell adherence and mobility to be characterized by a close cooperation of the two processes that may make it difficult to separate the two, particularly in adherence properties, and a mechanism for constantly changing the affinities to basement membrane to allow for attachment and release in an ordered, relatively smooth fashion.

It is rare, almost unscientific, to claim or argue that one molecular entity or protein is the sole agent for a biological function. Biological processes, perhaps more so than for non-biological phenomena, are summations of a dizzying array of events, controls, adaptations, and counter-adaptations. We would simply propose that the 67 kDa laminin receptor is a unique cell adhesion/motility factor in that its synthesis depends on a post-translational transpeptidation reaction to form a homodimer from an abundant acidic ribosomal protein. This synthetic pathway would be more responsive since it does not have to wait for signals to be trans-mitted to the nucleus to induce transcription and/or to await translation into a protein that has to be transmitted to the cell surface. Cell surface signals calling for more cell adhesion/motility factors need to be answered in a way that allows for a more rapid and variable response required for modulating cell motility appro-priate to the dynamic circumstances a cell constantly experiences. Applied to the intestine, our data suggest that few LR messages are transcribed by the mature enterocyte. Thus, one must postulate that there is sufficient excess of the 32–40 kDa acidic ribosomal protein to serve both functions and/or that the process of cell mobility requires the reactivation and reuse of the 67 kDa LR, possibly by rerouting it back into the cell. It would be unlikely and wasteful if it were to be shed by the normal enterocyte, as has been shown for human cancer cells in a tissue culture system[79]. (This shedding, however, may be important to metastasis if it can be shown that cancer cells, in situ, shed the 67 kDa LR.) Our finding of decreased levels of the 67 kDa LR in villus tip cells is compatible with the increase of apoptotic cells at the villus tip with their consequent decrease in adhesive strength and mobility. However, there are cells at the villus tip still capable of repairing injury by spreading to cover a wound[80–82]; do these cells have an increase of the 67 kDa protein at the cell surface?

In summary, we have reviewed the data that implicate the 67 kDa LR as an important laminin-binding protein on the cell surface of many cell types, including the intestinal enterocyte. Confusion regarding the relationship of the 67 kD LR with an acidic ribosomal protein of 33–40 kDa has been clarified by a report showing that the 67 kDa LR is formed post-translationally, probably enzymatically, by the transpeptidation of two 33–40 kDa ribosomal proteins to make a fatty acid acylated homodimer. Evidence is reviewed that indicates that the 67 kDa LR for laminin depends on still other factors yet to be defined. It is proposed that the 67 kDa LR, working in concert with integrins and other cell adhesive forces, is more critical to cell spreading and motility than to cell adhesion. This concept may be particularly applicable to the enterocyte as it progresses through its life-cycle moving from crypt to villus tip in 3 to 5 days.

References

1. Potten CS, Loeffler M. A comprehensive model of the crypts of the small intestine of the mouse provides insight into the mechanisms of cell migration and the proliferation hierarchy. J Theor Biol. 1987;127:381–91.
2. Weiser MM, Sykes DE, Killen PD. Rat intestinal basement membrane synthesis, epithelial vs non-epithelial contribution. Lab Invest. 1990;62:325–30.
3. Panayotou G, End P, Aumailley M, Timpl R, Engel J. Domains of laminin with growth-factor activity. Cell. 1989;56:93–101.
4. Grant DS, Tashiro K, Segui-Real B, Yamada Y, Martin GR, Kleinman HK. Two different laminin domains mediate the differentiation of human endothelial cells into capillary-like structures in vitro. Cell. 1989;58:933–43.
5. Tashiro K, Sechel GC, Weeks B et al. A synthetic peptide containing the IKVAV sequence from the A chain of laminin mediates cell attachment, migration, and neurite outgrowth. J Biol Chem. 1989;264:16174–82.
6. Haffen KM, Kedinger MK, Simon-Assmann P. Mesenchyme-dependent differentiation of epithelial progenitor cells in the gut. J Pediatr Gastroenterol Nutr. 1987;6:14–23.
7. Helaakoski T, Pajunen L, Kivirikko KI, Pihlajaniemi T. Increase in mRNA concentrations of the α and β subunits of prolyl 4-hydroxylase accompany increased gene expression of type IV collagen during differentiation of mouse F9 cells. J Biol Chem. 1990;265:11413–16.
8. Gatmaitan Z, Jefferson DM, Ruiz-Opazo N et al. Regulation of growth and differentiation of a rat hepatoma cell line by the synergistic interactions of hormones and collagenous substrata. J Cell Biol. 1983;97:1179–90.
9. Wicha MS, Lowrie G, Kohn E, Bagavandoss P, Mahn T. Extracellular matrix promotes mammary epithelial growth and differentiation in vitro. Proc Natl Acad Sci USA. 1982;79:3213–17.
10. Simon-Assmann P, Bouziges F, Arnold C, Haffen K, Kedinger M. Epithelial-mesenchymal inter-actions in the production of basement membrane components in the gut. Development. 1988; 102:339–47.
11. Simon-Assmann P, Bouziges F, Freund JN, Perrin-Schmitt F, Kedinger M. Type IV collagen mRNA accumulates in the mesenchymal compartment at early stages of murine developing intestine. J Cell Biol. 1990;110:849–57.
12. Weiser MM, Ryzowicz S, Soroka CJ, Albini B. In vitro translation of rat intestinal RNA prepared from isolated villus and crypt cells and from the epithelium-denuded intestine. Synthesis of intestinal basement membrane. Trans Assoc Am Phys. 1987;100:316–28.
13. Beaulieu J, Vachon PH. Reciprocal expression of laminin A-chain isoforms along the crypt-villus axis in the human small intestine. Gastroenterology. 1994;106:829–39.
14. Perreault N, Vachon PH, Beaulieu J. Appearance and distribution of laminin A chain isoforms and integrin alpha 2, alpha 3, alpha 6, beta 1, and beta 4 subunits in the developing human small intestinal mucosa. Anat Rec. 1995;242:242–50.
15. Trier JS, Allan CH, Abrahamson DR, Hagen SJ. Epithelial basement membrane of mouse jejunum. Evidence for laminin turnover along the entire crypt-villus axis. J Clin Invest. 1990;86:87–95.
16. Goodman SL, Deutzmann R, von der Mark K. Two distinct cell-binding domains in laminin can independently promote nonneuronal cell adhesion and spreading. J Cell Biol. 1987;105:589–98.
17. Hall DE, Reichardt LF, Crowley E et al. The α_1/β_1 and α_6/β_1 integrin heterodimers mediate cell attachment to distinct sites on laminin. J Cell Biol. 1990;110:2175–84.
18. Sakamoto N, Iwahana M, Tanaka NG, Osada Y. Inhibition of angiogenesis and tumor growth by a synthetic laminin peptide. Cancer Res. 1991;51:903–6.

19. Sariola H, Aufderheide E, Bernhard H, Henke-Fahle S, Dippold W, Ekblom P. Antibodies to cell surface ganglioside G_{q3} perturb inductive epithelial-mesenchymal interactions. Cell. 1988;54: 235–45.
20. Shaw LM, Messier JM, Mercurio AM. The activation dependent adhesion of macrophages to laminin involves cytoskeletal anchoring and phosphorylation of the $\alpha_6\beta_1$ integrin. J Cell Biol. 1990;110:2167–74.
21. Mecham RP. Laminin receptors. In: Palade GE, Alberts BM, Spudich JA, editors. Annual review of cell biology. 7th edn. Palo Alto: Annual Reviews Inc. 1991:71–91.
22. Boller K, Vestweber D, Kemler R. Cell adhesion molecule uvomorulin is localized in the intermediate junctions of adult intestinal epithelial cells. J Cell Biol. 1985;100:327–32.
23. Madara JL. Loosening tight junctions. Lessons from the intestine. J Clin Invest. 1989;83:1089–94.
24. Drenckhahn D, Groschel-Stewart U. Localization of myosin, actin, and tropomyosin in rat intestinal epithelium: immunohistochemical studies at the light and electron microscope levels. J Cell Biol. 1980;86:475–82.
25. Hagen SJ, Trier JS. Immuncytochemical localization of actin in epithelial cells of rat small intestine by light and electron microscopy. J Histochem Cytochem. 1988;36:717–27.
26. Wilson JR, Weiser MM. Rat small intestinal laminin-binding proteins. Digestion. 1990;46: 22–30.
27. Malinoff HL, Wicha MS. Isolation of a cell surface receptor protein for laminin from murine fibrosarcoma cells. J Cell Biol. 1983;96:1475–9.
28. Terranova VP, Rao CN, Kalebic T, Margulies IM, Liotta LA. Tumor receptor on human breast carcinoma cells. Proc Natl Acad Sci USA. 1983;80:444–8.
29. Ruoslahti E. Fibronectin and its receptors. In: Richardson CC, Boyer PD, Dawid IB, Meister A, editors. Annual review of biochemistry. 57th edn. Palo Alto: Annual Reviews Inc. 1988:375–413.
30. Horwitz A, Duggan K, Greggs R, Decker C, Buck C. The cell substrate attachment (CSAT) antigen has properties of a receptor for laminin and fibronectin. J Cell Biol. 1985;101:2134–44.
31. Ruoslahti E. Integrins. Cell. 1991;87:1–5.
32. Albelda SM, Buck CA. Integrins and other cell adhesion molecules. FASEB J. 1990; 4:2868–80.
33. Beaulieu J. Differential expression of the VLA family of integrins along the crypt-villus axis in the human small intestine. J Cell Sci. 1992;102:427–36.
34. Felsenfeld DP, Choquet D, Sheetz MP. Ligand binding regulates the directed movement of β1 integrins on fibroblasts. Nature. 1996;383:438–40.
35. Rao CN, Barsky SH, Terranova VP, Liotta LA. Isolation of a tumor cell laminin receptor. Biochem Biophys Res Commun. 1983;111:804–8.
36. Davis CM, Papadopoulos V, Jia MC, Yamada Y, Kleinman HK, Dym M. Identification and partial characterization of laminin binding proteins in immature rat sertoli cells. Exp Cell Res. 1991;193:262–73.
37. Huard TK, Malinoff HL, Wicha MS. Macrophages express a plasma membrane receptor for basement membrane laminin. Am J Pathol. 1986;123:365–70.
38. Douville PJ, Harvey WJ, Carbonetto S. Isolation and partial characterization of high affinity laminin receptors in neural cells. J Biol Chem. 1988;263:14964–9.
39. Graj J, Iwamoto Y, Saski M et al. Identification of an amino acid sequence in laminin mediating cell attachment, chemotaxis, and receptor binding. Cell. 1987;48:989–96.
40. Graf J, Ogle RC, Robey FA et al. A pentapeptide from the laminin B1 chain mediates cell adhesion and binds the 67,000 laminin receptor. Biochemistry. 1987;26:6896–900.
41. Bushkin-Harav I, Garty NB, Littauer UZ. Down-regulation of a 67-kDa YIGSR-binding protein upon differentiation of neuroblastoma cells. J Biol Chem. 1995;270:13422–8.
42. Stallmach A, Riecken EO. Laminin-cell binding proteins in small intestinal epithelial cells. Digestion. 1990;46:31–9.
43. Sykes DE, Weiser MM. The identification of genes specifically expressed in epithelial cells of the rat intestinal crypts. Differentiation. 1992;50:41–6.
44. Rao CN, Castronovo V, Schmitt MC et al. Evidence for a precursor of the high-affinity metastasis-associated murine laminin receptor. Biochemistry. 1989;28:7476–86.
45. Rao M, Manishen WJ, Maheshwari Y et al. Laminin receptor expression in rat intestine and liver during development and differentiation. Gastroenterology. 1994;107:764–72.
46. Quaroni A, May RJ. Establishment and characterization of intestinal epithelial cell cultures. Methods Cell Biol. 1980;21:403–27.
47. Wewer UM, Liotta LA, Jaye M et al. Altered levels of laminin receptor mRNA in various human

carcinoma cells that have different abilities to bind laminin. Proc Natl Acad Sci USA. 1986; 83:7137–41.

48. Yow H, Wong JM, Chen HS, Lee C, Steele GD Jr, Chen LB. Increased mRNA expression of a laminin-binding protein in human colon carcinoma: Complete sequence of a full-length cDNA encoding the protein. Proc Natl Acad Sci USA. 1988;85:6394–8.

49. Makrides S, Chitpatima ST, Bandyopadhyay R, Brawerman G. Nucleotide sequence for a major messenger RNA for a 40 kilodalton polypeptide that is under translational control in mouse tumor cells. Nucleic Acids Res. 1988;16:2349.

50. Auth D, Brawerman G. A 33-kDa polypeptide with homology to the laminin receptor: component of translation machinery. Proc Natl Acad Sci USA. 1992;89:4368–72.

51. Hand PH, Thor A, Schlom J, Liotta L. Expression of laminin receptor in normal and carcinomatous human tissues as determined by a monoclonal antibody. Cancer Res. 1985;45:2713–19.

52. Barsky SH, Rao CN, Hyams D, Liotta LA. Characterization of a laminin receptor from human breast carcinoma tissue. Breast Cancer Res Treat. 1984;4:181–8.

53. Mafune K, Ravikumar TS, Wong JM, Yow H, Chen LB, Steele GDJ. Expression of a Mr 32,000 laminin-binding protein messenger RNA in human colon carcinoma correlates with disease progression. Cancer Res. 1990;50:3888–91.

54. Jun SH, Thompson EW, Gottardis M et al. Laminin adhesion-selected primary human colon cancer cells are more tumorigenic than the parental and non adherent cells. Int J Oncol. 1994; 4:55–60.

55. Yamamura K, Kibbey MC, Kleinman HK. Melanoma cells selected for adhesion to laminin peptides have different malignant properties. Cancer Res. 1993;53:423–8.

56. Piscatelli JJ, Cohen SA, Berenson CS, Lance P. Determinants of differential liver-colonizing potential of variants of the MCA-38 murine colon cancer cell line. Clin Exp Metastasis. 1995; 13:141–50.

57. Taraboletti G, Belotti D, Giavazzi R, Sobel ME, Castronovo V. Enhancement of metastatic potential of murine and human melanoma cells by laminin receptor peptide G: Attachment of cancer cells to subendothelial matrix as a pathway for hematogenous metastasis. J Natl Cancer Inst. 1993;85:235–40.

58. Yudoh K, Matsui H, Kanamori M, Ohmori K, Tsuji H. Tumor cell attachment to laminin promotes degradation of the extracellular matrix and cell migration in high-metastatic clone cells of RCT sarcoma in vitro. Jpn J Cancer Res. 1995;86:685–90.

59. Yannariello-Brown J, Wewer UM, Liotta L, Madri JA. Distribution of a 69-kD laminin-binding protein in aortic and microvascular endothelial cells: modulation during cell attachment, spreading, and migration. J Cell Biol. 1988;106:1773–86.

60. Massia SP, Rao SS, Hubbell JA. Covalently immobilized laminin peptide Tyr-Ile-Gly-Ser-Arg (YIGSR) supports cell spreading and co-localization of the 67-kilodalton laminin receptor with a-actinin and vinculin. J Biol Chem. 1993;268:8053–9.

61. Castronovo V, Taraboletti G, Sobel ME. Functional domains of the 67-kDa laminin receptor precursor. J Biol Chem. 1991;266:20440–6.

62. Grosso LE, Park PW, Mecham RP. Characterization of a putative clone for the 67-kilodalton elastin/laminin receptor suggests that it encodes a cytoplasmic protein rather than a cell surface receptor. Biochemistry. 1991;30:3346–50.

63. Davis SC, Tzagoloff A, Ellis SR. Characterization of a yeast mitochondrial ribosomal protein structurally related to the mammalian 68-kDa high affinity laminin receptor. J Biol Chem. 1992; 267:5508–14.

64. García-Hernández M, Davies E, Staswick PE. Arabidopsis p40 homologue: a novel acidic protein associated with the 40 S subunit of ribosomes. J Biol Chem. 1994;269:20744–9.

65. Damianova M, Formosa TG, Ellis SR. Yeast proteins related to the p40/laminin receptor precursor are essential components of the 40 S ribosomal subunit. J Biol Chem. 1996;271:11383–91.

66. Landowski TH, Dratz EA, Starkey JR. Studies of the structure of the metastasis-associated 67 kDa laminin binding protein: fatty acid acylation and evidence supporting dimerization of the 32 kDa gene product to form the mature protein. Biochemistry. 1995;34:11276–87.

67. Rich BE, Steitz JA. Human acidic ribosomal phosphoproteins P0, P1 and P2: analysis of cDNA clones, in vitro synthesis, and assembly. Mol Cell Biol. 1987;7:4065–74.

68. Uchiumi T, Komonami R. Direct evidence for interaction of conserved GTP-ase domain with 28S RNA with mammalian ribosomal acidic phosphoprotein and L12. J Biol Chem. 1992;267: 19179–85.

69. Maheshwari Y, Rao M, Sykes DE, Tyner AL, Weiser MM. Changes in ribosomal protein and

ribosomal RNA synthesis during rat intestinal differentiation. Cell Growth Diff. 1993;4:745–52.

70. Castronovo V, Claysmith AP, Barker KT, Cioce V, Krutzsch HC, Sobel ME. Biosynthesis of the 67 kDa high affinity laminin receptor. Biochem Biophys Res Commun. 1991;177:177–83.

71. Romanov VI, Wrathall LS, Simmons TD, Pinto da Silva P, Sobel ME. Protein synthesis is required for laminin-induced expression of the 67-kDa laminin receptor and its 37-kDa precursors. Biochem Biophys Res Commun. 1995:208:637–43.

72. Guo N, Krutzsch HC, Vogel T, Roberts DD. Interactions of a laminin-binding peptide from a 33-kDa protein related to the 67-kDa laminin receptor with laminin and melanoma cells are heparin-dependent. J Biol Chem. 1992;267:17743–7.

73. Yurchenco PD, Cheng YS, Colognato H. Laminin forms an independent network in basement membrane. J Cell Biol. 1992;117:1119–33.

74. Sung U, O'Rear JJ, Yurchenco PD. Cell and heparin binding in the distal long arm of laminin: identification of active and cryptic sites with recombinant and hybrid glycoprotein. J Cell Biol. 1993;123:1255–68.

75. Yurchenco PD, Cheng Y, Schittny JC. Heparin modulation of laminin polymerization. J Biol Chem. 1990;265:3981–91.

76. Cioce V, Margulies IMK, Sobel ME, Castronovo V. Interaction between the 67 kilodalton metastasis-associated laminin receptor and laminin. Kidney Int. 1993;43:30–7.

77. Romanov V, Sobel ME, Pinto da Silva P, Menard S, Castronovo V. Cell localization and redistribution of the 67 kD laminin receptor and α6β1 integrin subunits in response to laminin stimulation: an immunogold electron microscopy study. Cell Adhesion Commun. 1994;2:201–9.

78. Pellegrini R, Martignone S, Ménard S, Colnaghi MI. Laminin receptor expression and function in small-cell lung carcinoma. Int J Cancer. 1994;8(Suppl.):116–20.

79. Karpatova M, Tagliabue E, Castronovo V et al. Shedding of the 67-kD laminin receptor by human cancer cells. J Cell Biochem. 1996;60:226–34.

80. Nusrat A, Delp C, Madara JL. Intestinal epithelial restitution. Characterization of a cell culture model and mapping of cytoskeletal elements in migrating cells. J Clin Invest. 1992;89:1501–11.

81. Moore R, Madri J, Carlson S, Madara JL. Collagens facilitate epithelial migration in restitution of native guinea pig intestinal epithelium. Gastroenterology. 1992;102:119–30.

82. Nusrat A, Parkos CA, Bacarra AE et al. Hepatocyte growth factor/scatter factor effects on epithelia. Regulation of intercellular junctions in transformed and nontransformed lines, basolateral polarization of c-met receptor in transformed and natural intestinal epithelia and induction of rapid wound repair in a transformed model epithelium. J Clin Invest. 1994;93:2056–65.

83. Sykes DE, Weiser MM. Rat intestinal crypt cell replication factor with homology to early S-phase proteins required for cell division. Gene. 1995;163:243–7.

15
Recent work with migration/patterns of expression: cell–matrix interactions in human intestinal cell differentiation

J.-F. BEAULIEU

INTRODUCTION

The intestinal epithelium represents an attractive system in which to study cell–matrix interactions in relation to growth and cytodifferentiation. The interest in this organ first comes from the fact that during development, the process of endodermal differentiation into a functional epithelium is closely related to intestinal morphogenesis. Indeed, as reviewed elsewhere[1-3], the ontogenic appearance of the main epithelial cell types takes place precisely at the time short villi begin to form while a gradual confinement of the proliferative cell population occurs with crypt formation. Second is the fact that the epithelium is in constant and rapid renewal in the mature intestine. Its functional unit, the crypt-villus axis, consists of spatially separated proliferative and differentiated cell populations located respectively in the crypt and on the villi[1,4,5].

As in many other organs, the intestinal epithelium lies on a thin and continuous sheet of specialized extracellular matrix, the basement membrane (BM), which separates parenchymal cells from the interstitial connective tissue. It is now recognized that the BM composition defines the necessary microenvironment required for multiple cellular functions during development and at maturity such as proliferation, migration, and anoikis as well as tissue-specific gene expression[6-9]. These functions are themselves mediated by various cell membrane receptors, many of which are members of the integrin superfamily[10-14].

In this chapter, after a brief update on the functional aspects of the crypt-villus unit in the human small intestine, I will summarize our current knowledge concerning BM composition and expression of integrins in relation to the cell state in human intestinal cells (see Ref. 3 for a more comprehensive review). Analysing the distribution of these functional molecules in a spatially well organized structure such as the intact intestinal epithelium represents a powerful approach to evaluate the potential implication of individual components in a normal environment. Furthermore, with the availability of well established in vitro models, in concert with recent developments in the generation of human normal intestinal cell lines, it has also become possible to investigate these cell–matrix interactions more directly in order to define cause–effect relationships with intestinal cell differentiation.

THE CRYPT-VILLUS FUNCTIONAL UNIT IN THE HUMAN SMALL INTESTINE

The crypt-villus functional unit, which develops relatively early during human ontogeny (being established by mid-pregnancy), can be defined by typical morphological and functional properties displayed by the mature villus enterocytes that distinguish them from crypt cells. Indeed, the villi are mainly lined by functional absorptive cells and goblet cells while the crypts contain stem cells and the proliferative and poorly differentiated cells as well as a subset of differentiated secretory cells, namely Paneth, goblet and enteroendocrine cells. The differentiation of each cell type take place as the cells move either upwards towards the villus (adsorptive, mucus and endocrine cell) or downwards to concentrate at the bottom of the crypt (Paneth cells). The compartmentalization of distinct cell populations according to their functional state is a well documented phenomenon which can be exemplified by the analysis of the localization of various markers along the crypt-villus axis (Figure 1). It is noteworthy that in all species studied, the crypt-villus junction represents a physical limit from which enterocytes acquire their final functional characteristics. For instance, immunostaining for the detection of maltase-glucoamylase, a marker of the functional enterocyte, is restricted to villus cells while MIM-1/39, a specific marker for secretory granules, is expressed only by crypt cells. However, it appears more and more evident that in the human, in contrast with the situation observed in laboratory animals, some of the classical enterocytic markers can be expressed by immature cells located below this border. For instance, aminopeptidase N has been found constitutively expressed by both proliferative and differentiated intestinal cells while immature forms of sucrase-isomaltase and apolipoprotein B are present in crypt cells. These differences have to be considered when choosing markers to study human intestinal cell differentiation both in situ and in vitro. More importantly, they point out that the regulation of gene expression along the crypt-villus axis[1,2,15] fundamentally differs between man and animal models.

EPITHELIAL BASEMENT MEMBRANE COMPOSITION

The epithelial BM of the human intestine contains all the major components specific to most BMs (see Refs. 3 and 16 for recent reviews). Surprisingly, it was some of the BM-associated macromolecules such as tenascin and fibronectin which were first identified to be differentially expressed along the crypt-villus axis in both the adult (Figure 2) and developing small intestine[17–23]. BM components such as the classical type IV collagen, heterotrimeric laminin and various proteoglycans,

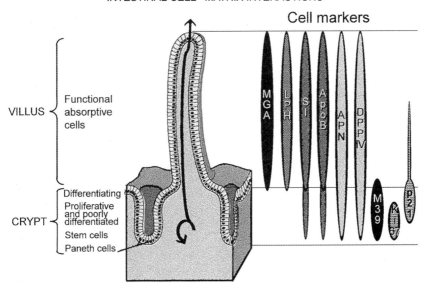

Figure 1 The crypt-villus axis of the human adult small intestine. While maltase-glucoamylase (MGA) and lactase-phlorizin hydrolase (LPH) complexes are exclusively expressed by the functional entero-cytes of the villus, immature forms of sucrase-isomaltase (SI) and apolipoprotein B (ApoB) are also detected in crypts cells. Aminopeptidase N (APN) and dipeptidylpeptidase IV (DPPIV) are expressed by all enterocytes. The MIM-1/39 antigen (M39) is expressed only by immature enterocytes. The proliferating antigen Ki67 is expressed by the proliferating epithelial cells of the crypt while the cyclin dependent protein tyrosine kinase inhibitor p21/WAF-1/Cip1 (p21) is detected in committed cells. Adapted from Refs. 1 and 3

were detected at the base of all epithelial cells[18,21,23–25], while some of their receptors were found to be expressed under distinctive crypt-villus gradients[23,26]. However, the identification of new, genetically distinct laminin and type IV collagen chains prompted many laboratories to re-investigate the expression of these BM molecules in the small intestine over the last few years.

Identification of the newly discovered $\alpha 5$(IV) and $\alpha 6$(IV) chains of collagen

The study of the type IV collagen $\alpha 1$(IV) to $\alpha 6$(IV) chains[27] in the adult human small intestine (Figure 3) revealed a clear predominance of the $\alpha 1$ and $\alpha 2$ chains, which assemble as a $[\alpha 1(IV)]_2\alpha 2(IV)]$ complex, at the epithelial BM, while the $\alpha 3$(IV) and $\alpha 4$(IV) chains were not detected. However, the $\alpha 5$(IV) chain was found to be expressed, although with relatively low amounts of both protein and tran-script, in the adult in comparison to the fetal small intestine[28]. Interestingly, in contrast to the $\alpha 1$(IV) and $\alpha 2$(IV) chains which originate from the mesenchymal compartment, the $\alpha 5$(IV) chain was found to be produced by both epithelial and mesenchymal cells[3,29]. This minor chain was also found to be expressed by colon carcinoma cell lines (Simoneau et al., unpublished) suggesting a possible relation-ship between $\alpha 5$(IV) expression by intestinal cells and fetal development and

167

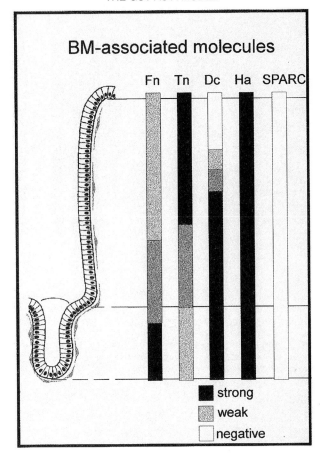

Figure 2 Patterns of distribution for some basement membrane-associated molecules along the crypt-villus axis in the human adult small intestine. In contrast to hyaluronan (hyaluronic acid, hyaluronan; Ha) which is uniformly present at the base of all epithelial cells and SPARC (secreted protein acidic and rich in cysteine, also known as osteonectin or BM40) which is not detected, the cellular fibro-nectin (Fn), tenascin (Tn) and decorin (Dc) extracellular macromolecules were found expressed according to specific gradients of expression. Adapted from Ref. 3

cancer progression. Furthermore, recent evidence[30] (Simoneau et al., unpublished data) suggests that $\alpha6(IV)$, which presumably associates with $\alpha5(IV)$, is also expressed in both the developing and adult small intestinal BM.

Differential expression of laminin chains along the crypt-villus axis and functional significance

Laminin, initially thought to be a unique heterotrimeric molecule formed by one heavy A chain and two distinct light B chains[31,32], has been redefined as a multigene family of related proteins[33,34]. In light of this complexity, a new nomenclature has

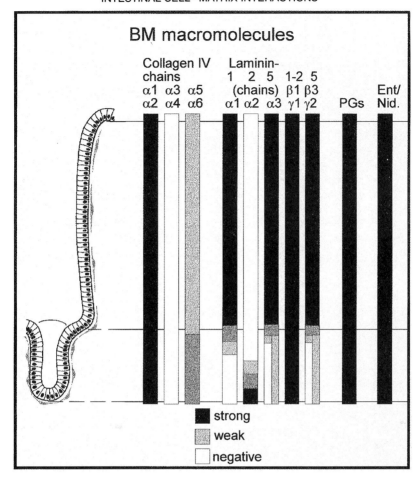

Figure 3 Patterns of distribution of basement membrane macromolecules along the crypt-villus axis in the human adult small intestine. Type IV collagen α1, α2, α5 and α6 chains, laminin-1 (α1β1γ1), laminin-2 (α2β1γ1) and laminin-5 (α3β3γ2), heparan sulphate proteoglycans (PGs), and entactin/nidogen (Ent./Nid.) were found in the epithelial basement membrane. Mainly laminins are differentially expressed, laminin-1 and 5 being principally detected at the base of villus cells and laminin-2 being confined at the bottom of the glands. Adapted from Ref. 3

been proposed where the designated A, B1 and B2 chains have been replaced by α, β and γ, respectively, and the identification of isoforms is distinguished by arabic numbers[35]. This nomenclature, although somewhat confusing with the integrin classification, has been largely adopted. Functionally, laminins have been shown to mediate several cellular activities, namely the promotion of adhesion, growth, polarization and differentiation, depending on the cell type studied[9,36,37]. Variability in spatial and temporal expression of a number of these laminin chains[38–41] suggests that different heterotrimeric forms of laminin could perform distinct functions.

The expression of laminin variants in the small intestinal BM received a great deal of attention since reciprocal expression of laminin-1 ($\alpha1\beta1\gamma1$) and laminin-2 ($\alpha2\beta1\gamma1$) along the crypt-villus axis was reported by two independent groups[42–44]. The occurrence of laminin-1 as a villus form and laminin-2 as a crypt form (Figure 3) suggested for the first time a possible relationship between laminin expression and functional intestinal cell differentiation. In further investigating this relationship in the Caco-2/15 cell model, our laboratory provided evidence that enterocytic differentiation-related gene expression is specifically promoted by laminins, and is susceptible to a differential modulation by variant forms of this family[45] (Desloges et al., unpublished). Indeed, a close relationship between laminin-1 deposition and sucrase-isomaltase expression was demonstrated at the cell level, suggesting that the well established potential of Caco-2/15 cells to differentiate in vitro[46–48] could be related to their potential to synthesize and accumulate functional laminin-1 at their basal pole. For instance, subclones of the Caco-2/15 cell line in which laminin-1 deposition is impaired were found to express considerably less sucrase-isomaltase at their apical pole[45]. Furthermore, growth of Caco-2/15 cells on purified human laminin-1 and laminin-2 revealed that both substrates can promote intestinal cell marker expression but that only laminin-1 has the ability to induce precocious functional differentiation markers such as sucrase-isomaltase and lactase-phlorizin hydrolase[45]. Finally, additional evidence that laminin-1 plays an important role in regulating cell differentiation was recently obtained by transfecting Caco-2 cells with an antisense laminin α1-chain cDNA fragment[49].

In this context, the recent observation showing an increasing gradient of expression of laminin-5 ($\alpha3\beta3\gamma2$) from the upper crypt to the villus tip in the human small intestine[50,51] (Figure 3) is of interest since this laminin has previously been reported only in BMs of stratified epithelia, in association with anchoring filaments of hemidesmosomes. It is noteworthy that hemidesmosomes have not been observed in the human small intestinal epithelium[52] and that type VII collagen and major hemidesmosomal proteins are lacking[53,54]. Although the functional role for laminin-5 in the intestinal epithelium remains to be determined, a possible involvement of this molecule in intestinal cell migration has been proposed, based on the promoting effect of laminin-5 on the migration of certain types of cells[55,56].

INTEGRINS AS MAJOR CELL RECEPTORS FOR BASEMENT MEMBRANE MOLECULES

Integrins are a large family of transmembrane $\alpha\beta$ heterodimeric glycoproteins which are the primary mediators of extracellular matrix molecule–cell interactions and signalling[10–14,57,58]. So far, 16 α subunits and eight β subunits have been identified which can form more than 20 different heterodimers. It is mainly the integrins that belong to the β1 class, also known as the very late antigens or VLAs, that bind to BM molecules such as laminin, type IV collagen and fibronectin. The β1 integrins are widely distributed and numerous, as the β1 subunit can form heterodimers with any of the $\alpha1 - \alpha9$ and αv subunits. A subset of β1 integrins is constitutively present in virtually all epithelial cells, the most ubiquitous being $\alpha2\beta1$ and $\alpha3\beta1$. In general, β1 integrin binding to BM molecules is relatively selective. For example, the $\alpha5\beta1$ and $\alpha6\beta1$ integrins have been found to specifically interact with fibronectins and laminins, respectively, while $\alpha3\beta1$ has been found to respond to a broad spectrum of extracellular ligands, although it seems to primarily mediate adhesion to laminin-5. In contrast to $\beta1$ integrins, the only α subunit known to associate with $\beta4$ is $\alpha6$. This particular $\alpha6\beta4$ heterodimer is found in a number of epithelia and functions exclusively as a laminin-specific binding integrin.

Interestingly, $\beta1$ and $\beta4$ integrins exhibit major structural differences but, as demonstrated recently, share also some of their functional characteristics[11–14,58–60]. From a structural point of view, the $\beta4$ subunit, because of its unique and very large cytoplasmic domain that can associate with keratin filaments, differs fundamentally from the other β subunits, including $\beta1$, which possess a short cytoplasmic domain that associates with actin-based filaments. Interactions with actin or keratin to form focal adhesion complexes or hemidesmosomes, respectively, seem to depend on their unique ability to associate with intermediate proteins such as focal adhesion proteins, including α-actinin, talin and FAK for $\beta1$, or hemidesmosomal proteins for $\beta4$. However, more importantly from a functional point of view, both sets of integrins can transduce signals across the plasma membrane through their association with cytoplasmic tyrosine kinases and can thus, ultimately, regulate growth, apoptosis and tissue-specific gene expression[9,60,61].

Integrin expression in the human small intestinal epithelium

Based on the fact that it may provide important information relative to the potential involvement of integrins in cell–matrix interactions in situ, the distribution of most $\beta1$ and $\beta4$ integrins has been determined along the intestinal crypt-villus axis. As summarized in Figure 4 for the human small intestine, the principal integrin subunits present in epithelial cells include $\beta1$ and $\beta4$ as well as $\alpha2$, $\alpha3$, $\alpha6$ and $\alpha7$, all of which are among the subgroup of the laminin-binding integrins[3,13]. The $\alpha5$ subunit, which associates with $\beta1$ to act as a fibronectin receptor, was detected at the base of crypt and villus cells according to a faint and punctuated pattern of staining reminiscent of that observed for its ligand in the BM[23] while the $\alpha1$, $\alpha4$, $\alpha9$ and αv subunits were only weakly expressed or absent from the normal adult epithelium[23,26,63] (Desloges et al., unpublished). Up to now most of these studies have been performed on human tissues. Although data are beginning to accumulate for laboratory animals as specific antibodies become available, patterns of integrin expression differ substantially in many instances between man and rodents[43,62] and thus, for more simplicity, will not be considered here.

The analysis of the laminin-binding integrins along the crypt-villus axis revealed interesting features. The $\alpha2$ and $\alpha3$ subunits were found at the basal domain of intestinal cells according to strict complementary staining patterns along the crypt-villus axis, the $\alpha2$ subunit being predominant in the crypts and $\alpha3$ on the villus[3,23,44,51]. It is noteworthy that both of these subunits were also localized at the lateral domain of enterocytes, where they can serve as mediators of intercellular adhesion[64], and that the population of cells exhibiting this lateral staining extends beyond the crypt and villus compartments for the $\alpha2$ and $\alpha3$ subunits,

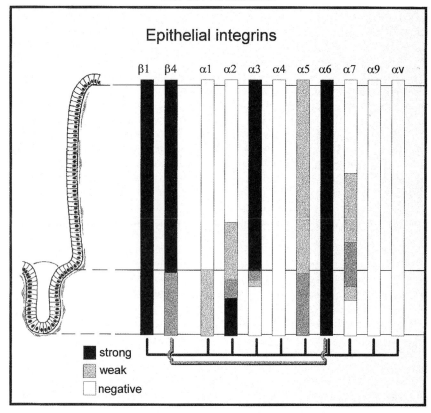

Figure 4 Patterns of expression of epithelial integrin subunits along the crypt-villus axis in the human adult small intestine. The main integrin subunits present in intestinal cells are $\alpha2$, $\alpha3$, $\alpha5$, $\alpha6$, $\alpha7$ and $\beta1$ and $\beta4$. The $\alpha4$, $\alpha9$ and αv subunits are not detected in the epithelium. Besides $\alpha5\beta1$ which acts exclusively as a fibronectin receptor, $\alpha2\beta1$ can bind both laminins and collagens while $\alpha3\beta1$, $\alpha7\beta1$ and $\alpha6\beta4$ serve as specific receptors for laminins. Adapted from Ref. 3

respectively[3]. On the other hand, the $\alpha6$ subunit was uniformly distributed at the base of epithelial cells from the bottom of the crypt to the tip of the villus[23,42–44,65]. However, difficulties in interpreting the widespread distribution of this subunit arise from the ability of $\alpha6$ to form two distinct integrin complexes by combining with either $\beta1$ or $\beta4$, depending on the cell type[66,67], and the existence of variants, referred to as $\alpha6$A and $\alpha6$B, which can combine with either $\beta1$ or $\beta4$[68]; there are also multiple variants for $\beta1$[69–72] and $\beta4$[73–75]. At the present time, the expression of $\alpha6$, $\beta1$ and $\beta4$ variants and their $\alpha\beta$ association have not been investigated in normal human enterocytes. Finally, the expression of the $\alpha7$ subunit has only recently been reported[62,76]. In the adult, only the $\alpha7$B isoform is detected in the epithelium and it is present under a unique pattern of expression, being restricted to the upper part of the crypt and the lower villus region (Basora et al., unpublished).

Taken together, the observations showing the expression of a number of primary laminin-binding integrins in the intestinal epithelium and their differential localization along the crypt-villus axis, in concert with compositional changes in laminin-1, 2 and 5 (see above), delineate the potential complexity of epithelial cell–laminin interactions involved in the maintenance of a relatively simple system such as the human intestinal epithelium. Analysing the distribution of these functional molecules in a spatially well organized structure such as the crypt-villus axis represents a powerful method of estimating the potential implication of individual components in a normal environment. Nevertheless, to recapitulate the mechanisms in play, several questions pertaining to the basic organization of integrin subunits (exact form(s)/variant(s) expressed, relative quantitative importance, association with β1 or β4, ligand specificity) and, more importantly, their precise involvement in the regulation of specific cell functions such as proliferation, polarization, adhesion, migration, apoptosis and differentiation, also needs to be addressed by means of more direct approaches.

Functional relevance of laminin-binding integrins in the regulation of intestinal functions

The expression and potential roles of a number of laminin-binding integrins have been investigated in various intestinal cell lines. Although mostly of colon adenocarcinoma origin, these human cell lines have been used to study integrin-mediated intestinal cell adhesion. In relatively good agreement with the in vivo situation where the expression of α2, α6, β1 and β4 is generally maintained and α3 is reduced or absent in colorectal carcinoma cells[77–79], the predominant integrins expressed in colon cancer cell lines and involved in cell adhesion, spreading and migration appear to be α2β1 and α6β4.

The α2β1 integrin has been shown to be involved in intestinal cell adhesion to both laminin and collagen in clone A cells[80]. The α2β1 binding capacity for laminin-1 appears substantially greater than for laminin-2, although much lower than for collagen[81], but recent studies suggest that α2β1 may act in cooperation with α6β4 for attachment to laminin-1[13]. There is also evidence that this receptor may be involved in EGF-mediated Caco-2 cell migration on laminin[82]. On the other hand, the promoting effect of transforming growth factor-α on glandular differentiation of SW1222 cells grown in a three-dimensional collagen gel was shown to be primarily mediated by the α2β1 integrin[83]. Interestingly, this latter observation is reminiscent of the situation during gland formation in the developing fetal small intestine[44]. In the adult, α2β1 is predominantly associated with crypt cells which exhibit a BM containing type IV collagens but which lack laminin-1 and 5 (see above). Taken together, these observations would suggest that in the intestinal epithelium, the α2β1 integrin may act primarily as a collagen receptor involved in gland morphogenesis and maintenance, rather than as a laminin receptor.

The α6β4 integrins were first reported as a laminin receptor in intestinal cells working in cooperation with another β1 integrin, most likely α2β1[80,84,85]. In hemidesmosome-expressing cells such as those at the epidermal–mesenchymal interface, α6β4 plays an essential role in the assembly and for the stability of hemidesmosomes while it mediates anchorage on laminin-5 in cooperation with α3β1[86,87]. However, as mentioned in a previous section, intestinal cells do not possess hemidesmosomes but express these receptors. Interestingly, most colon

173

cancer cell lines tested that express $\alpha6\beta4$ (e.g. clone A, differentiated HT29 and LoVo clone E2) adhere better to laminin than their counterparts which express lower levels of intact $\alpha6\beta4$ or $\alpha6$ predominantly as the $\alpha6\beta1$ form (e.g. undifferentiated HT29, LoVo clone C5, and RKO)[3,84,85,88,89]. Furthermore, as well illustrated in RKO cells, the low avidity for laminin-1 in cells that express $\alpha6\beta1$ can be reversed after transfection with full-length $\beta4$ cDNA[75], showing that $\alpha6\beta4$, but not $\alpha6\beta1$, is a high affinity receptor for laminin-1 and that in the presence of $\beta1$ and $\beta4$, the $\alpha6$ subunit associates preferentially with $\beta4$ to act as a specific laminin-1 and 5 receptor[85,90]. Whether the same phenomenon occurs in vivo has not been verified but is suggested by the fact that at least some forms of the $\beta4$ subunit are expressed in both crypt and villus cells[3,42,43,51] although $\alpha6$ and $\beta1$ are present in all intestinal cells. Interestingly, the forced expression of $\beta4$ in RKO cells induces, in a laminin-1 or laminin-5 substrate-independent manner, expression of p21/Cip1/WAF-1, an inhibitor of cyclin-dependent kinases, and apoptosis[75]. Although further work is required to verify to which extent the phenomenon can be extrapolated to the in vivo situation, it is pertinent to note that the intestinal epithelium of newborn mice deficient for $\beta4$ expression was found recently to be susceptible to degeneration and loss of cell–substratum adhesion, suggesting that $\alpha6\beta4$ interacts with laminin-5 to mediate a signal essential for cell survival in the animal[91]. Mice lacking the $\alpha6$ subunit develop until birth but die soon after with severe blistering of the skin and other epithelia[92]. Finally, there is also evidence that $\alpha6\beta4$ plays a key role in the modulation of adhesion properties in the human[86]. The suggestion that $\alpha6\beta4$ primarily serves as a high affinity receptor for cell adhesion to laminin-1 and laminin-5, and as a regulator of the p21-related growth control mechanism, would appear to be in good agreement with the distribution of these molecules along the crypt-villus axis in the intact intestinal epithelium[42,43,51,93] (Quaroni and Beaulieu, unpublished data).

Much less is known about the implication of integrins as mediators of extracellular matrix-regulated cell-specific gene expression[9,52,94]. Although it is still to be better documented in other systems, studying of the role of integrins in human intestinal cells has been further complicated by the lack of normal cell models in which the differentiation process can be initiated under in vitro conditions. In light of this, the finding that laminin-1 plays a key role in the establishment and maintenance of functional differentiation in the enterocytic-like Caco-2 cell line[45,49] is of importance by providing for the first time evidence that a BM molecule, in particular laminin-1, is directly involved in the modulation of the expression of enterocytic functions, and a suitable model in which to analyse laminin–cell interactions in the context of intestinal differentiation. At first glance, the potential role of integrins in this phenomenon may appear relatively complicated to investigate, in light of the numerous laminin-binding integrins expressed in the small intestinal epithelium, namely $\alpha3\beta1$, $\alpha7\beta1$ and $\alpha6\beta4$ as well as $\alpha1\beta1$ and $\alpha2\beta1$. However, few appear to be good candidates for mediating the effects of laminin-1 on intestinal functional cell differentiation[3]. Indeed, $\alpha1\beta1$ and $\alpha2\beta1$, as mentioned above for $\alpha2\beta1$, are confined to the crypts, which are devoid of laminin-1. Furthermore, the widespread expression of $\alpha6\beta4$ by both crypt and villus cells in the adult as well as during fetal development and in most colon cancer cells suggests that this integrin may not be responsible for triggering terminal differentiation in the intestinal epithelium. The predominant expression of $\alpha3\beta1$ at the

174

base of villus cells in both the developing and adult small intestine may indicate a role for this integrin. However, there is good evidence that epithelial cells, including intestinal ones, use primarily $\alpha3\beta1$ as a high affinity laminin-5 receptor[13,95,96], a laminin form also predominantly expressed in the BM of villus cells in both the developing and adult small intestine. On the other hand, the integrin $\alpha7\beta1$ has only been reported recently in epithelial cells. In muscle, this integrin was first identified as a laminin-1 receptor[97,98] mediating laminin functions during myogenic differentiation[99–101]. The particular distribution of the $\alpha7B$ variant, at the upper crypts and lower villus region, in concert with its regulated expression in Caco-2 cells and its absence in HIEC cells, a human intestinal crypt like cell line[102], suggests that the $\alpha7B\beta1$ integrin plays a role in the regulation of laminin-1-mediated enterocytic differentiation[76].

Although a cause–effect relationship between $\alpha7\beta1$, and/or any other of these integrins, and laminin-mediated intestinal cell differentiation still remains to be directly demonstrated, these studies illustrate well the use of intestinal epithelial cells, both in the intact organ and in vitro, as an integrated model to investigate cell–matrix interactions and define their significance in the regulation of functional gene expression.

Acknowledgements

I would like to thank the members of my laboratory for their contribution to the original research and their suggestions to the manuscript: Nuria Basora, Isabelle Bélanger, Yamina Bouatrouss, Nathalie Deslosges, Elizabeth Herring-Gillam, Sophie Jutras, Aneil Mujumdar, Nathalie Perreault, Aline Simoneau, and Pierre H. Vachon. I would also like to thank Drs Raymond Calvert, Daniel Ménard and Andrea Quaroni for their constant support, Drs Stephen Akiyama, Martin E. Hemler, Eva Engvall, Andrea Quaroni, Erkki Ruoslahti, Dean Sheppard, Jaro Sodek, Dallas M. Swallow, Karl Tryggvason, Effie C. Tsilibary, Jörgen Wieslander, Kenneth M. Yamada and Peter D. Yurchenco who generously provided key antibodies and/or probes, Drs Alain Bilodeau, Claude Poulin, Martine Morin and Francis Jacot of the Département de santé communautaire, and Dr Jacques Poisson of the Département de chirurgie générale as well as the members of the Département de pathologie, Centre Universitaire de Santé de l'Estrie, for their excellent cooperation in providing tissue specimens for these investigations, and N. Basora and F.E. Herring-Gillam for reviewing the manuscript. The original work and the preparation of this review was supported by grants MT-11289 and MT-12904 from the Medical Research Council of Canada and from the 'Fonds pour la Formation de Chercheurs et l'Aide à la Recherche'. The author was a chercheur boursier of the 'Fonds de la rechereche en santé du Québec'.

References

1. Ménard D, Beaulieu J-F. Human intestinal brush border membrane hydrolases. In: Bkaily G, editor, Membrane Physiopathology. Norwell: Kluwer Academic Publishers, 1994:319–41.
2. Podolsky DK, Babyatsky MW. Growth and development of the gastrointestinal tract. In: Yamada T, editor, Textbook of Gastroenterology, 2nd edn. Philadelphia: JB Lippincott, 1995:546–77.

3. Beaulieu J-F. Extracellular matrix components and integrins in relationship to human intestinal epithelial cell differentiation. Prog Histochem Cytochem. 1997;31:1–76.
4. Leblond CP. The life history of cells in renewing systems. Am J Anat. 1981;160:114–59.
5. Louvard D, Kedinger M, Hauri HP. The differentiating intestinal epithelial cell: establishment and maintenance of functions through interactions between cellular structures. Annu Rev Cell Biol. 1992;8:157–95.
6. Adams JC, Watt FM. Regulation of development and differentiation by the extracellular matrix. Development. 1993;117:1183–98.
7. Juliano RL, Haskill S. Signal transduction from the extracellular matrix. J Cell Biol. 1993;120: 577–85.
8. Lin QC, Bissell MJ. Multi-faceted regulation of cell differentiation by extracellular matrix. FASEB J. 1993;7:737–43.
9. Rosekelly CD, Desprez PY, Bissell MJ. A hierarchy of ECM-mediated signaling regulates tissue-specific gene expression. Curr Opin Cell Biol. 1995;7:736–47.
10. Ruoslahti E. Integrins. J Clin Invest. 1991;87:1–5.
11. Hynes RO. Integrins: versatility, modulation, and signaling in cell adhesion. Cell. 1992;69:11–25.
12. Sonnenberg A. Laminin receptors in the integrin family. Pathol Biol. 1992;40:773–78.
13. Mercurio AM. Laminin receptors: achieving specificity through cooperation. Trends Cell Biol. 1995;5:419–23.
14. Sheppard D. Epithelial integrins. BioEssays. 1996;18:655–60.
15. Boyle WJ, Brenner DA. Molecular and cell biology of the small intestine. Curr Opin Gastroenterol. 1995;11:121–7.
16. Simon-Assmann P, Kedinger M, De Archangelis A, Rousseau V, Simo P. Extracellular matrix components in intestinal development. Experientia. 1995;51:883–900.
17. Quaroni A, Isselbacher KJ, Ruoslahti E. Fibronectin synthesis by epithelial crypt cells of rat small intestine. Proc Natl Acad Sci USA. 1978;75:5548–52.
18. Simon-Assmann P, Kedinger M, Haffen K. Immunocytochemical localization of extracellular matrix proteins in relation to rat intestinal morphogenesis. Differentiation. 1986;32:59–66.
19. Aufderheide E, Ekblom P. Tenascin during gut development: appearance in the mesenchyme, shift in molecular forms, and dependence on epithelial-mesenchymal interactions. J Cell Biol. 1988; 107:2341–9.
20. Probstmeier R, Martini R, Schachner M. Expression of J1/tenascin in the crypt-villus unit of adult mouse small intestine: implication for its role in epithelial cell shedding. Development. 1990;109:313–21.
21. Beaulieu JF, Vachon PH, Chartrand A. Immunolocalization of extracellular matrix components during organogenesis in the human small intestine. Anat Embryol. 1991;1983:363–9.
22. Beaulieu JF, Jutras S, Durand J, Vachon PH, Perreault N. Relationship between tenascin and α-smooth muscle actin expression in the developing human small intestinal mucosa. Anat Embryol. 1993;188:149–58.
23. Beaulieu JF. Differential expression of the VLA family of integrins along the crypt-villus axis in the human small intestine. J Cell Sci. 1992;102:427–36.
24. Laurie GW, Leblond CP, Martin GR. Localization of type IV collagen, laminin, heparan sulfate proteoglycan and fibronectin to the basal lamina of basement membranes. J Cell Biol. 1982;95: 340–4.
25. Trier JS, Allan CH, Abrahamson DR, Hagen SJ. Epithelial basement membrane of mouse jejunum. Evidence for laminin turnover along the entire crypt-villus axis. J Clin Invest. 1990;86:87–95.
26. MacDonald TT, Horton MA, Choy MY, Richman PI. Increased expression of laminin/collagen receptor (VLA-1) on epithelium of inflamed human intestine. J Clin Pathol. 1990;43:313–15.
27. Hudson BG, Reeders ST, Tryggvason K. Type IV collagen: Structure, gene organization, and role in human diseases. J Biol Chem. 1993;268:26033–6.
28. Beaulieu JF, Vachon PH, Herring-Gillam E et al. Expression of the $\alpha5(IV)$ collagen chain in the fetal human small intestine. Gastroenterology. 1994;107:957–67.
29. Vachon PH, Durand J, Beaulieu JF. Basement membrane formation and re-distribution of β_1 integrins in a human intestinal co-culture system. Anat Rec. 1993;236:567–76.
30. Peissel B, Geng L, Kalluri R et al. Comparative distribution of the $\alpha1(IV)$ and $\alpha6(IV)$ collagen chains in normal adult and fetal tissues and in kidney from X-linked Alport syndrome patients. J Clin Invest. 1995;96:1948–57.
31. Beck K, Hunter I, Engel J. Structure and function of laminin: anatomy of a multidomain glycoprotein. FASEB J. 1990;4:148–60.

32. Engel J. Laminins and other strange proteins. Biochemistry. 1992;31:10643–51.
33. Weiver UM, Engvall E. Laminins. Methods Enzymol. 1994;245:85–104.
34. Beck K, Gruber T. Structure and assembly of basement membrane and related extracellular matrix proteins. In: Richardson PD, Steiner M, editors, Principles of Cell Adhesion. Boca Raton: CRC Press, 1995:219–52.
35. Burgeson RE, Chiquet M, Deutzmann R et al. A new nomenclature for the laminins. Matrix Biol. 1994;14:209–11.
36. Paulsson M. Basement membrane proteins: Structure, assembly, and cellular interactions. Crit Rev Biochem Mol Biol. 1992;27:93–127.
37. Engvall E. Laminin variants: why, where and when? Kidney Int. 1993;43:2–6.
38. Engvall E, Earwicker D, Haaparanta T, Ruoslahti E, Sanes SR. Distribution and isolation of four laminin variants: Tissue restricted distribution of heterotrimers assembled from five different subunits. Cell Reg. 1990;1:731–40.
39. Sanes JR, Engvall E, Butkowski R, Hunter DD. Molecular heterogeneity of basal laminae: isoforms of laminin and collagen IV at the neuromuscular junction and elsewhere. J Cell Biol. 1990;111:1685–99.
40. Weiver UM, Engvall E, Paulsson M, Yamada Y, Albrechtsen R. Laminin A, B1, B2, S and M subunits in the postnatal rat liver development and after partial hepatectomy. Lab Invest. 1992; 66:378–89.
41. Vuolteenaho R, Nissinen M, Sainio K et al. Human laminin M chain (merosin): Complete primary structure, chromosomal assignment, and expression of the M and A chain in human fetal tissues. J Cell Biol. 1994;124:381–94.
42. Beaulieu J-F, Vachon PH. Reciprocal expression of laminin A-chain isoforms along the crypt-villus axis in the human small intestine. Gastroenterology. 1994;106:829–39.
43. Simon-Assmann P, Duclos B, Orian-Rousseau V et al. Differential expression of laminin isoforms and $\alpha6$-$\beta4$ integrins subunits in the developing human and mouse intestine. Dev Dynamics. 1994; 201:71–85.
44. Perreault N, Vachon PH, Beaulieu J-F. Appearance and distribution of laminin A chain isoforms and integrin $\alpha2$, $\alpha3$, $\alpha6$, $\beta1$, and $\beta4$ subunits in the developing human small intestinal mucosa. Anat Rec. 1995;242:242–50.
45. Vachon PH, Beaulieu J-F. Extracellular heterotrimeric laminin promotes differentiation in human enterocytes. Am J Physiol. 1995;268:G857–67.
46. Beaulieu J-F, Quaroni A. Clonal analysis of sucrase-isomaltase expression in the human colon adenocarcinoma Caco-2 cells. Biochem J. 1991;280:599–608.
47. Vachon PH, Beaulieu J-F. Transient mosaic patterns of morphological and functional differentiation in the Caco-2 cell line. Gastroenterology. 1992;103:414–23.
48. Vachon PH, Perreault N, Magny P, Beaulieu J-F. Uncoordinated, transient mosaic patterns of intestinal hydrolases expression in differentiating human enterocytes. J Cell Physiol. 1996;166: 198–207.
49. De Archangelis A, Neuville P, Boukamel R, Lefebvre O, Kedinger M, Simon-Assmann P. Inhibition of laminin $\alpha1$-chain expression leads to alteration of basement membrane assembly and cell differentiation. J Cell Biol. 1996;133:417–30.
50. Orian-Rousseau V, Aberdam D, Fontano L et al. Developmental expression of laminin-5 and HD1 in the intestine – epithelial to mesenchymal shift for the laminin $\gamma2$ chain subunit deposition. Dev Dynamics. 1996;206:12–23.
51. Leivo I, Tani T, Laitinen L et al. Anchoring complex components laminin-5 and type VII collagen in the intestine: Association with migration and differentiating enterocytes. J Histochem Cytochem. 1996;44:1267–77.
52. Jones JCR, Asmuth J, Baker SE, Langhofer M, Roth SI, Hopkinson SB. Hemidesmosomes: Extracellular matrix/intermediate filament connectors. Exp Cell Res. 1994;213:1–11.
53. Leigh IM, Purkis PE, Bruckner-Tuderman L. LH7.2 monoclonal antibody detects type VII collagen in the sublamin densa zone of ectodermally-derived epithelia, including skin. Epithelia. 1987;1:17–29.
54. Owaribe K, Kartenbeck J, Stumpp S et al. The hemidesmosomal plaque. I. Characterization of a major constituent protein as a differentiation marker for certain forms of epithelia. Differentiation. 1990;45:207–20.
55. Nishiyama T, Tsunenaga M, Akutsu N et al. Laminin-5 (kalinin) promotes human keratinocyte migration. J Invest Dermatol. 1995;104:589a.

56. Pyke C, Romer J, Kallunki P et al. The γ2 chain of kalinin/laminin 5 is preferentially expressed in invading malignant cell in human cancers. Am J Pathol. 1994;145:782–91.

57. Akiyama SK, Nagata K, Yamada KM. Cell surface receptors for extracellular matrix components. Biochim Biophys Acta. 1990;1031:91–110.

58. Clark EA, Brugge JS. Integrin and signal transduction pathways: The road taken. Science. 1995; 268:233–9.

59. Parson JT. Integrin-mediated signaling: regulation by protein tyrosine kinases and small GTP-binding proteins. Curr Opin Cell Biol. 1996;8:146–52.

60. Giancotti FG. Signal transduction by the $\alpha6\beta4$ integrin: charting the path between laminin binding and nuclear events. J Cell Sci. 1996;109:1165–72.

61. Craig SW, Johnson RP. Assembly of focal adhesions: progress, paradigms, and portents. Curr Opin Cell Biol. 1996;8:74–85.

62. Vachon PH, Basora N, Xu N, Beaulieu J-F, Engvall E. Species-specific patterns of laminin variants and laminin-binding integrins in murine and adult small intestine. Proc Seventh Int Symp Basem Memb. 1995:87.

63. Palmer EL, Rüegg C, Ferrando R, Rytela R, Sheppard D. Sequence and tissue distribution of the integrin $\alpha9$ subunit, a novel partner of $\beta1$ that is widely distributed in epithelia and muscle. J Cell Biol. 1993;123:1289–97.

64. Symington BE, Takada Y, Carter WG. Interaction of integrin $\alpha3\beta1$ and $\alpha2\beta1$: Potential role in keratinocyte intercellular adhesion. J Cell Biol. 1993;120:523–35.

65. Choy MY, Richman PI, Horton MA, MacDonald TT. Expression of the VLA family of integrins in human intestine. J Pathol. 1990;160:35–40.

66. Hemler ME, Crouse C, Sonnenberg A. Association of the VLA alpha subunit with a novel protein. A possible alternative to the common VLA beta 1 subunit on certain cell line. J Biol Chem. 1989; 264:6529–35.

67. Sonnenberg A, Linders CJT, Daams JH, Kennel SJ. The $\alpha6\beta1$ (VLA-6) and $\alpha6\beta4$ protein complexes: tissue distribution and biochemical properties. J Cell Sci. 1990;96:207–17.

68. Hogervorst F, Admiraal LG, Niessen C et al. Biochemical characterization and tissue distribution of the A and B variants of the integrin $\alpha6$ subunit. J Cell Biol. 1993;121:179–91.

69. Altruda F, Cervella P, Tarone G et al. A human integrin $\beta1$ subunit with a unique cytoplasmic domain generated by alternative mRNA processing. Gene. 1990;95:261–6.

70. Languino LR, Ruoslahti E. An alternative form of the integrin $\beta1$ subunit with a variant cytoplasmic domain. J Cell Biol. 1992;267:7116–20.

71. Meredith J Jr, Takada Y, Fornaro M, Languino LR, Schwartz MA. Inhibition of cell cycle progression by the alternative spliced integrin $\beta1C$. Science. 1995;269:1570–2.

72. Zhidkova N, Belkin AM, Mayne R. Novel isoform of $\beta1$ integrin expressed in skeletal and cardiac muscle. Biochem Biophys Res Commun. 1995;214:279–85.

73. Tamura RN, Rozzo C, Starr L et al. Epithelial integrin $\alpha6\beta4$: complete primary structure of $\alpha6$ and variant forms of $\beta4$. J Cell Biol. 1990;111:1593–604.

74. Hogervorst F, Kuikman I, Kr von dem Borne AEG, Sonnenberg A. Cloning and sequence analysis of $\beta4$ cDNA; an integrin subunit that contains a unique 118kD cytoplasmic domain. EMBO J. 1990;9:765–70.

75. Clarke AS, Lotz MM, Mercurio AM. A novel structural variant of the human $\beta4$ integrin cDNA. Cell Adhesion Commun. 1994;2:1–6.

76. Basora N, Perreault N, Vachon PH, Engvall E, Beaulieu J-F. Restricted expression of the $\alpha7B\beta1$ integrin, a laminin receptor, in human intestinal epithelial cells. Gastroenterology. 1996;110: A791.

77. Koretz K, Schlag P, Boumsell L, Moller P. Expression of VLA-$\alpha2$, VLA-$\alpha6$ and VLA-$\beta1$ chains in normal mucosa and adenomas of the colon, and in colon carcinomas and their liver metastases. Am J Pathol. 1991;138:741–50.

78. Stallmach A, v Lampe B, Matthes H, Bornhöft G, Riecken EO. Diminished expression of integrin adhesion molecules on human colonic epithelial cells during the benign to malign tumor transformation. Gut. 1992;33:342–6.

79. Falcioni R, Turchi V, Vitullo P et al. Integrin $\beta4$ expression in colorectal cancer. Int J Oncol. 1994;5:573–8.

80. Lotz MM, Korzelius CA, Mercurio AM. Human colon carcinoma cells use multiple receptors to adhere to laminin: involvement of $\alpha6\beta4$ and $\alpha2\beta1$ integrins. Cell Reg. 1990;1:249–57.

81. Pfaff M, Gohring W, Brown JC, Timpl R. Binding of purified collagen receptors (alpha 1 beta 1,

alpha 2 beta 2) and RGD-dependent integrins to laminin and laminin fragments. Eur J Biochem. 1994;225:975–84.

82. Basson MD, Modlin IM, Madri JA. Human enterocyte (Caco-2) migration is modulated in vitro by extracellular matrix composition and epidermal growth factor. J Clin Invest. 1992;90:15–23.

83. Liu D, Gagliardi G, Nasim MM et al. TGF-alpha can act as a morphogen and/or mitogen in a colon-cancer cell line. Int J Cancer. 1994;56:603–8.

84. Schreiner C, Bauer J, Margolis M, Juliano RL. Expression and role of integrins in adhesion of human colonic carcinoma cells to extracellular matrix components. Clin Exp Metastasis. 1991; 9:163–78.

85. Lee EC, Lotz MM, Steel GD Jr, Mercurio AM. The integrin $\alpha6\beta4$ is a laminin receptor. J Cell Biol. 1992;117:671–8.

86. Niessen CM, van der Raaij-Hemler LMH, Hulsman EHM, van der Neut R, Jonkman MF, Sonnenberg A. Deficiency of the integrin $\beta4$ subunit in junctional epidermolysis bullosa with pyloric atrasia: consequences for hemidesmosome formation and adhesion properties. J Cell Sci. 1996;109:1695–706.

87. Xia Y, Gil SG, Carter WG. Anchorage mediated by integrin $\alpha6\beta4$ to laminin 5 (epiligrin) regulates tyrosine phosphorylation of a membrane-associated 80-kD protein. J Cell Biol. 1996; 132:727–40.

88. Simon-Assmann P, Leberquier C, Molto N, Uezato T, Bouziges F, Kedinger M. Adhesion properties and integrin expression profiles in two colonic cancer populations differing by their spreading on laminin. J Cell Sci. 1994;107:577–87.

89. Daemi N, Valet T, Thomasset N et al. Expression of the alpha 6, beta 1 and beta 4 integrin subunits, basement membrane organization and proteolytic capacities in low and high metastatic human colon carcinoma xenografts. Invas Metastasis. 1995;15:103–15.

90. Niessen CM, Hogervorst F, Jaspars LH et al. The integrin $\alpha6\beta4$ is a receptor for both laminin and kalinin. Exp Cell Res. 1994;211:360–7.

91. Dowling J, Yu Q-C, Fuchs E. $\beta4$ integrin is required for hemidesmosome formation, cell adhesion and cell survival. J Cell Biol. 1996;134:559–72.

92. Georges-Labouesse E, Messaddeq N, Yehia G, Cadalbert L, Dierich A, Le Meur M. Absence of integrin $\alpha6$ leads to epidermolysis bullosa and neonatal death in mice. Nature Genet. 1996; 13:370–3.

93. Gartel AL, Serfas MS, Gartel M et al. p21 (WAF1/CIP1) expression is induced in newly non-dividing cells in diverse epithelia and during differentiation of the Caco-2 intestinal cell line. Exp Cell Res. 1996;227:171–81.

94. Ruoslahti E, Obrink B. Common principles in cell adhesion. Exp Cell Res. 1996;227:1–11.

95. Carter WG, Ryan MC, Gahr PJ. Epliligrin, a new cell adhesion ligand for integrin $\alpha3\beta1$ in epithelial basement membranes. Cell. 1991;65:599–610.

96. Delwel G, de Melker AA, Hogervost F et al. Distinct and overlapping ligand specificities of the $\alpha3A\beta1$ and $\alpha3B\beta1$ integrins: recognition of laminin isoforms. Mol Biol Cell. 1994;5:203–15.

97. Kramer RH, Vu NM. Laminin-binding integrin $\alpha7\beta1$: functional characterization and expression in normal and malignant melanocytes. Cell Reg. 1991;2:805–17.

98. Von der Mark H, Dürr J, Sonnenberg A, Von der Mark K. Skeletal myoblasts utilize a novel $\beta1$-series integrin and not $\alpha6\beta1$ for binding to the E8 and T8 fragments of laminin. J Biol Chem. 1991;266:23593–601.

99. Song WK, Wang W, Sato H, Bielser DA, Kaufman SJ. Expression of $\alpha7$ integrin cytoplasmic domains during skeletal muscle development: alternate forms, conformational change, and homologies with serine/threonine kinases and tyrosine phosphatases. J Cell Sci. 1993;106: 1139–52.

100. Collo G, Starr L, Quaranta V. A new isoform of the laminin receptor integrin $\alpha7\beta1$ is developmentally regulated in skeletal muscle. J Biol Chem. 1993;268:19019–24.

101. Vachon PH, Loechel F, Xu H, Wever UM, Engvall E. Merosin and laminin in myogenesis; specific requirement for merosin in myotube stability and survival. J Cell Biol. 1996;134: 1483–97.

102. Perreault N, Beaulieu J-F. Use of the dissociating enzyme thermolysin to generate viable human normal intestinal epithelial cell cultures. Exp Cell Res. 1996;224:354–64.

16
Recent work with hepatocyte growth/scatter factor

A. SCHMASSMANN, C. HIRSCHI, C. STETTLER, R. POULSOM and F. HALTER

INTRODUCTION

After partial hepatectomy, cells in the remaining liver rapidly proliferate and original liver weight and liver-specific functions are re-established in approximately 10 days[1]. The presence of a blood-borne hepatotropic factor, a potent initiator of liver regeneration, was proposed more than 30 years ago[2]. The existence of a factor that serves as a signal for liver regeneration was verified in 1984: parallel studies have been performed in three different laboratories[3-5]. Hepatocyte growth factor (HGF) was originally purified from serum and platelets. By 1989, the amino acid sequence of HGF was known, the encoding cDNA was cloned, and the gene for human HGF was localized on chromosome 7[6,7]. In 1991, another fibroblast-derived factor, described earlier and called scatter factor (SF) for its ability to disperse tightly packed mammary epithelial cells, was also sequenced and found to be identical to HGF[7,8].

CHARACTERIZATION, DISTRIBUTION, AND REGULATION OF HGF/SF AND ITS RECEPTOR c-met

Characterization of HGF/SF

HGF/SF is translated from a single mRNA, as a single chain prepro-HGF/SF. Prepro-HGF/SF consists of 728 amino acids and is extracellularly cleaved by HGF/SF specific serine protease, HGF/SF activator or converting enzyme to produce the mature heterodimer[6,10-12]. Mature HGF/SF is a large molecule made up of a heavy α chain and a light β chain (Figure 1). It has a 38% sequence homology to plasminogen. The heavy chain has four kringle domains reminiscent of the five kringle domains in plasminogen and those in several other fibrinolytic and coagulation-related proteins. They play an important role in protein–protein interactions. The β chain contains the consensus sequence for serine proteases and has a 37% homology with the β chain of plasmin[13].

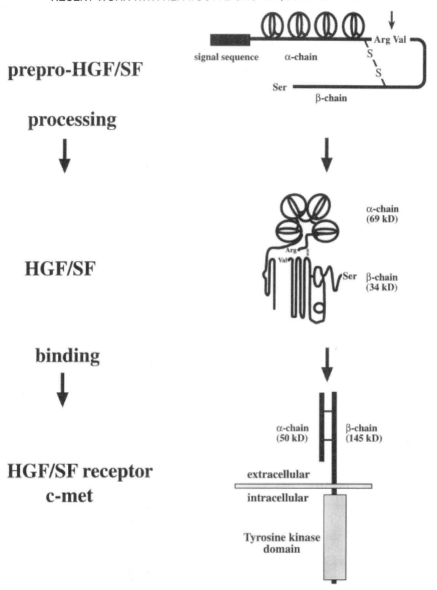

prepro-HGF/SF

processing

HGF/SF

binding

**HGF/SF receptor
c-met**

Figure 1 Schematic structure of prepro-HGF/SF, mature HGF/SF and HGF/SF receptor c-met. HGF/SF is translated from a single mRNA, as a single chain prepro-HGF/SF. The biologically inactive prepro-HGF/SF is extracellularly processed by a converting enzyme to active mature HGF/SF. Mature HGF/SF is a heterodimer with an α-chain and a β-chain, linked by a single disulphide bridge. The α-chain contains four homologous 'kringle domains' and the β-chain has serine protease-like motif. HGF/SF binds to its high affinity receptor c-met. The HGF/SF c-met receptor is a heterodimer composed of an α-chain and a membrane spanning β-chain which contains the intracellular tyrosine kinase domain

Distribution of HGF/SF

HGF/SF is predominantly produced by cells of mesodermal origin, such as fibroblasts, endothelial cells, Kupffer's cells and fat-storing cells in the liver. In addition, HGF/SF is produced by some epithelial cells and malignant cells such as lung, pancreatic cancer and leukaemic cell lines. HGF/SF mRNA was found in human placenta, and rat liver, lung, kidney, stomach and brain. HGF/SF protein was found in liver parenchymal cells, exocrine pancreas, throughout the gastrointestinal tract mucosa and in all squamous epithelia and lining glandular epithelia. However, it is not clear whether all of these cells produce HGF/SF or whether its presence indicates passive uptake, because not all were found to contain HGF/SF mRNA[10–12,14].

Factors regulating production and activation of HGF/SF

Expression of HGF/SF is regulated by various factors. Interleukin-1, platelet-derived growth factor, acidic and basic fibroblast growth factor, epidermal growth factor, prostaglandins and heparin are potent inducers of HGF/SF expression[12,15]. In contrast, transforming growth factor β-1 and glucocorticoids have an inhibitory effect on HGF/SF release from fibroblasts. Injurin, a humeral substance that increases after partial hepatectomy, induces expression of HGF/SF mRNA in intact lungs of rats. Although these regulatory molecules are likely to have distinct roles, the regulatory network for expression of HGF/SF may be involved not only in organ regeneration but also in epithelia–mesenchymal and tumour–stromal interactions during organogenesis and tumour progression, respectively. The liver is especially important in the clearance and subsequent proteolytic activation of HGF/SF[16–18].

Scatter factor

In 1985 Stocker and Perryman[8] reported that conditioned medium from embryo fibroblasts was able to disburse tightly packed mammary epithelial cells. Because of its 'scattering' effect this protein, which was able to induce disassociation and increase local cell motility of a variety of epithelial cells, including some cancer cells and endothelial cells, was termed scatter factor[19]. The standard assay uses the Madin-Darby canine kidney (MDCK) cell line. When SF is added to MDCK cell cultures, these cells change their morphology and cell–cell junctions are disrupted. SF shows both chemotactic and chemokinetic activities. However, SF is not mitogenic to MDCK cells. When the complete amino acid sequences of HGF and SF were obtained it was a surprise to find that SF and HGF are identical[9].

HGF/SF receptor c-met

HGF/SF binds to epithelial and other cells via the high-affinity HGF/SF receptor c-met, a transmembrane tyrosine kinase[20,21]. This transmembrane protein is encoded by a c-met proto-oncogene and consists of a light α-chain and a heavy transmembrane β-chain. The intracellular domain for the β subunit has tyrosine kinase activity and transduces all the effects of HGF/SF (Figure 1). The receptor is expressed on the surface of hepatocytes, gastric epithelial cells, fibroblasts, keratinocytes, and can be detected in the kidney, lung, spleen and some haemopoietic cells[10–12].

The c-met oncogene was originally identified in HOS cells that had been transformed by treatment with a carcinogen[22]. High affinity sites for HGF/SF with a Kd of 20–30 pM was first demonstrated in rat hepatocytes and plasma membranes of the rat liver[23]. The HGF/SF receptor was subsequently shown to be the c-met proto-oncogene product, and conclusive evidence was obtained in expression experiments[24]. Similar to mature hepatocytes, high affinity receptors for HGF/SF with a Kd of 20–30 pM were expressed at 20–1500 sites/cell, predominantly in various types of epithelial cells, but not in fibroblasts[25]. However, target cells of HGF/SF are not exclusively epithelial cells. HGF/SF exerts biological activity on microvascular endothelial cells and some non-differentiated lymphoblasts and monocytes[26,27].

Signal transduction

Signalling by tyrosine kinase receptors is mediated by selective interactions between individual Src homology 2 (SH2) domains of cytoplasmic effectors and specific phosphotyrosine residues in the activated receptor. Signal transduction by the HGF/SF receptor c-met is likely to involve the integration of multiple pathways given the complex biological response that the ligand evokes in epithelial cells[28]. Ponzetto reported the existence in the HGF/SF receptor c-met of a multifunctional docking site made of the tandemly arranged degenerate sequence YVH/NV. Phosphorylation of this site mediates intermediate- to high-affinity interactions with multiple SH2-containing signal transducers, including phosphatidylinositol 3-kinase, phospholipase Cγ, pp60[c-src], and the GRB-2-Sos complex. Mutation of the two tyrosines results in loss of biological function[29].

Transduction of the HGF/SF signal results in either increased division/differentiation of the cells or in cell dissociation and increased motility with loss of adhesion and junctional communication. The type of response seems to depend on the target cell, the culture conditions or cellular microenvironment or structural alterations in HGF/SF or HGF/SF receptor c-met[30].

BIOLOGICAL ACTIVITY OF HGF/SF

HGF/SF was initially considered to have a narrow target cell specificity and to act only as a mitogen. Further studies, however, have shown that HGF/SF exerts multiple biological activities as a mitogen, motogen and morphogen for various types of cells (Table 1)[10–12,31,32]. HGF/SF has mitogenic activity for epithelial cells, endothelial cells, some stromal cells, and various species of carcinoma cells. HGF/SF has an angiogenic activity when implanted in vivo. Recent studies revealed that HGF/SF is also involved in haematopoiesis, chondrogenesis and bone remodelling[12]. HGF/SF stimulates proliferation of haematopoietic progenitor cells and enhances the formation of colonies toward erythroid lineage or granulocyte–erythroid–megakaryocyte lineage. HGF/SF enhances growth and differentiation of osteoclastic cells at the terminal stage. Articular chondrocytes are target cells of HGF/SF and HGF/SF mRNA is expressed at presumptive articular regions during development.

HGF/SF has been involved in organ regeneration including liver, kidney, lung and gastrointestinal tract as well as in fetal organ development. Because of its impact on cell proliferation and motility, HGF/SF may influence tumour propagation and development of distant metastases.

Mitogenic activity of HGF/SF

HGF/SF is the single most potent in vitro mitogen for hepatocytes, being 100-fold more active than transforming growth factor α or epidermal growth factor[31]. it is species indiscriminate. However, the stimulatory effect is restricted to normal hepatocytes; in the presence of HGF/SF, growth of hepatoma cell lines is inhibited[33]. HGF/SF also stimulates growth of other target cells, as summarized in Table 1.

Motogenic activity of HGF/SF

Cell movement is an important process during embryogenesis, wound healing and tumour invasion. Although some growth factors are known to enhance cell motility, HGF is one of the most potent motogens, inducing dissociation and movement in various types of cells. HGF/SF stimulates the motility of various cells in monolayer culture, including MDCK canine kidney epithelial cells, epidermal keratinocytes, HepG2 hepatoma cells, A431 and KB human squamous cell carcinoma cells, and PAM 212 murine keratinocytes and others (Table 1). It does not stimulate motility of cells such as human epidermal melanocytes and various fibroblasts (Table 1)[19,25,34].

From the results on effects of HGF/SF on cell growth and cell motility or scattering in various cell species, it is concluded that cell growth and cell motility/scattering are independently regulated by HGF/SF. HGF/SF induces marked scattering of MDCK cells yet it has no effect on growth of MDCK cells. On the other hand, cell growth stimulation by HGF/SF in PAM212 cells, A4341 cells and Lu99 cells is linked to cell scattering, whereas cell scattering by HGF/SF in KB cells and HepG2 cells is linked to inhibition of cell growth.

The motogenic activity of HGF is mediated by activation of small GTP-binding proteins, Rho, Ras and Rac. Disruption and regulation of cell–cell and cell–matrix interactions are related to the phosphorylation of E-cadherin-associated molecules (β-catenin, plakoglobin and p120) and focal adhesion kinase (p125[FAK]), respectively. HGF also disrupts intercellular communications mediated by gap junctions[12].

Morphogenic activity of HGF/SF

Among the multipotent characteristics of HGF/SF, the morphogenic activity is notable and unique and is not mimicked by any other known growth factors[36–39].

Table 1 Biological activities of HGF and target cells

Mitogenic
  Hepatocytes and hepatic ductular epithelial cells
  Renal tubular cells
  Gastric epithelial cells
  Mammary gland epithelial cells
  Vascular endothelial cells
  Bronchial and alveolar type II epithelial cells
  Thyroid cells, pancreatic β cells
  Keratinocytes, hair cells, melanocytes
  Schwann cells
  Placental cytotrophoblasts
  Prostate epithelial cells
  Osteoclast-like cells, articular chondrocytes
  Haemopoietic progenitor cells, etc.

Motogenic
  Renal epithelial cells
  Hepatic ductular epithelial cells
  Keratinocytes
  Thyroid cell
  Mammary gland epithelial cells
  Vascular endothelial cells
  Articular chondrocytes
  Myogenic precursor cells
  Oral squamous carcinoma cells, etc.

Morphogenic
  Renal epithelial cells
  Hepatic epithelial cells
  Gastric epithelial cells
  Mammary gland epithelial cells
  Colon carcinoma cells, etc.

Tumour inhibition
  Hepatoma cells (HepG2, etc.)
  B6/F1 melanoma cells
  KB squamous carcinoma cells, etc.

Montensano et al.[36] showed that MDCK renal epithelial cells grown in collagen gel matrix in the presence of conditioned medium of fibroblasts such as MRC-5 form branching tubules, instead of the spherical cysts that develop in the absence of the conditioned medium. The fibroblast-derived molecule responsible for epithelia tubulogenesis was identified as HGF/SF[27]. As HGF/SF is synthesized by mesenchymal cells and potently induces epithelial morphogenesis by several epithelial cells (Table 1), it is one of the long-sought paracrine mediators of morphogenetic epithelial–mesenchymal interactions[36,37].

HGF/SF in epithelial–mesenchymal interactions and development

Interactions between epithelium and mesenchyme mediate crucial aspects of normal development, affecting tissue induction, organogenesis and morphogenesis of specific multicellular structures (Table 2). Development and morphogenesis of various organs and tissues, including kidney, lung, liver, pancreas, limb, tooth,

Table 2 Pleiotropic roles of HGF during embryo-genesis, organ regeneration and tumour progression

---

Embryogenesis in fetus
  Branching morphogenesis
    Kidney
    Lung
    Liver
    Gastrointestinal tract, etc.
  Skeletal morphogenesis
  Cell migration
    Migration of myogenic precursor cells, etc.

Organ regeneration in adults
  Liver
  Kidney
  Lung
  Gastrointestinal tract

Tumour invasion in adults
  Tumour growth
  Tumour invasion and metastasis

---

mammary gland and hair follicle depend on epithelial – mesenchymal interactions. Localization of HGF/SF and c-met receptor mRNA in various tissues indicates that functional coupling between HGF/SF and the c-met receptor is important for development, morphogenesis and migration of cells in other tissues, including limb, branchial arches, lung, tooth and bone[10–12,40–50].

TISSUE REPAIR AND REGENERATION

Interactions between epithelium and mesenchyme also mediate crucial aspects of organ regeneration after tissue injury (Table 2). Initially, HGF/SF was studied for its role in liver regeneration; however, further studies revealed that HGF/SF is also a key molecule in regeneration of kidney and lung and in gastrointestinal wound healing.

Liver regeneration

The role of HGF/SF in liver regeneration was suggested by its potent mitogenic effect on mature hepatocytes. Apart from inducing rapid cell division of paren-chymal cells, HGF/SF also stimulates biliary epithelial cell proliferation, and thereby affects the entire organ[51].

Damage to the liver (e.g. CCl_4 administration) causes a rapid increase of DNA synthesis with a peak after 24–72 h. HGF/SF activity in the liver of rats increased markedly 12 h after CCl_4 administration and was 20 times higher than normal after 30 h. HGF/SF mRNA markedly and rapidly increased in the liver. HGF/SF mRNA increased as early as 5 h after injury and reached a maximum after 10 h[52]. Growth of hepatocytes during liver regeneration following liver injury which accompanies direct hepatocellular damage seems to be mainly regulated by HGF/SF, which seems to act at least in part through a paracrine mechanism.

After partial hepatectomy, there is no direct damage to hepatocytes in the remnant liver, unlike the situation following administration of CCl_4. HGF/SF activity increases rapidly in the blood of rats after partial hepatectomy or unilateral nephrectomy. An increased concentration of mRNA coding for HGF/SF was detected in the lung and spleen; this observation emphasizes the regulation of HGF/SF production by humeral factors such as injurin[18]. Additional observations suggest that HGF/SF is an important player in liver regeneration. Labelled exogenous HGF/SF binds strongly to the remaining hepatocytes after liver resection, and infusion of HGF/SF greatly accelerates repair in the organ[53,54]. In transgenic mice that express HGF/SF under the control of albumin regulatory sequences, hepatocytes expressed high concentrations of HGF/SF as an autocrine growth factor. HGF/SF was a strong stimulus for liver regeneration; the livers of these transgenic mice recovered more quickly than did those of the wild-type after partial hepatectomy.

HGF/SF causes liver regeneration through at least two mechanisms: one is a paracrine mechanism in which HGF/SF is rapidly produced by Kupffer cells, Ito cells and sinusoidal endothelial cells in the liver. The other is an endocrine mechanism through which HGF/SF is supplied from extrahepatic organs, through blood circulation. In the case of direct hepatocellular injury, HGF/SF supplied by a paracrine mechanism is more predominant, while following partial hepatectomy, HGF/SF supplied by an endocrine mechanism is more important[10-12].

Kidney and lung regeneration

HGF/SF mRNA is rapidly increased in the remaining tissues after unilateral nephrectomy[55,56]. There is also a pronounced increase in circulating HGF/SF concentrations after renal injury. In vitro HGF/SF stimulates DNA synthesis in renal tubular cells, and also increases epithelial tubule formation. Recently, HGF/SF was shown to ameliorate acute renal injury in several animal models. Thus, in rats treated with GF/SF, renal function was better after bilateral renal artery occlusions than in non-treated animals, and in mice, cisplatin-mediated acute renal failure was prevented by intravenous HGF/SF[57,58]. These new data indicate that HGF/SF may be a crucial renotropic factor. Further studies have also shown that HGF/SF has a relevant role in lung regeneration after injury[10-12].

Gastrointestinal wound healing

HGF/SF has a relevant role in gastrointestinal wound repair[59-64]. Artificial gastric wounds in rabbits heal faster with administration of HGF/SF[63]. SGF/SF reduces transepithelial resistance to passive ion flow when added to T84 intestinal epithelial cell monolayers. This effect results from a specific alteration of paracellular junction resistance. HGF/SF also enhances the closure of intestinal epithelial wounds by influencing migratory and spreading responses[59-64].

HGF/SF mRNA could only be detected in minimal amounts of the intact gastrointestinal wall but is found in abundance during gastric ulcer healing, assessed by in situ hybridization in our laboratories. HGF/SF mRNA were detected between

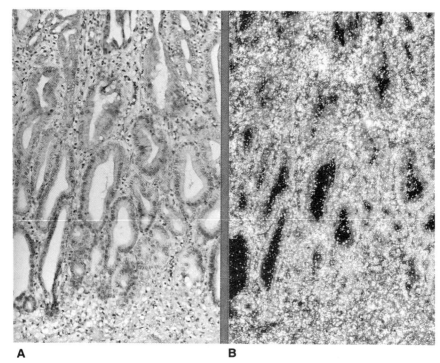

A   **B**

Figure 2   Regenerative glands in the mucosal ulcer scar of the stomach, 15 days after injury. (A) Regenerative glands in mucosal ulcer scar (Giemsa staining, light field illumination, original magnification, × 100). (B) In situ hybridization for HGF/SF using dark field illumination: HGF/SF mRNA was detected in numerous cells scattered in the stromal compartment between regenerative glands. HGF/SF which is secreted in the stromal compartment stimulates epithelial cells in the mucosal ulcer scar which express the HGF/SF c-met receptor

epithelial glands probably in fibroblasts both in the early phase in the ulcer margin as well as in the late phase between remodelled epithelial glands (Figure 2). In addition, HGF/SF mRNA was detected in cells associated with vessels in the submucosa[65].

HGF/SF c-met receptor mRNA was detected in low concentrations in the mucous neck cells in the intact mucosa. After injury, c-met receptor mRNA was increased in epithelial cells adjacent to the ulcer margin (Figure 2)[66,67]. In contrast, c-met protein was nearly absent on day 3, reappeared on day 8, and was over-expressed on day 15. The down-regulation of c-met receptor protein in the early healing phase is probably due to HGF/SF binding and internalization of the receptor (Figure 2). These combined data suggest HGF/SF in the healing of gastric ulcers.

In vivo administration of HGF/SF

Direct confirmation for the organotrophic roles of HGF/SF has been acquired from in vivo studies and these studies suggested potential therapeutic strategies using recombinant HGF/SF. Administration of HGF to experimental animals with liver injury strongly enhanced liver regeneration and, importantly, suppressed the onset of hepatic dysfunction. Furthermore, HGF/SF prevented the onset of liver fibrosis/cirrhoses and abrogated lethal hepatic dysfunction due to chronic liver injury. HGF/SF enhances renal regeneration and suppresses the onset of acute renal failure caused by renal toxins, renal ischaemia or unilateral nephrectomy. Mitogenic, motogenic and morphogenic activities, all of which are required for reconstruction of tissue architecture, are responsible for the organotrophic functions of HGF/SF[12]. During gastric ulcer healing, the morphogenic properties of HGF/SF are particularly important in the late healing phase, when formation of gland lumen, branching and reconstruction of glandular structure occur.

HGF/SF AND MALIGNANCY

Because of its significant impact on growth and motility, HGF/SF may well be an important factor in tumour propagation and development of distant metastases. Thus, transfection of c-met receptor-negative cells with receptor cDNA resulted in increased motility and tumorigenicity.

Both malignant and normal cells can over-express HGF/SF receptor. Hepatocytes show increased c-met receptor expression after liver and kidney resection or injury, but the level of expression returns to normal shortly afterwards. Normal cells therefore control their proliferative response to HGF/SF by lowering the number of receptors. Expression of c-met receptor on malignant cells does not change; this property might contribute to their invasive nature.

Experiments with transfected NIH 3T3 cells, which produced HGF/SF but do not stimulate their own growth unless transfected the c-met receptor, suggest a possible role for autocrine and paracrine stimulation of tumour growth[68]. Because HGF/SF stimulates endothelial cell proliferation, another possible regulatory effect on tumour growth is angiogenesis – i.e. induction of neovasculature by modulation of the tumour matrix. Ingrowth of new blood vessels has been induced in mouse subcutaneous tissue and rat cornea by HGF/SF-containing implants.

A great surprise in the HGF/SF story so far has been the recognition that a cytotoxic factor produced by IMR-90 human fibroblasts, which is toxic to most sarcoma cells and cytostatic to a number of other cell lines, is also identical to HGF/SF[69]. Subsequent work has shown that HGF/SF inhibits the growth of other cell lines such as certain hepatoma cell lines, including HepG2[70]. The mechanism underlying this effect is uncertain. Intracellular signals for HGF/SF stimulation in normal and malignant hepatocytes are not alike: HGF/SF induces tyrosine phosphorylation of the phospholipase C in normal cells but not in hepatoma cells. Similar growth inhibition has been observed with other malignant cell lines.

PERSPECTIVE AND FUTURE DIRECTIONS

It is now well accepted that HGF/SF is a pleiotropic factor whose biological role is not entirely clear. The biological and physiological functions of HGF/SF have been much greater than expected. However, much work remains in order to determine how HGF/SF exerts its highly diversified activities and how it is involved in construction of organized multicellular tissue structures.

HGF/SF regulates cell proliferation, motility and morphogenesis and has an important role in embryonic development. HGF/SF plays a significant part in regeneration of liver, kidney and lung and regulates wound healing in the gastro-intestinal tract. By influencing the growth and invasiveness of malignant cells, HGF/SF is a relevant regulator of metastasis formation.

Because of its organotrophic functions, HGF/SF may well have therapeutic potential for disorders of the liver, kidney and lung. HGF/SF is highly effective for chronic and often incurable hepatic disease, such as liver fibrosis/cirrhosis. Use of the HGF/SF gene as a therapeutic for chronic diseases may be feasible. The generation and application of antagonistic molecules of HGF/SF may prove to be therapeutic in inhibiting tumour invasion and metastasis.

References

1. Higgins GM, Anderson RM. Experimental pathology of the liver: I. Restoration of the liver of the white rat following partial surgical removal. Arch Pathol. 1931;12:186–202.
2. Bucher NLR. Regeneration of mammalian liver. Int Rev Cytol. 1963;15:245–300.
3. Nakamura T, Nawa K, Ichihara A. Partial purification and characterization of hepatocyte growth factor from serum of hepatectomized rats. Biochem Biophys Res Commun. 1984;122:1450–9.
4. Michalopoulos GK, Houck KA, Dolan ML, Luetteke NC. Control of hepatocyte replication by two serum factors. Cancer Res. 1984;44:4414–19.
5. Russel WE, McGowan JA, Bucher NLR. Partial characterization of a hepatocyte growth factor from rat platelets. J Cell Physiol. 1984;119:183–92.
6. Nakamura T, Nishizawa T, Hagiya M et al. Molecular cloning and expression of human hepatocyte growth factor. Nature. 1989;342:440–3.
7. Zarnegar R, Peterson B, DeFrances MC, Michalopoulos G. Localization of hepatocyte growth factor (HGF) gene on human chromosome 7. Genomics. 1992;12:147–50.
8. Stocker M, Perryman M. An epithelial scatter factor released by embryo fibroblasts. J Cell Sci. 1985;77:209–23.
9. Weidner KM, Arakaki N, Hartmann G et al. Evidence for the identity of human scatter factor and human hepatocyte growth factor. Proc Natl Acad Sci USA. 1991;88:7001–5.
10. Matsumoto K, Nakamura T. In: Goldberg ID, Rosen EM, editors. Hepatocyte growth factor scatter factor (HGF-SF) and c-MET receptor. Basel: Birkhauser Verlag 1993:225–49.
11. Boros P, Miller CM. Hepatocyte growth factor: a multifunctional cytokine. Lancet. 1995;345: 293–5.
12. Matsumoto K, Nakamura T. Emerging multipotent aspects of hepatocyte growth factor. J Biochem. 1996;119:591–600.
13. Tashiro K, Hagiya M, Nishizawa T et al. Deduced primary structure of rat hepatocyte growth factor and expression of the mRNA in rat tissues. Proc Natl Acad Sci USA. 1990;87:3200–4.
14. Wolf HK, Zarnegar R, Michalopoulos GK. Localization of hepatocyte growth factor in human and rat tissues: an immunohistochemical study. Hepatology. 1991;14:488–94.
15. Tamura M, Arakaki N, Tsubouchi H, Takada H, Daikuhara Y. Enhancement of human hepatocyte growth factor production by interleukin-1 alpha and -1 beta and tumor necrosis factor-alpha by fibroblasts in culture. J Biol Chem. 1993;268:8140–5.
16. Miyazawa K, Shimomura T, Kitamura N. Activation of hepatocyte growth factor in the injured tissues is mediated by hepatocyte growth factor activator. J Biol Chem. 1996;271:3615–18.
17. Zioncheck TF, Richardson L, DeGuzman GG, Modi NB, Hansen SE, Godowski PJ. The pharma-cokinetics, tissue localization, and metabolic processing of recombinant human hepatocyte growth factor after intravenous administration in rats. Endocrinology. 1994;134:1879–87.
18. Matsumoto K, Tajima H, Hamanoue M, Kohno S, Kinoshita T, Nakamura T. Identification and characterization of 'injurin' an inducer of expression of the gene for hepatocyte growth factor. Proc Natl Acad Sci USA. 1992;89:3800–4.

19. Gherardi E, Gray J, Stoker M, Perryman M, Furlong R. Purification of scatter factor, a fibroblast-derived basic protein that modulates epithelial interactions and movement. Proc Natl Acad Sci USA. 1989;86:5844–8.

20. Bottaro DP, Rubin JS, Faletto DL *et al.* Identification of the hepatocyte growth factor receptor as the c-met proto-oncogene product. Science. 1991;251:802–4.

21. Naldini L, Vigna E, Narsimhan RP *et al.* Hepatocyte growth factor (HGF) stimulates the tyrosine kinase activity of the receptor encoded by the proto-oncogene c-MET. Oncogene. 1991; 6:501–4.

22. Rhim JA, Park DK, Arnstein P, Huebner RJ, Weisburger EK. Transformation of human cells in culture in culture by *N*-methyl-*N'*-nitro-*N*-nitrosoguanidine. Nature. 1975;256:751–3.

23. Higuchi O, Nakamura T. Identification and change in the receptor for hepatocyte growth factor in rat liver after partial hepatectomy or induced hepatitis. Biochem Biophys Res Commun. 1991; 176:599–607.

24. Higuchi O, Mizuno K, Vande Woude GF, Nakamura T. Expression of c-met proto-oncogene in COX cells induces the signal transducing high-affinity receptor for hepatocyte growth factor. FEBS Lett. 1992;301:282–6.

25. Tajima H, Matsumoto K, Nakamura T. Regulation of cell growth and motility by hepatocyte growth factor and receptor expression in various cell species. Exp Cell Res. 1992;202:423–31.

26. Morimoto A, Okamura K, Hamanaka R *et al.* Renotropic functions of hepatocyte growth factor in renal regeneration after unilateral nephrectomy. J Biol Chem. 1991;266:22781–4.

27. Hayashi S, Morishita R, Higaki J *et al.* Autocrine-paracrine effects of overexpression of hepatocyte growth factor gene on growth of endothelial cells. Biochem Biophys Res Commun. 1996; 220:539–45.

28. Zhu H, Naujokas MA, Fixman ED, Torossian K, Park M. Tyrosine 1356 in the carboxyl terminal tail of the HGF/SF receptor is essential for the transduction of signals for cell motility and morphogenesis. J Biol Chem. 1994;269:29943–8.

29. Ponzetto C, Bardelli A, Zhen Z *et al.* A multifunctioning docking site mediates signalling and transformation by the hepatocyte growth factor/scatter factor receptor family. Cell. 1994;77: 261–71.

30. Hartmann G, Naldini L, Weidner KM *et al.* A functional domain in the heavy chain of scatter factor/hepatocyte growth factor binds the cMet receptor and induces cell dissociation but not mitogenesis. Proc Natl Acad Sci USA. 1992;89:11574–8.

31. Nakamura T, Teramoto H, Ichihara A. Purification and characterization of a growth factor from rat platelets for mature parenchymal hepatocytes in primary cultures. Proc Natl Acad Sci USA. 1986;83:6489–93.

32. Weidner KM, Sachs M, Birchmeier W. The Met receptor tyrosine kinase transduces motility, proliferation, and morphogenic signals of scatter factor/hepatocyte growth factor in epithelial cells. J Cell Biol. 1993;121:145–54.

33. Tajima H, Matsumoto K, Nakamura T. Hepatocyte growth factor has a potent anti-proliferative activity for various tumor cell lines. FEBS Lett. 1991;291:229–32.

34. Matsumoto K, Hashimoto K, Yoshikawa K, Nakamura T. Marked stimulation of growth and motility of human keratinocytes by hepatocyte growth factor. Exp Cell Res. 1991;196:114–20.

35. Montesano R, Schaller G, Orci L. Induction of epithelial tubular morphogenesis in vitro by fibroblast-derived soluble factors. Cell. 1991;66:697–711.

36. Montesano R, Matsumoto K, Nakamura T, Orci L. Identification of a fibroblast-derived epithelial morphogen as hepatocyte growth factor. Cell. 1991;67:901–8.

37. Barros EJ, Santos OF, Matsumoto K, Nakamura T, Nigam SK. Differential tubulogenic and branching morphogenetic activities of growth factors: implications for epithelial tissue development. Proc Natl Acad Sci USA. 1995;92:4412–16.

38. Nishikawa Y, Yokusashi Y, Kadohama T, Nishimori H, Ogawa K. Hepatocytic cells form bile duct-like structures within a three-dimensional collagen gel matrix. Exp Cell Res. 1996;223:357–71.

39. Tsarfaty I, Resau JH, Rulong S, Keydar I, Faletto DL, Vande-Woude GF. The met proto oncogene receptor and lumen formation. Science. 1992;257:1258–61.

40. Sonnenberg E, Meyer D, Weidner KM, Birchmeier C. Scatter factor/hepatocyte growth factor and its receptor the c-met tyrosine kinase can mediate a signal exchange between mesenchymal and epithelia during mouse development. J Cell Biol. 1993;123:223–35.

41. Santos OF, Barros EJ, Yang X-M, Matsumoto K, Nakamura T, Nigam SK. Involvement of hepatocyte growth factor in kidney development. Dev Biol. 1994;163:525–9.

42. Woolf AS, Kolatsi-Joannou M, Hardman P *et al*. Role of hepatocyte growth factor/scatter factor and the Met receptor in the early development of the metanephros. J Cell Biol. 1995;128:171–84.
43. Schmidt C, Bladt F, Goedecke S *et al*. Scatter factor/hepatocyte growth factor is essential for liver development. Nature. 1995;373:699–702.
44. Uehara Y, Minowa O, Mori C *et al*. Placental defect and embryonic lethality in mice lacking hepatocyte growth factor/scatter factor. Nature. 1995;373:702–5.
45. Soriano JV, Pepper MS, Nakamura T, Orci L, Montesano R. Hepatocyte growth factor stimulates extensive development of branching duct-like structures by cloned mammary gland epithelia cells. J Cell Sci. 1995;108:413–30.
46. Niranjan B, Biuluwela L, Yant J *et al*. HGF/Sf: A potent cytokine for mammary growth morphogenesis and development. Development. 1995;121:2897–908.
47. Yang YM, Spitzer E, Meyer D *et al*. Sequential requirement of hepatocyte growth factor and neuregulin in the morphogenesis and differentiation of the mammary gland. J Cell Biol. 1995; 131:215–26.
48. Tabata MJ, Kim K, Liu J *et al*. Hepatocyte growth factor involved in the morphogenesis of tooth germ in murine molars. Development, in press.
49. Myokai F, Washio N, Asahara Y *et al*. Expression of the hepatocyte growth factor gene during chick limb development. Dev Dynamics. 1995;202:80–90.
50. Thery C, Sharpe MJ, Batley SJ, Stern CD, Gherardi E. Expression of HGF/Sf, HGF1/MSP, and c-met suggests new functions during early chick development. Dev Genet. 1995;17:90–101.
51. Joplin R, Hishida T, Tsubouchi H *et al*. Human intrahepatic biliary epithelia cells proliferate in vitro in response to human hepatocyte growth factor. J Clin Invest. 1992;9:1284–9.
52. Kinoshita T, Tashiro K, Nakamura T. Marked increase of HGF mRNA in non-parenchymal liver cells of rats treated with hepatotoxins. Biochem Biophys Res Commun. 1989;165:1229–34.
53. Kobayashi Y, Hamanoue M, Ueno S *et al*. Induction of hepatocyte growth by intraportal infusion of HGF into beagle dogs. Biochem Biophys Res Commun. 1996;220:7–12.
54. Liu KX, Kato Y, Narukawa M *et al*. Importance of the liver in plasma clearance of hepatocyte growth factors in rats. Am J Physiol. 1992;263:G642–9.
55. Ishibashi K, Sasaki S, Sakamoto H, Hoshino Y, Nakamura T, Marumo F. Expressions of receptor gene for hepatocyte growth factor in kidney after unilateral nephrectomy and renal injury. Biochem Biophys Res Commun. 1992;187:1454–9.
56. Joannidis M, Spokes K, Nakamura T, Faletto D, Cantley LG. Regional expression of hepatocyte growth factor/c-met in experimental renal hypertrophy and hyperplasia. Am J Physiol. 1994;267: F231–6.
57. Igawa T, Matsumoto K, Kanda S, Saito Y, Nakamura T. Hepatocyte growth factor may function as a renotropic factor for regeneration in rats with acute renal injury. Am J Physiol. 1993;265: F61–9.
58. Miller SB, Martin DR, Kissane J, Hammerman MR. Hepatocyte growth factor accelerates recovery from acute ischemic renal injury in rats. Am J Physiol. 1994;266:F129–34.
59. Dignass AU, Lynch-Devaney K, Podolsky DK. Hepatocyte growth factor/scatter factor modulates intestinal epithelial cell proliferation and migration. Biochem Biophys Res Commun. 1994;202: 701–9.
60. Fukamachi H, Ichinose M, Tsukada S *et al*. Hepatocyte growth factor region specifically stimulates gastrointestinal epithelial growth in primary culture. Biochem Biophys Res Commun. 1994; 205:1445–51.
61. Takahashi M, Ota S, Terano A *et al*. Hepatocyte growth factor induces mitogenic reaction to the rabbit gastric epithelial cells in primary culture. Biochem Biophys Res Commun. 1993;191: 528–34.
62. Watanabe S, Hirose M, Wang XE *et al*. Hepatocyte growth factor accelerates the wound repair of cultured gastric mucosal cells. Biochem Biophys Res Commun. 1994;199:1453–60.
63. Takahashi M, Ota S, Shimada T *et al*. Hepatocyte growth factor is the most potent endogenous stimulant of rabbit gastric epithelial cell proliferation and migration in primary culture. J Clin Invest. 1995;95:1994–2003.
64. Nusrat A, Parkos CA, Bacarra AE *et al*. Hepatocyte growth factor/scatter factor effects on epithelia. Regulation of intercellular junctions in transformed and nontransformed cell lines, basolateral polarization of c-met receptor in transformed and natural intestinal epithelia, and induction of rapid wound repair in a transformed model epithelium. J Clin Invest. 1994;93:2056–65.

65. Kinoshita Y, Nakata H, Hassan S *et al*. Gene expression of keratinocyte and hepatocyte growth factors during the healing of rat gastric mucosal lesions. Gastroenterology. 1995;109:1068–77.
66. Tsujii M, Kawano S, Tsuji S *et al*. Increased expression of c-met messenger RNA following acute gastric injury in rats. Biochem Biophys Res Commun. 1994;200:536–41.
67. Tsuji S, Kawano S, Tsujii M, Fusamoto H, Kamada T. Roles of hepatocyte growth factor and its receptor in gastric mucosa. A cell biological and molecular biological study. Dig Dis Sci. 1995; 40:1132–9.
68. Cooper CS. The met oncogene: from detection by transfection to transmembrane receptor for hepatocyte growth factor. Oncogene. 1992;7:3–7.
69. Higashio K, Shima N, Goto M *et al*. Identity of a tumor cytotoxic factor from human fibroblasts and hepatocyte growth factor. Biochem Biophys Res Commun. 1990;170:397–404.
70. Shiota G, Rhoads DB, Wang TC, Nakamura T, Schmidt EV. Hepatocyte growth factor inhibits growth of hepatocellular carcinoma cells. Proc Natl Acad Sci USA. 1992;89:373–7.

17
E-Cadherin/catenin complex in the gastrointestinal tract

M. PIGNATELLI, A. J. KARAYIANNAKIS, M. NODA, J. EFSTATHIOU
and W. KMIOT

E-CADHERIN/CATENIN COMPLEX

The cadherins constitute a large family of glycoproteins which mediate cell to cell adhesion through calcium-dependent, homotypic interactions[1]. To date, more than 16 cadherin molecules have been identified, among which are the classical E-cadherin (epithelial), N-cadherin (neural) found in muscle and neural tissues and P-cadherin, originally identified in mouse placenta but also expressed in some human epithelia[2]. Different cadherin molecules share common structural and functional features. They consist of an extracellular amino-terminal domain, a cell membrane spanning part and a carboxy-cytoplasmic domain. They show a high degree of sequence identity, especially in their cytoplasmic domain, while the extracellular domain exhibits less homology[2,3]. The extracellular domain of the classic cadherins is divided into five repeated domains, EC1–EC5. The first extracellular domain in the N-terminal region (EC1 domain) contains a highly conserved sequence between cadherin subclasses, the tripeptide His-Ala-Val, where cadherin-binding activity resides[4]. Nuclear magnetic resonance spectroscopy analysis and X-ray crystallography have provided insights into the three-dimensional structure of the cadherin molecule[5,6]. Results from these studies suggested that two extracellular domain monomers are arranged in parallel to form a dimer. The cadherin dimers from interacting cell surfaces bind in such a way that they form a linear 'zipper' at the intercellular contact space[6].

Adhesion between epithelial cells is mediated mainly by E-cadherin[7,8]. This 120 kDa transmembrane glycoprotein, known also as L-CAM, uvomorulin, ARC-1 and cell-CAM 120/80, is constitutively expressed in all epithelia with endo-, meso- and ectodermal origin and its gene has been mapped to chromosome 16q.22.1[1,9,10]. E-cadherin is localized mainly in the zonula adherens junctions. Its extracellular part consists of three domains which in the presence of calcium ions interact with the E-cadherin molecule of the neighbouring cell to form a tight cell–cell adhesion. The cytoplasmic domain (15 kDa) is associated with a group of closely related but distinct undercoat proteins, termed catenins (α-, β- and γ-

catenin)[1,11]. α-Catenin is a 102 kDa protein homologous to the focal contact associated protein vinculin[12,13]; β-catenin (88 kDa) shows homology to the *Drosophila* segment polarity gene protein *armadillo* and to plakoglobin[14,15], while γ-catenin (82 kDa) is identical to plakoglobin, a major component of desmosomal and zonula adherens junctions[15,16]. Catenins play an essential role in cadherin-mediated cell adhesion. Both β-catenin and γ-catenin are capable of direct binding to the cytoplasmic domain of E-cadherin while α-catenin links the bound β-catenin or γ-catenin to the actin microfilament network of the cellular cytoskeleton. This binding is essential for the adhesive function of E-cadherin and for establishment of tight physical cell–cell adhesion[17–21].

A number of studies have shown that the E-cadherin/catenin complex plays a key role in cell adhesion and that structural and functional integrity of the components of this complex are necessary for this purpose. Exposure to E-cadherin neutralizing antibodies or deletion of its encoding gene causes cells to dissociate from each other[22,23]. Truncated cadherin molecules whose cytoplasmic domain is deleted cannot bind to catenins and lose their adhesive capacity, even though the extracellular domain is expressed on the cell surface[18,19]. Similarly, loss of the extracellular E-cadherin domain also perturbs cell adhesion[24,25], as does point mutation in the calcium binding site of E-cadherin[26,27]. Reduced or absent E-cadherin expression is also associated with increased motility in several carcinoma cells lines[22,23]. Conversely, transfection of E-cadherin cDNA into poorly differentiated carcinoma cell lines increases cellular adhesion and inhibits their invasive phenotype. This effect was reversed after treatment of the transfected cells with anti-E-cadherin antibodies[28–31]. In vitro studies also provided direct evidence for the requirement of α-catenin and β-catenin for proper cell–cell adhesion. Cells expressing E-cadherin and β-catenin but lacking α-catenin show minimal intercellular cohesion[32], whereas after transfection with α-catenin cDNA they acquire strong intercellular adhesiveness[33]. Similarly, cells expressing E-cadherin, α- and γ-catenins but lacking β-catenin do not aggregate; their non-adhesiveness is reversed after transfection with β-catenin cDNA[34].

Despite the evidence that catenins are necessary for the establishment of cell –cell adhesion, the underlying mechanisms by which they regulate and/or modulate cadherin function are not known. However, there is some evidence that cadherin adhesion may be regulated by tyrosine phosphorylation. In cells transfected with the v-*src* oncogene, increased tyrosine phosphorylation of β-catenin and E-cadherin was observed and this resulted in functional changes such as decreased adhesion, increased migration and increased invasiveness, without affecting the overall expression of either the catenins or the cadherins[35,36]. Recently it was found that β-catenin associates with the epidermal growth factor receptor (EGFR)[37]. It is well established that EGFR has tyrosine kinase activity, which is activated through autophosphorylation upon its binding to epidermal growth factor (EGF). This event induces several cellular changes, including alteration of cellular morphology, cell proliferation and induction of cell motility in certain epithelial cells, through tyrosine phosphorylation of other intracellular proteins[37–39]. Indeed, EGF as well as hepatocyte growth factor have been found to induce tyrosine phosphorylation of β-catenin and γ-catenin[37,40]. Interestingly, this was associated with redistribution of E-cadherin from the intercellular junction to the apical surface of cell membrane, resulting in increased cell dissociation, increased motility and invasion[41]. Further evidence for the possible role of tyrosine phosphorylation as the mechanism by which cadherin/catenin function is modulated comes from the finding that the intracellular domain of E-cadherin can also associate with the p120 protein[42]. This protein, which is homologous to β-catenin and γ-catenin, is a substrate of several receptor tyrosine kinases and is phosphorylated after treatment with several growth factors, including EGF[36,42].

Another recent important finding was that β-catenin associates also with the adenomatous polyposis coli (APC) gene product[43,44] and that E-cadherin and APC directly compete for binding to β-catenin. Plakoglobin (γ-catenin) also binds directly to APC, suggesting that the APC protein can form distinct complexes containing combinations of α-catenin, β-catenin and γ-catenin which are independent from the cadherin–catenin complexes, and through them bind to the cytoskeleton[45,46]. These findings suggest that tyrosine phosphorylation of β-catenin might be a significant mechanism that modulates E-cadherin/catenin mediated cell adhesion. Moreover, it also raises the possibility that β-catenin participates in several important cellular functions such as cell growth and differentiation.

E-CADHERIN/CATENIN COMPLEX IN MORPHOGENESIS AND DIFFERENTIATION

The expression of cadherins is developmentally regulated. Differential expression of several cadherins and distinct spatiotemporal changes in their expression occur during embryogenesis in association with a variety of morphological events that involve cell aggregation[9].

The role of the cadherins and catenins in embryonic development and epithelial morphogenesis has been evaluated in vivo by gene targeting experiments in mouse embryonic stem cells and subsequent generation of transgenic or chimeric animals. Studies on E-cadherin gene knockout mice revealed that E-cadherin mediated cell adhesion is essential for the compaction of mesenchymal cells and their transition into a polarized epithelium. Homologous deletion of E-cadherin was associated with lack of trophoectodermal epithelium or a blastocyst cavity formation and with early embryonic death[47,48]. Similarly, deletion of β-catenin resulted in absence of mesoderm formation, disturbed ectoderm development and caused early death[49].

In a chimeric-transgenic animal model, a dominant negative N-cadherin mutant was expressed in mouse intestinal epithelial cells. Expression of this construct in the villous enterocytes alone resulted in disruption of cell–cell and cell–matrix adhesion. Perturbation of cell–cell adhesion was associated with increased enterocyte migration rate along the crypt-villus axis, loss of their differentiated polarized phenotype and increased apoptosis[50]. When the dominant negative N-cadherin mutant was expressed along the entire crypt-villus axis, disrupted cell–cell adhesion resulted in increased cell proliferation and apoptosis in the crypts and increased cell migration in the villi. Altered cell cycle in the crypts resulted in adenoma formation[51]. In contrast, forced expression of E-cadherin in the same model resulted in decreased cell proliferation and migration and increased cell apoptosis in the upper part of the intestinal crypt[52].

The importance of E-cadherin and the catenins in tissue development and morphogenesis is also evident from studies on other developmental systems. In *Drosophila*, mutation in the β-catenin homologue, *Armadillo*, results in defective segment polarity[53]. Expression of a dominant negative cadherin mutant in embryos of the frog *Xenopus laevis* resulted in perturbations of cell adhesion and tissue morphogenesis[54,55]. Ectopic over-expression of β-catenin[56] or γ-catenin[57] induces duplication of the body axis in *Xenopus* embryos. Depletion of β-catenin by injection of antisense oligonucleotides[58] or anti-β-catenin antibodies[59] also causes defective dorsal development.

E-CADHERIN/CATENIN COMPLEX IN INFLAMMATORY BOWEL DISEASE

Mucosal ulceration and chronic inflammation of the intestinal wall are common pathological features in ulcerative colitis and Crohn's disease. Immediately after ulceration of the intestinal mucosa a reparative mechanism called epithelial restitution is induced. This early response consists in rapid migration of viable epithelial cells from the ulcer margins over the denuded area in order to cover the defect and to restore the structural and functional integrity of the mucosa[60–62]. During this phase there is no cell proliferation, but cell migration is the essential factor contributing to mucosal repair.

Cell migration requires a dynamic interaction between cells, their extracellular substratum and the cytoskeletal network. Spatial and temporal changes in cell–cell and cell–matrix interactions occur during cell migration[63]. We have recently shown that perturbation of E-cadherin/catenin mediated cell–cell adhesion is associated with cell migration and epithelial restitution in an in vitro model of epithelial injury. In vivo, using immunohistochemical and in situ hybridization techniques, we have shown that in Crohn's disease the regenerating epithelium over ulcerated mucosa shows altered cellular localization and decreased levels of E-cadherin expression[64]. Loss of normal membranous α-catenin immunoreactivity and cytoplasmic localization were also found in vivo in inflammatory bowel disease (unpublished observations).

Several soluble factors, such as various growth factors and the recently recognized trefoil peptides, are involved in mucosal repair. In vitro, both EGF and transforming growth factor α (TGF-α) promote cell migration of colonic epithelial cells growing on laminin and collagen[65,66]. Hepatocyte growth factor/scatter factor (HGF/SF) has a potent proliferative effect on gastric epithelial cells in vitro but also promotes cell migration and epithelial restitution, an action which can be reversed by using anti-HGF antibodies[67]. The trefoil peptides have also been shown to stimulate cell migration and promote epithelial restitution in in vitro models of epithelial injury[68–70]. The EGF receptor binds to β-catenin and induces its tyrosine phosphorylation, leading to suppression of E-cadherin function in vitro[37]. EGF and HGF/SF have been shown to induce tyrosine phosphorylation of β-catenin and γ-catenin[37,40]. This was associated with cellular redistribution of E-cadherin, resulting in increased cell motility[41]. The motogenic effect of the trefoil peptide human spasmolytic polypeptide in vitro was also associated with perturbation of E-cadherin expression and cellular localization (unpublished data). Therefore, it is quite possible that the stimulatory effect of these factors on epithelial restitution and regeneration requires the modulation of the E-cadherin/catenin expression and/or function.

The importance of cadherin-mediated cell adhesion in intestinal epithelium is evident from studies using chimeric-transgenic mice in which islets of enterocytes transfected with truncated N-cadherin lacking the extracellular domain, can be generated alongside the normal intestinal mucosa[51]. In this experimental model, disruption of cadherin-mediated cell–cell adhesion in the crypt epithelial cells resulted in an altered cell cycle, perturbed mucosal barrier function and induced progressive inflammatory changes with features of Crohn's disease. Histopathological changes included lymphoid aggregates, cryptitis and crypt abscesses, goblet depletion, Paneth cell hyperplasia, and aphthoid and linear mucosal ulcers.

E-CADHERIN/CATENIN COMPLEX IN GASTROINTESTINAL NEOPLASIA

Altered cell adhesion has long been implicated in the neoplastic process. Loss of function and/or expression of any of the E-cadherin/catenin complex components perturbs intercellular cohesion, leading to loss of epithelial differentiation and normal architecture and the acquisition of an invasive potential.

In vitro studies have shown that loss of E-cadherin-mediated intercellular adhesion is associated with an invasive and poorly differentiated cell phenotype in several human carcinoma cell lines[22,23,29,70]. Down-regulation of the E-cadherin protein after E-cadherin antisense RNA transfection induces invasiveness in otherwise non-invasive cells[2,30]. Conversely, transfection of E-cadherin cDNA into dedifferentiated carcinoma cells[29,30] including poorly differentiated colon carcinoma cell lines, increases intercellular adhesion and inhibits their invasive phenotype[31,72]. This effect was reversed after treatment with anti-E-cadherin antibodies. Non-transformed Madin-Darby canine kidney epithelial cells[22], as well as a well-differentiated colon carcinoma cell line[23], acquire a dedifferentiated and invasive phenotype when intercellular adhesion is inhibited by anti-E-cadherin monoclonal antibodies.

In vitro studies also provided evidence for the possible role of α-catenin and β-catenin in the neoplastic process. Lung carcinoma PC9 cells and poorly differentiated colon carcinoma cell lines lacking α-catenin cannot aggregate tightly and grow as single cells despite their expression of E-cadherin and β-catenin[32,73]. Transfection with α-catenin cDNA restores intercellular adhesion and the ability of these cells to form epithelioid aggregates[33,73]. Similarly, the HSC-39 gastric cancer cells express E-cadherin, α- and γ-catenins but do not aggregate due to mutated β-catenin; their non-adhesiveness is reversed after transfection with β-catenin cDNA[34].

Expression of E-cadherin has been evaluated in vivo in a variety of human malignancies including oesophageal[74–76], gastric[78–80] and colonic[81–87] adenocarcinomas. In these studies reduced or absent E-cadherin expression was associated with poorly differentiated phenotype. Although in most studies there was no correlation between altered E-cadherin expression and tumour metastasis, in oesophageal[75,76] and gastric[79] adenocarcinomas down-regulation of E-cadherin was associated with infiltrative growth and lymph node involvement and in colonic cancer[83] with advanced stage. Despite the well established role of E-cadherin as a tumour differentiation marker its role as a prognostic factor in gastrointestinal malignancies is unclear. In gastric cancer, low E-cadherin expression was associated with tumour recurrence and mortality[80]. In colonic cancer, Dorudi et al.[88] have shown that patients with Dukes' stage B colorectal cancers surviving more than 5 years have higher E-cadherin mRNA levels than those who survive for less than 5 years.

Immunohistochemical studies have shown that α-catenin expression is also reduced in oesophageal, gastric and colonic cancers[76,89,90]. In oesophageal and gastric cancer the reduction of α-catenin expression was associated with tumour dedifferentiation, infiltrative growth, and lymph node and liver metastasis[76,90]. Furthermore, reduction of α-catenin expression was a better predictor of local spread or distant metastasis compared with E-cadherin expression.

β-Catenin expression is also frequently reduced in oesophageal, gastric and colonic cancers[91,92]. In colorectal and gastric cancer, reduced β-catenin expression is associated with high tumour grade (poorly differentiated morphology). In addition, we have recently shown that β-catenin expression in gastric cancer is a prognostic factor independent of tumour type, grade and stage[92].

Qualitative changes in E-cadherin cellular localization appear to occur also in dysplastic lesions of the oesophagus (Barrett's metaplasia)[74], stomach[92] and colon[87]. E-cadherin/catenin complex may be required for the initiation of tumorigenesis in the gastrointestinal tract as shown by Hermiston and Gordon[51] in the dominant N-cadherin mutant mice. Interestingly, mutation of the APC gene is an early event in the development of human colonic, oesophageal and gastric neoplasms[93-95]. In vitro, mutant APC protein has been shown to bind more avidly to β-catenin than wild-type APC[96]. It is conceivable that in dysplastic lesions of the gastrointestinal tract in which there is APC mutation, a shift in the equilibrium towards β-catenin–APC complex may occur. This may result in decreased E-cadherin-β-catenin binding, loss of E-cadherin-mediated adhesion, increased proliferation and promotion of cell migration.

In conclusion, the E-cadherin/catenin complex appears to function as a master molecule in the regulation of cell adhesion, polarity, differentiation, migration, proliferation and survival of gastrointestinal epithelial cells. Its fundamental role in embryogenesis has been clearly defined by the lethality seen in the E-cadherin/catenin knockout mice. In addition, loss of E-cadherin/catenin function appears to be an important step in the development of inflammatory and neoplastic lesions of the gastrointestinal tract. Elucidation of the mechanisms underlying the changes in E-cadherin and catenin function may lead to the development of novel therapeutic approaches based on its modulation at the genetic and biochemical levels.

References

1. Takeichi M. Cadherin cell adhesion receptors as a morphogenetic regulator. Science. 1991;251: 1451–5.
2. Kemler R. Classical cadherins. Semin Cell Biol. 1992;3:149–55.
3. Grunwald GB. The structural and functional analysis of cadherin calcium-dependent cell adhesion molecules. Curr Opin Cell Biol. 1993;5:797–805.

4. Nose A, Tsuji K, Takeichi M. Localization of specificity determining sites in cadherin cell adhesion molecules. Cell. 1990;61:147–55.
5. Overduin M, Harvey TS, Bagby S *et al*. Solution structure of the epithelial cadherin domain responsible for selective cell adhesion. Science. 1995;267:386–9.
6. Shapiro L, Fannon AM, Kwong PD *et al*. Structural basis of cell-cell adhesion by cadherins. Nature. 1995;374:327–37.
7. Duband J-L, Dufour S, Hatta K, Takeichi M, Edelman GM, Thiery JP. Adhesion molecules during somitogenesis in the avian embryo. J Cell Biol. 1987;104:1361–74.
8. Takeichi M. Cadherins: a molecular family important in selective cell-cell adhesion. Annu Rev Biochem. 1990;59:237–52.
9. Takeichi M. The cadherins: cell–cell adhesion molecules controlling animal morphogenesis. Development. 1988;102:639–55.
10. Berx G, Staes K, van Hengel J *et al*. Cloning and characterization of the human invasion suppressor gene E-cadherin (CDH1). Genomics. 1995;26:281–9.
11. Gumbiner BM, McCrea PD. Catenins as mediators of the cytoplasmic functions of cadherins. J Cell Sci. 1993;Suppl. 17:155–8.
12. Herrenknecht K, Ozawa M, Eckerskorn C, Lottspeich F, Lenter M, Kemler R. The uvomorulin-anchorage protein α-catenin is a vinculin homologue. Proc Natl Acad Sci USA. 1991;88:9156–60.
13. Nagafuchi A, Takeichi M, Tsukita S. The 102 kd cadherin-associated protein: similarity to vinculin and posttranscriptional regulation of expression. Cell. 1991;65:849–57.
14. McCrea PD, Turck CW, Gumbiner B. A homolog of the armadillo protein in Drosophila (plako-globin) associated with E-cadherin. Science. 1991;254:1359–61.
15. Butz S, Stappert J, Weissig H, Kemler R. Plakoglobin and β-catenin: Distinct but closely related. Science. 1992;257:1142–4.
16. Knudsen KA, Wheelock MJ. Plakoglobin, or an 83-kD homologue distinct from β-catenin, inter-acts with E-cadherin and N-cadherin. J Cell Biol. 1992;118:671–9.
17. Wachsstock DH, Wilkins JA, Lin S. Specific interaction of vinculin with α-actinin. Biochem Biophys Res Commun. 1987;146:554–60.
18. Nagafuchi A, Takeichi M. Cell binding function of E-cadherin is regulated by the cytoplasmic domain. EMBO J. 1988;7:3679–84.
19. Ozawa M, Ringwald M, Kemler R. Uvomorulin-catenin complex formation is regulated by a specific domain in the cytoplasmic region of the cell adhesion molecule. Proc Natl Acad Sci USA. 1990;87:4246–50.
20. Tsukita SH, Tsukita SA, Nagafuchi A, Yonemura S. Molecular linkage between cadherins and actin filaments in cell-cell adherens junctions. Curr Opin Cell Biol. 1992;4:834–9.
21. Näthke IS, Hinck L, Swedlow JR, Papkoff J, Nelson WJ. Defining interactions and distributions of cadherin and catenin complexes in polarized epithelial cells. J Cell Biol. 1994;125:1341–52.
22. Behrens J, Mareel MM, Van Roy FM, Birchmeier W. Dissecting tumor cell invasion: epithelial cells acquire invasive properties after the loss of uvomorulin-mediated cell-cell adhesion. J Cell Biol. 1989;108:2435–47.
23. Pignatelli M, Liu D, Nasim MM, Stamp GWH, Hirano S, Takeichi M. Morphoregulatory activities of E-cadherin and beta-1 integrins in colorectal tumour cells. Br J Cancer. 1992;66:629–34.
24. Kintner C. Regulation of embryonic cell adhesion by the cadherin cytoplasmic domain. Cell. 1992;69:225–36.
25. Fujimori T, Takeichi M. Disruption of epithelial cell-cell adhesion by exogenous expression of a mutated nonfunctional N-cadherin. Mol Biol Cell. 1993;4:37–47.
26. Ozawa M, Engel J, Kemler R. Single amino acid substitutions in one Ca^{2+} binding site of uvomorulin abolish the adhesive function. Cell. 1990;63:1033–8.
27. Buxton RS, Magee AI. Structure and interactions of desmosomal and other cadherins. Semin Cell Biol. 1992;3:157–67.
28. Nagafuchi A, Shirayoshi Y, Okazaki K, Yasuda K, Takeichi M. Transformation of cell adhesion properties by exogenously introduced E-cadherin cDNA. Nature. 1987;329:341–3.
29. Frixen UH, Behrens J, Sachs M *et al*. E-cadherin-mediated cell–cell adhesion prevents invasive-ness of human carcinoma cells. J Cell Biol. 1991;113:173–85.
30. Vleminckx K, Vakaet L Jr, Mareel M, Fiers W, Van Roy F. Genetic manipulation of E-cadherin expression by epithelial tumor cells reveals an invasion suppressor role. Cell. 1991;66:107–19.
31. Liu D, Nigam AK, Lalani EN, Stamp GWH, Pignatelli M. Transfection of E-cadherin into a human colon carcinoma cell line induces differentiation and inhibits growth in vitro. Gut. 1993;34(Suppl 4):S27.

32. Hirano S, Kimoto N, Shimoyama Y, Hirohashi S, Takeichi M. Identification of a neural α-catenin as a key regulator of cadherin function and multicellular organization. Cell. 1992;70:293–301.
33. Shimoyama Y, Nagafuchi A, Fujita S et al. Cadherin dysfunction in a human cancer cell line: possible involvement of loss of α-catenin expression in reduced cell-cell adhesiveness. Cancer Res. 1992;52:5770–4.
34. Kawanishi J, Kato J, Sasaki K, Fujii S, Watanabe N, Niitsu Y. Loss of E-cadherin-dependent cell-cell adhesion due to mutation of the β-catenin gene in a human cancer cell line, HSC-39. Mol Cell Biol. 1995;15:1175–81.
35. Matsuyoshi N, Hamaguchi M, Taniguchi S, Nagafuchi A, Tsukita S, Takeichi M. Cadherin-mediated cell-cell adhesion is perturbed by v-src tyrosine phosphorylation in metastatic fibroblasts. J Cell Biol. 1992;118:703–14.
36. Behrens J, Vakaet L, Friis R et al. Loss of epithelial differentiation and gain of invasiveness correlates with tyrosine phosphorylation of the E-cadherin/β-catenin complex in cells transformed with a temperature-sensitive v-src gene. J Cell Biol. 1993;120:757–66.
37. Hoschuetzky H, Aberle H, Kemler R. β-Catenin mediates the interaction of the cadherin–catenin complex with epidermal growth factor receptor. J Cell Biol. 1994;127:1375–80.
38. Barrandon Y, Green H. Cell migration is essential for sustained growth of keratinocyte colonies: The roles of transforming growth factor-α and epidermal growth factor. Cell. 1987;50:1131–7.
39. Lund-Johansen M, Bjerkvig R, Humphrey PA, Bigner SH, Bigner DD, Laerum O-D. Effect of epidermal growth factor on glioma cell growth, migration, and invasion in vitro. Cancer Res. 1990;50:6039–44.
40. Shibamoto S, Hayakawa M, Takeuchi K et al. Tyrosine phosphorylation of β-catenin and plakoglobin enhanced by hepatocyte growth factor and epidermal growth factor in human carcinoma cells. Cell Adhes Commun. 1994;1:295–305.
41. Shiozaki H, Kadowaki T, Doki Y et al. Effect of epidermal growth factor on cadherin-mediated adhesion in a human oesophageal cancer cell line. Br J Cancer. 1995;71:250–8.
42. Shibamoto S, Hayakawa M, Takeuchi K et al. Association of p120, a tyrosine kinase substrate, with E-cadherin/catenin complexes. J Cell Biol. 1995;128:949–57.
43. Rubinfeld B, Souza B, Albert I et al. Association of the APC gene product with β-catenin. Science. 1993;262:1731–4.
44. Su L-K, Vogelstein B, Kinzler KW. Association of the APC tumor suppressor protein with catenins. Science. 1993;262:1734–7.
45. Hülsken J, Birchmeier W, Behrens J. E-cadherin and APC compete for the interaction with β-catenin and the cytoskeleton. J Cell Biol. 1994;127:2061–9.
46. Rubinfeld B, Souza B, Albert I, Munemitsu S, Polakis P. The APC protein and E-cadherin form similar but independent complexes with α-catenin, β-catenin, and plakoglobin. J Biol Chem. 1995;270:5549–55.
47. Larue L, Ohsugi M, Hirchenhain J, Kemler R. E-cadherin null mutant embryos fail to form a trophectoderm epithelium. Proc Natl Acad Sci USA. 1994;91:8263–7.
48. Riethmacher D, Brinkmann V, Birchmeier C. A targeted mutation in the mouse E-cadherin gene results in defective preimplantation development. Proc Natl Acad Sci USA. 1995;92:855–9.
49. Haegel H, Larue L, Ohsugi M, Fedorov L, Herrenknecht K, Kemler R. Lack of beta-catenin affects mouse development at gastrulation. Development. 1995;121:3529–37.
50. Hermiston ML, Gordon JI. In vivo analysis of cadherin function in the mouse intestinal epithelium: essential roles in adhesion, maintenance of differentiation, and regulation of programmed cell death. J Cell Biol. 1995;129:489–506.
51. Hermiston ML, Gordon JI. Inflammatory bowel disease and adenomas in mice expressing a dominant negative N-cadherin. Science. 1995;270:1203–7.
52. Hermiston ML, Wong MH, Gordon JI. Forced expression of E-cadherin in the mouse intestinal epithelium slows cell migration and provides evidence for nonautonomous regulation of cell fate in a self-renewing system. Genes Dev. 1996;10:985–96.
53. Peifer M, Orsulic S, Sweeton D, Wieschaus E. A role for the Drosophila segment polarity gene armadillo in cell adhesion and cytoskeletal integrity during oogenesis. Development. 1993;118:1191–207.
54. Levine E, Lee CH, Kintner C, Gumbiner BM. Selective disruption of E-cadherin function in early Xenopus embryos by a dominant negative mutant. Development. 1994;120:901–9.
55. Dufour S, Saint-Jeannet JP, Broders F, Wedlich D, Thiery JP. Differential perturbations in the morphogenesis of anterior structures induced by overexpression of truncated XB- and N-cadherins in Xenopus embryos. J Cell Biol. 1994;127:521–35.

56. Funayama N, Fagotto F, McCrea P, Gumbiner BM. Embryonic axis induction by the armadillo repeat domain of beta-catenin: evidence for intracellular signaling. J Cell Biol. 1995;128:959–68.

57. Karnovsky A, Klymkowsky MW. Anterior axis duplication in *Xenopus* induced by the overexpression of the cadherin-binding protein plakoglobin. Proc Natl Acad Sci USA. 1995;92: 4522–6.

58. Heasman J, Crawford A, Goldstone K *et al*. Overexpression of cadherins and underexpression of beta-catenin inhibit dorsal mesoderm induction in early *Xenopus* embryos. Cell. 1994;79: 791–803.

59. McCrea PD, Brieher WM, Gumbiner BM. Induction of a secondary body axis in *Xenopus* by antibodies to beta-catenin. J Cell Biol. 1993;123:477–84.

60. Buck RC. Ultrastructural features of rectal epithelium of the mouse during the early phases of migration to repair a defect. Virchows Arch (B). 1986;51:331–40.

61. Waller DA, Thomas NW, Self TJ. Epithelial restitution in the large intestine of the rat following insult with bile salts. Virchows Arch (A) Pathol Anat. 1988;414:77–81.

62. Feil W, Lacy ER, Wong Y-MM *et al*. Rapid epithelial restitution of human and rabbit colonic mucosa. Gastroenterology. 1989;97:685–701.

63. Huttenlocher A, Sandborg RR, Horwitz AF. Adhesion in cell migration. Curr Opin Cell Biol. 1995;7:697–706.

64. Hanby AM, Chinery R, Poulsom R, Playford RJ, Pignatelli M. Downregulation of E-cadherin in the reparative epithelium of the human gastrointestinal tract. Am J Pathol. 1996;148:723–9.

65. Basson MD, Modlin IM, Madri JA. Human enterocytes (Caco-2) migration is modulated *in vitro* by extracellular matrix composition and epidermal growth factor. J Clin Invest. 1992;90:15–23.

66. Liu D, Gagliardi G, Nasim MM *et al*. TGF-α can act as morphogen and/or mitogen in a colorectal carcinoma cell line. Int J Cancer. 1994;56:603–8.

67. Takahashi M, Ota S, Shimada T *et al*. Hepatocyte growth factor is the most potent endogenous stimulant of rabbit gastric epithelial cell proliferation and migration in primary culture. J Clin Invest. 1995;95:1994–2003.

68. Dignass A, Lynch-Devaney K, Kindon H, Thim L, Podolsky DK. Trefoil peptides promote epithelial migration through a transforming growth factor β-independent pathway. J Clin Invest. 1994;94:376–83.

69. Kindon H, Pothoulakis C, Thim L, Lynch-Devaney K, Podolsky DK. Trefoil peptide protection of intestinal epithelial barrier function: cooperative interaction with mucin glycoprotein. Gastroenterology. 1995;109:516–23.

70. Playford RJ, Marchbank T, Chinery R *et al*. Human spasmolytic polypeptide is a cytoprotective agent that stimulates cell migration. Gastroenterology. 1995;108:108–16.

71. Doki Y, Shiozaki H, Tahara H *et al*. Correlation between E-cadherin expression and invasiveness *in vitro* in a human esophageal cancer cell line. Cancer Res. 1993;53:3421–6.

72. Breen E, Steele G Jr, Mercurio AM. Role of the E-cadherin/alpha-catenin complex in modulating cell-cell and cell-matrix adhesive properties of invasive colon carcinoma cells. Ann Surg Oncol. 1995;2:378–85.

73. Breen E, Clarke A, Steele G Jr, Mercurio AM. Poorly differentiated colon carcinoma cell lines deficient in alpha-catenin expression express high levels of surface E-cadherin but lack Ca(2+)-dependent cell-cell adhesion. Cell Adhes Commun. 1993;1:239–50.

74. Jankowski JA, Newham PM, Kandemir O, Hirano S, Takeichi M, Pignatelli M. Differential expression of E-cadherin in normal, metaplastic and dysplastic oesophageal mucosa: a putative biomarker. Int J Oncol. 1994;4:441–8.

75. Miyata M, Shiozaki H, Iihara K, Shimaya K, Oka H, Kadowaki T. Relationship between E-cadherin expression and lymph node metastasis in human esophageal cancer. Int J Oncol. 1994;4:61–5.

76. Kadowaki T, Shiozaki H, Inoue M *et al*. E-cadherin and α-catenin expression in human esophageal cancer. Cancer Res. 1994;54:291–6.

77. Shimoyama Y, Hirohashi S. Expression of E- and P-cadherin in gastric carcinomas. Cancer Res. 1991;51:2185–92.

78. Matsuura K, Kawanishi J, Fujii S *et al*. Altered expression of E-cadherin in gastric cancer tissues and carcinomatous fluid. Br J Cancer. 1992;66:1122–30.

79. Oka H, Shiozaki H, Kobayashi K *et al*. Immunohistochemical evaluation of E-cadherin adhesion molecule expression in human gastric cancer. Virchows Arch (A) Pathol Anat Histopathol. 1992; 421:149–56.

80. Mayer B, Johnson JP, Leitl F *et al*. E-cadherin expression in primary and metastatic gastric cancer: down-regulation correlates with cellular dedifferentiation and glandular disintegration. Cancer Res. 1993;53:1690–5.

81. Van der Wurff AA, ten Kate J, van der Linden EP, Dinjens WN, Arends JW, Bosman FT. L-CAM expression in normal, premalignant, and malignant colon mucosa. J Pathol. 1992;168:287–91.

82. Van der Wurff AA, Arends JW, van der Linden EP, ten Kate J, Bosman FT. L-CAM expression in lymph node and liver metastases of colorectal carcinomas. J Pathol. 1994;172:177–81.

83. Dorudi S, Sheffield JP, Poulsom R, Northover JM, Hart IR. E-cadherin expression in colorectal cancer. An immunocytochemical and in situ hybridization study. Am J Pathol. 1993;142:981–6.

84. Kinsella AR, Green B, Lepts GC, Hill CL, Bowie G, Taylor BA. The role of the cell–cell adhesion molecule E-cadherin in large bowel tumour cell invasion and metastasis. Br J Cancer. 1993; 67:904–9.

85. Nigam AK, Savage FJ, Boulos PB, Stamp GW, Liu D, Pignatelli M. Loss of cell-cell and cell-matrix adhesion molecules in colorectal cancer. Br J Cancer. 1993;68:507–14.

86. Van Aken J, Cuvelier CA, De Wever N, Roels J, Gao Y, Mareel MM. Immunohistochemical analysis of E-cadherin expression in human colorectal tumours. Pathol Res Pract. 1993;189: 975–8.

87. Gagliardi G, Kandemir O, Liu D *et al*. Changes in E-cadherin immunoreactivity in the adenoma-carcinoma sequence of the large bowel. Virchows Arch. 1995;426:149–54.

88. Dorudi S, Hanby AM, Poulsom R, Northover J, Hart IR. Level of expression of E-cadherin mRNA in colorectal cancer correlates with clinical outcome. Br J Cancer. 1995;71:614–16.

89. Shiozaki H, Iihara K, Oka H *et al*. Immunohistochemical detection of α-catenin expression in human cancers. Am J Pathol. 1994;144:667–74.

90. Matsui S, Shiozaki H, Inoue M *et al*. Immunohistochemical evaluation of alpha-catenin expression in human gastric cancer. Virchows Arch. 1994;424:375–81.

91. Takayama T, Shiozaki H, Shibamoto S *et al*. β-Catenin expression in human cancers. Am J Pathol. 1995;148:39–46.

92. Jawhari A, Jordan S, Poole S, Browne P, Pignatelli M, Farthing MJG. Abnormal immuno-reactivity of the E-cadherin-catenin complex in gastric carcinoma: relationship with patient survival. Gastroenterology. 1997;112:46–54.

93. Tamura G, Maesawa C, Suzuki Y *et al*. Mutations of the APC gene occur during early stages of gastric adenoma development. Cancer Res. 1994;54:1149–51.

94. Powell SM, Papadopoulos N, Kinzler KW, Smolinski KN, Meltzer SJ. APC gene mutations in the mutation cluster region are rare in esophageal cancers. Gastroenterology. 1994;107:1759–63.

95. Powell SM, Zilz N, Beazer-Barclay Y *et al*. APC mutations occur early during colorectal tumori-genesis. Nature. 1992;359:235–7.

96. Munemitsu S, Albert I, Souza B, Rubinfeld B, Polakis P. Regulation of intracellular β-catenin levels by the adenomatous polyposis coli (APC) tumor-suppressor protein. Proc Natl Acad Sci USA. 1995;92:3046–50.

18
Molecular aspects of restitution

R. POULSOM

RESTITUTION AND REPAIR OF MUCOSAL INTEGRITY

Maintaining the integrity of the gastrointestinal mucosal barrier is essential to ameliorate damage brought about by a broad range of damaging agents from acids, detergent-like salts, enzymes and drugs to bacteria, yeast and parasites. This defence must still, however, allow appropriate absorption to occur. Secreted mucus contributes to the barrier, but the principal active role is played by the surface epithelial cells, which show a remarkable restitutive ability to realign and reconnect themselves rapidly with new neighbouring cells when cells are lost.

Restitution of mucosal integrity in human gastric epithelium[1] appears to be essentially the same process in other species[2,3]; cells adjacent to damage lose some features of their differentiated appearance (e.g. discharge mucus), loosen their attachment to underlying basement membrane and migrate at about $2-5\,\mu m/$ min. If, however, the area of denudation is large, some epithelial cells resemble those seen at the margins of chronic ulcers, with sheets of attenuated cells still connected to neighbours but maximizing the surface covered. Once this restitutive phase of repair has been accomplished, later phases of mucosal or even submucosal remodelling may be needed.

In studying chronic ulceration, even if serial biopsies were taken, it is difficult to know how recently a partially healed lesion has suffered a setback in repair: the morphology of the repair epithelium thus cannot indicate whether it has recently started to migrate or if it has been in position for several days. Restitutive and repair epithelium may be different[4], but they cannot easily be distinguished in real ulcerated tissues. Accordingly, several model systems have been used in which discrete lesions are produced and the rate of healing followed in diverse ways. These range from assays in vitro in which monolayers of epithelial cells are damaged and the rate of migration/repair is determined[5-10], through to in vivo models[4,11] where the rate of healing of cryoprobe-induced ulcers is measured by video endoscopy (and later histology) and the effects of anti-ulcer drugs assessed[12].

Motogens, mitogens and morphogens

One of the most interesting concepts central to the healing process is that a variety of agents is secreted or activated in the local environment of these cells which promote restitution, repair and remodelling to restore glandular architecture. Cell movement alone may be sufficient for restitution of small lesions[1], and this can be promoted by a class of agents termed motogens that increase the rate of migration of epithelial cells without the need for cell proliferation, which would take too long. Several of the peptides available to wound epithelia are motogens, including epidermal growth factor (EGF)[13], transforming growth factor-α (TGF-α)[8], basic fibroblast growth factor (bFGF) and IGF[14], and interestingly TGF-β which is both a mediator of the motogenic effects of some peptides[6,8] and anti-proliferative[15].

Migration of cells for restitution needs to occur without losing cell–cell attachments (otherwise barrier functions such as those monitored electrically in vitro[2] would not improve). The migrating epithelium over chronic gastric ulcers or ulcers in the small intestine of patients with Crohn's disease shows altered expression of E-cadherin, as detected by immunohistochemistry[16]. Reduced and patchy expression of this calcium-dependent cell–cell adhesion protein is seen at the basolateral aspects of the cells and stronger intracellular pools of immunoreactivity are seen, indicative of reduced cell–cell attachment[16]. This is not the only likely consequence of decreased basolateral localization, as E-cadherin localization to specific sites on a cell surface appears able to trigger changes in gene expression and cell phenotype[17].

Repair of larger lesions will benefit from epithelial proliferation as well: some peptides, including EGF[18], are mitogens as well as motogens, depending on their concentrations. Hepatocyte growth factor/scatter factor (HGF/SF) acts as both for gastric epithelium[10,19], and can also be a morphogen. HGF is able to promote tubulogenesis of MDCK cells in vitro, and just one receptor (c-met) appears necessary for all the effects of HGF to be mediated[20]. There could well be a hierarchy regulating the effectiveness of the various agents present at the wound monolayer; e.g. HGF seems able to over-rule TGF-β-mediated growth arrest[15].

Interactions with the extracellular matrix

A further component of the repair environment is the extracellular matrix on or within which epithelial cells must migrate and divide in an orderly manner, in concert with the repair of the lamina propria. Restitution of experimental lesions in human stomach appears to rely on there being an intact basement membrane[1], as if the rapid movement of these cells depends upon specific matrix molecules being present. In this context, laminin-1 the major glycoprotein of basement membranes, is an excellent substratum for rapid migration of cells[21], and transfection of cells normally immobile on laminin with integrin α-7 confers motility[22]. In contrast, serum fibronectin and stromal collagens, which are found in granulation tissue, are poor substrates for epithelial migration[21]. Migration of non-epithelial cells into the wound is also important for remodelling of granulation tissue and re-establishing vascularity. This is also affected by extracellular matrix: the preferred direction of migration of fibroblasts is affected by the accessibility and orientation of collagen fibrils[23], which in turn will have been affected by proteolytic attack from the lumen and from neighbouring or preceding cells. The cells populating the stroma express both matrix degrading enzymes and their inhibitors in a variety of activation states. Even the wound epithelium is not neutral because it expresses matrilysin (MMP-7)[24], a metalloproteinase that can be activated by trypsin and which is well suited to degrading basement membrane as well as activating MMPs in granulation tissue[25].

Recent studies indicate that tubule formation by MDCK cells can also be triggered by covering them with collagen I, provided that they have apical β1 integrins[26]. This might indicate that HGF is not necessary for tubulogenesis, but the picture will be less certain in vivo; alteration of wound epithelium morphology may release a specific protease[27] that activates deposits of HGF, and there are indications that endogenous expression of HGF increases in gastric ulcer tissues[19,28].

Thus ulcer healing occurs despite interactions between several complex systems, and it is challenging to try to identify which peptides are able to promote healing.

IDENTIFYING NATURAL ULCER REPAIR PEPTIDES

Until relatively recently, a peptide would have to be detected, purified and tested directly to establish whether it might naturally play any part in the process of ulcer healing. It is now possible to determine exactly where, when and to what level a gene is being expressed in an ulcer using immunohistochemistry together with molecular biology approaches such as in situ hybridization and RNA probe protection assays. This combination of techniques will help establish whether the pattern of expression, morphological and chronological, is relevant to the histological appearance of the lesion. In some cases it may be possible fairly easily to purify peptides or prepare them using recombinant DNA techniques, and then to look for biological activities relevant to repair. Three examples are discussed here: trefoil peptides, which have a substantial body of evidence supporting their involvement in restitution or repair; PSTI, which is localized appropriately and is able to promote cell migration; and the myeloic related proteins MRP8/14, the dimer of which is intriguingly elevated in serum during active episodes of inflammatory bowel disease. This protein is thought to be antimicrobial, and is reported to be present in epithelium adjacent to ulceration.

Trefoil peptides

The availability of partial cDNA and antibodies prepared against peptides whose sequences have been deduced was central to the many studies that implicated trefoil peptides as being actively involved in restitution and repair of chronic ulcers, although this was only circumstantial evidence (reviewed in Ref. 29). Subsequent studies in vitro and in vivo with recombinant peptides then established that they have diverse biological effects relevant to prevention and healing of ulcers, supporting the notion that they are expressed for this purpose normally.

In mammals three trefoil peptides are secreted by epithelial cells in specific

Table 1 Trefoil peptides

New name*	Synonyms	Locus	Principal sites of expression
TFF1	pS2, pNR-2	BCEI now TFF1* (34)	Surface epithelium of stomach, surface epithelium of Brunner's glands, some in large bowel, breast, many varied carcinomas
TFF2	spasmolytic polypeptide, SP	SML1 now TFF2* (34)	Surface epithelium and deep antral and pyloric gland epithelium of stomach, deep epithelium of Brunner's glands. Rarely in carcinomas
TFF3	intestinal trefoil factor, ITF, P1.B	TFF3 (35, 36)	Goblet cells throughout small and large bowel, breast, uterus, some carcinomas

*Nomenclature recommended by the organizing committee of the Conférences Philippe Laudat meeting 'Trefoil/P-domain peptides: from basic research to molecular medicine', Aix les Bains, France, 29 September–3 October 1996

patterns through the gastrointestinal tract (reviewed in Ref. 29) (Table 1). Expression is not confined to the gut but generally only TFF1 (the oestrogen- and EGF-inducible breast cancer associated peptide pS2[30]) and TFF3 (intestinal trefoil factor[31,32]) can be found in breast[33] and uterus[31]. In humans, the genes for all three peptides are clustered on chromosome 21[34-36] and appear to have evolved from a common precursor that bore the common TFF-domain shuffled module (previously termed a P-domain shuffled module[37]). These peptides have very compact structures in which the TFF-domain cores are made up of a short anti-parallel β-sheet and three disulphide bridges[38,39]. TFF2 contains two of these modules in tandem, linked by a further disulphide bond forming a structure that may be mimicked by dimerization of TFF1 and TFF3, which have free seventh cysteine residues near their C-termini[40-42].

Immunohistochemistry and in situ hybridization studies were able to define the normal sites of expression in gastrointestinal and other tissues with resolution and sensitivity impossible by Western or Northern blotting techniques, which require tissues to be homogenized before analysis. On the other hand, homogenization of specified areas of tissue allowed quantitation of the relative amounts of mRNAs present at the ulcer site at chosen times after creating a cryoprobe ulcer, revealing that specific induction of TFF2 occurs within 30 min[43].

Aberrant expression of TFF1 and TFF2 was detected in chronic ulceration, exemplified by that in the small bowel in Crohn's disease[44,45]. Normally, only TFF3 is expressed in most of the small bowel, but all three trefoil peptides were expressed by cells in glands of the ulceration-associated cell lineage (UACL). These glands presumably develop in response to chronic endodermal damage in many tissues[46]. The UACL glands resemble pyloric glands of the stomach and Brunner's glands of the duodenum, yet have certain differences in their phenotype. The glands were considered likely to be involved in ulcer repair because they expressed immunoreactive EGF[46], TGF-α[47], lysosome[48] (able to lyse bacteria;

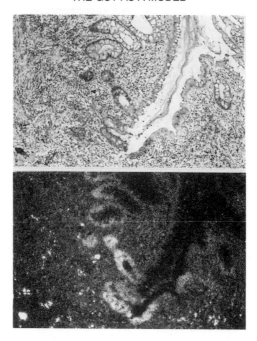

Figure 1 Paired bright field and reflected light dark field panels showing lysozyme mRNA expression in small intestinal Crohn's disease revealed by ^{35}S riboprobe in situ hybridization as described by Stamp and colleagues[48]. Clusters of autoradiographic grains appear white in dark field conditions and are present over the lower regions of some crypts and over the less differentiated surface epithelium at the lower edge of the image

Figure 1), and it was hypothesized that trefoil peptides were also expressed as part of this repair phenotype. The structure of these UACL glands indicated that their products would be secreted luminally. In addition some goblet cells adjacent to the UACL had also acquired the expression of TFF1, and occasionally TFF2, in addition to the normal expression of TFF3. Careful immunohistochemical studies, using double labelling and immunoelectron microscopy, revealed that many of the enteroendocrine cells that are present in increased numbers near the ulcers also expressed TFF1, co-packaged with the secretory granules and thus destined for release towards the local circulation rather than the lumen[44,49].

The ductular portion of the UACL opens out onto the villus surface and its cells appear to spread out as if displacing the indigenous population. These UACL surface cells express TFF1 but not TFF2, and subsequently the expression of TFF3 mRNA was detected in some but not all UACL glands[31,44]. Looking at single time points it is impossible to tell how well repair is progressing; the variable phenotype might be due to some maturation process, or there may be more than one type of repair epithelium present. Either way, these studies showed that putative repair epithelium expressed all three trefoil peptide mRNAs (Figure 2).

The availability of recombinant trefoil peptides allowed their biological activities to be studied. Purification from natural sources was difficult, and with the exception of porcine spasmolytic polypeptide (porcine TFF2[50]), yielded sub-milligram

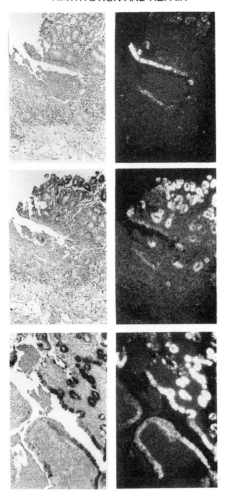

Figure 2   Paired bright field and reflected light dark field panels showing trefoil peptide mRNA expression in small intestinal Crohn's disease revealed by ^{35}S riboprobe in situ hybridization as described by Wright and colleagues[45] and Hauser et al.[31]. In the top pair, TFF1 (pS2) mRNA is conspicuous in most of the wound surface cells (possibly UACL surface cells) and also is being expressed ectopically in some goblet cells in adjacent crypts (right hand side). In the middle pair, TFF3 (intestinal trefoil factor) mRNA is seen in some wound surface cells, some acinar regions of the UACL (lower centre of image) and is expressed normally in goblet cells of adjacent crypts. In the lower pair, TFF2 (spasmolytic polypeptide) mRNA is seen to be expressed by wound surface epithelium, acinar regions of the UACL (lower centre of image) and by some goblet cells in adjacent crypts. Normally in the small bowel TFF2 mRNA is expressed only by Brunner's glands of the duodenum

amounts. TFF3[5,51] then TFF2[7,51] were found to reduce the extent of gastric or small intestinal damage resulting from indomethacin or even ethanol in some studies, but neither trefoil peptide was as effective as EGF. Oral or intraperitoneal doses were less effective than those given subcutaneously. Synergy between TFF3 and EGF was observed both against ulceration[5] and in electrophysiological studies of chloride secretion by cell monolayers[52]. In vitro, TFF2 and TFF3 were found to be motogens that act independently of TGF-β[6]. Transfection of a cell line with TFF1 caused spontaneous motility on type I collagen to increase from approximately 13 to 30 μm/h and result in a dispersed pattern of growth in three-dimensional culture[53].

TFF1 may also be able to prevent gastrointestinal damage. No experiments with recombinant TFF1 have been reported, but a transgenic mouse line has been made in which expression of human TFF1 was linked to the intestinal fatty acid binding protein promoter[54]. These mice showed increased resistance to indomethacin-induced damage in the jejunum (where the transgene was expressed) and no effect in the ileum.

Homologous recombination has been used by two groups to study the effects of knocking out TFF-domain genes. Deletion of intestinal trefoil factor (TFF3) is reported[55] to increase susceptibility to mucosal damage in the large bowel, and not to cause compensatory increases in expression of TFF1 or TFF2. Wound repair monolayers were not seen at the margins of ulcers in TFF1 null mice[55]. In contrast, deletion of TFF1[56] was associated with the early loss of mucous expression, development of dysplasia and increased mitotic rate in the antral and pyloric region of the stomach, and later to tumours in the antrum of 30% of homozygous null mice and loss of expression of gastric TFF2 in about 70%.

Taken together, these studies support strongly the notion that the trefoil peptides are involved directly in the healing process, at several levels.

Pancreatic secretory trypsin inhibitor (PSTI)

This too is a small peptide, resistant to proteolysis, normally expressed by several tissues including the gastrointestinal tract. Ulceration is associated with decreased expression, but the wound repair monolayer has high levels of the mRNA and peptide[57]. Further, purified PSTI increased cell migration in vitro three-fold by a mechanism that was blocked by antibodies neutralizing TGF-β or blocking EGF-receptor[57]. A considerable amount of further work is needed to define the role of PSTI in restitution and repair. One intriguing possibility is that PSTI expression by the wound monolayer would reduce activation of matrilysin by trypsin from the lumen and thereby affect remodelling of the basement membrane and granulation tissue (see above).

MRP8/14, Calprotectin

In the last few years there has been considerable interest in these myeloic related proteins (MRP) and the relevance of their expression to inflammatory bowel disease. Two MRPs of 8 and 14 kDa are known to form a complex termed variously MRP8/14, human leukocyte antigen L1-calprotectin, and cystic fibrosis antigen[58]. There are antisera specific to individual chains and to the complex (recognized by the monoclonal 27E10[59]). Immunohistochemistry supports the synthesis of chains and complex by some squamous epithelia, which can be supported by in situ hybridization evidence for synthesis rather than absorption (data not shown) and by a high proportion of granulocytes in various inflammatory conditions. Expression of the complex on the surface of macrophages is correlated with their activation on binding to fibronectin[60].

Serum levels of the complex are increased significantly in patients with active ulcerative colitis, and follow the current severity of disease[61]. The serum levels of complex attained appear high enough to be antimicrobial[58], which raises questions about their expression and function at the sites of ulceration.

Schmid and colleagues[59] presented strong immunohistochemical evidence for the complex being abundant in the inflammatory cell population in fissuring lesions of Crohn's disease whether in small or large bowel. In small bowel, and only in fissuring areas, the epithelium itself showed strong immunoreactivity for the MRP8/14 complex and only weak staining for the individual chains. This was taken as an indication that synthesis by fissure epithelium could contribute to increased serum levels in Crohn's disease. In a limited series however (Figure 3) expression of MRP8 or MRP14 mRNA was not detectable. This could mean that the fissure epithelium has acquired the complex from the adjacent granulocytes which express the mRNAs in abundance. In contrast, a sample of large bowel from a case of ulcerative colitis (Figure 4) reveals high level expression of MRP8 mRNA, yet the complex was not detected in epithelium of 23 cases of UC[61]. Immunohistochemistry and in situ hybridization often provide complementary information about the expression of genes.

How to identify new candidates?

The availability of reagents to characterize sites of expression of candidate genes is a limiting factor. Given adequate resources, a large number of candidates could be screened, but the likelihood of finding a relevant gene is low unless some pre-selection is carried out.

A molecular approach

Molecular biology offers differential display and subtractive hybridization techniques that might identify genes expressed specifically in response to ulceration, but these approaches may be limited by the lack of selectivity of early steps. A comparison of pools of cDNA from 'ulcerated' and 'control' tissues would be expected to select mainly for clones whose high level expression was simply consequent upon changes in the balance of cell types present. Genes expressed by normal epithelial cells would appear to be under-expressed, but large numbers of activated inflammatory cells, cells that are responding non-specifically to remodelling, hypoxic and dying cells, etc., would be present. Morphology-directed cloning, using microdissected regions of tissue[62] or even single cells[63], would generate greater specificity and reduced complexity of the cDNA pool to be screened. Of course, comparison of pools generated at various times following wounding of cultured epithelial cell lines in vitro could help identify genes expressed at different stages of response, but however identified, an early step in deciding whether to characterize the clones in detail would be to use in situ hybridization to see where the mRNA is expressed in real ulcers.

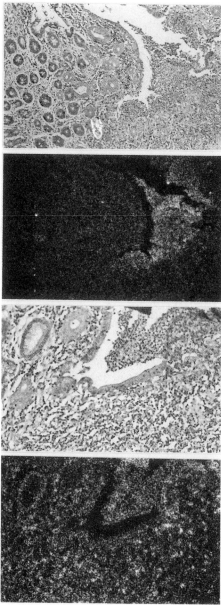

Figure 3   Paired bright field and reflected light dark field panels showing MRP mRNA expression in small intestinal Crohn's disease revealed by ^{35}S riboprobe in situ hybridization. In the top pair, MRP8 mRNA is seen to be abundant in most cells exuded into the fissure (reminiscent of the immunohistochemical staining pattern seen for the MRP8/14 complex in Figure 2 of Schmid and colleagues[59]). Note that neither the crypt epithelium, the UACL glands (centre), nor the sheet of wound monolayer lining the left hand side of the fissure has any perceptible MRP8 mRNA. In the lower pair MRP14 mRNA expression is shown in the base of the fissure at a higher magnification. Scattered inflammatory cells of indeterminate type give strong hybridization signals for MRP14 mRNA, but no expression is detectable over the epithelium

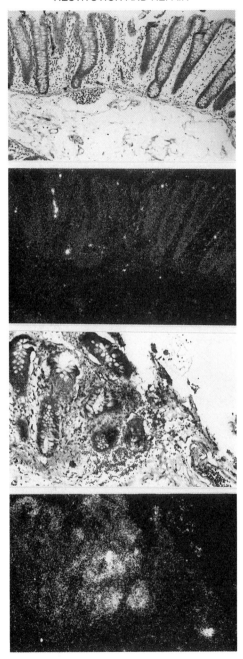

Figure 4   Paired bright field and reflected light dark field panels showing MRP mRNA expression in large bowel. The top pair shows a region of large bowel from a patient with Crohn's disease; there is some inflammation but MRP14 mRNA is detected only in scattered inflammatory cells, e.g. within a vessel in the lamina propria (left hand side). The lower pair shows MRP8 mRNA to be abundant in crypt epithelium and a few intravascular inflammatory cells in a case of ulcerative colitis

Acknowledgements

I am extremely grateful to Jan Longcroft, Rosemary Jeffery and Len Rogers of the ICRF In Situ Hybridization Service for skilful assistance with the in situ studies, to Professor Ray Playford and Dr Tania Marchbank for access to the PSTI clone, and to Drs Nancy Hogg and Paul Hessian of the ICRF Leukocyte Antigen Laboratory for advice and access to the MRP8/14 clones.

References

1. Lacy ER, Morris GP, Cohen MM. Rapid repair of the surface epithelium in human gastric mucosa after acute superficial injury. J Clin Gastroenterol. 1993;17(Suppl 1):S125–35.
2. Moore R, Carlson S, Madara JL. Rapid barrier restitution in an in vitro model of intestinal epithelial injury. Lab Invest. 1989;60:237–44.
3. Svanes K, Itoh S, Takeuchi K, Silen W. Restitution of the surface epithelium of the in vitro frog gastric mucosa after damage with hypermolar sodium chloride. Gastroenterology. 1982;82: 1409–26.
4. Szabo S, Kusstatscher S, Sandor Z, Sakoulos G. Molecular and cellular basis of ulcer healing. Scand J Gastroenterol. 1995;30(Suppl 208):3–8.
5. Chinery R, Playford R. Combined intestinal trefoil factor and epidermal growth factor is prophylactic against indomethacin-induced gastric damage in the rat. Clin Sci. 1995;88:401–3.
6. Dignass A, Lynch-Devaney K, Kindon H, Thim L, Podolsky DK. Trefoil peptides promote epithelial migration through a transforming growth factor beta-independent pathway. J Clin Invest. 1994;94:376–83.
7. Playford RJ, Marchbank T, Chinery R et al. Human spasmolytic polypeptide is a cytoprotective agent that stimulates cell migration. Gastroenterology. 1995;108:108–16.
8. Dignass AU, Podolsky DK. Cytokine modulation of intestinal epithelial cell restitution: central role of transforming growth factor β. Gastroenterology. 1993;105:1323–32.
9. Tsuji S, Kawano S, Tsujii M, Fusamoto H, Kamada T. Roles of hepatocyte growth factor and its receptor in gastric mucosa: a cell biological and molecular biological study. Dig Dis Sci. 1995; 40:1132–9.
10. Watanabe S, Hirose M, Wang X-E et al. Hepatocyte growth factor accelerates the wound repair of cultured gastric mucosal cells. Biochem Biophys Res Commun. 1994;199:1453–60.
11. Elson CO, Sartor RB, Tennyson GS, Riddell RH. Experimental models of inflammatory bowel disease. Gastroenterology. 1995;109:1344–67.
12. Schmassmann A, Tarnawski A, Peskar B, Varga L, Flogerzi B, Halter F. Influence of acid and angiogenesis on kinetics of gastric ulcer healing in rats: interaction with indomethacin. Am J Physiol. 1995;268:G276–85.
13. Miller CA, Debas HT. Epidermal growth factor stimulates the restitution of rat gastric mucosa in vitro. Exp Physiol. 1995;80:1009–18.
14. Kato K, Chen MC, Lehman F et al. Trefoil peptides, IGF-I and basic FGF stimulate restitution in primary cultures of canine oxyntic mucosal cells. Gastroenterology. 1995;108:A130.
15. Taipale J, Keski-Oja J. Hepatocyte growth factor releases epithelial and endothelial cells from growth arrest induced by transforming growth factor beta1. J Biol Chem. 1996;271:4342–8.
16. Hanby AM, Chinery R, Poulsom R, Playford RJ, Pignatelli M. Downregulation of E-cadherin in the reparative epithelium of the human gastrointestinal tract. Am J Pathol. 1996;148:723–9.
17. Marrs JA, Andersson-Fisone C, Jeong MC et al. Plasticity in epithelial cell phenotype: modulation by expression of different cadherin cell adhesion molecules. J Cell Biol. 1995;129:507–19.
18. Walker-Smith JA, Phillips AD, Walford N et al. Intravenous EGF/URO increases small intestinal cell proliferation in congenital microvillous atrophy. Lancet. 1985;ii:1239–40.
19. Kinoshita Y, Nakata H, Hassan S et al. Gene expression of keratinocyte and hepatocyte growth factors during the healing of rat gastric mucosal lesions. Gastroenterology. 1995;109:1068–77.
20. Weidner KM, Sachs M, Birchmeier W. The Met receptor tyrosine kinase transduces motility, proliferation, and morphogenesis signals of scatter factor/hepatocyte growth factor in epithelial cells. J Cell Biol. 1993;121:145–54.

21. Ohtaka K, Watanabe S, Iwazaki R, Hirose M, Sato N. Role of extracellular matrix on colonic cancer cell migration and proliferation. Biochem Biophys Res Commun. 1996;220:346–52.
22. Echtermeyer F, Schöber S, Pöschl E, von der Mark H, von der Mark K. Specific induction of cell motility on laminin by alpha7 integrin. J Biol Chem. 1996;271:2071–5.
23. Dickinson RB, Guido S, Tranquillo RT. Biased cell migration of fibroblasts exhibiting contact guidance in oriented collagen gels. Ann Biomed Eng. 1994;22:342–56.
24. Saarialho-Kere UK, Vaalamo M, Puolakkainen P, Airola K, Parks WC, Karjalainen-Lindsberg M-L. Enhanced expression of matrilysin, collagenase and stromelysin-1 in gastrointestinal ulcers. Am J Pathol. 1996;148:519–26.
25. Imai K, Yokohama Y, Nakanishi I et al. Matrix metalloproteinase 7 (matrilysin) from human rectal carcinoma cells. J Biol Chem. 1995;270:6691–7.
26. Zuk A, Matlin KS. Apical beta-1 integrin in polarized MDCK cells mediates tubulocyst formation in response to type I collagen overlay. J Cell Sci. 1996;109:1875–89.
27. Miyazawa K, Shimomura T, Kitamura N. Activation of hepatocyte growth factor in the injured tissues is mediated by hepatocyte growth factor activator. J Biol Chem. 1996;271:3615–18.
28. Stettler C, Hirschi C, Schmassmann A et al. Role of hepatocyte growth factor (HGF) and trefoil peptides in experimental gastric ulcer healing. Regul Pept. 1996;64:183.
29. Poulsom R. Trefoil peptides. Bailliére's Clin Gastroenterol. 1996;10:113–34.
30. Rio M, Chambon P. The pS2 gene, mRNA, and protein: a potential marker for human breast cancer. Cancer Cells. 1990;2:269–74.
31. Hauser F, Poulsom R, Chinery R et al. hP1.B, a human P-domain peptide homologous with rat intestinal trefoil factor, is expressed in the ulcer associated cell lineage and the uterus. Proc Natl Acad Sci USA. 1993;90:6961–5.
32. Podolsky DK, Lynch-Devaney K, Stow JL et al. Identification of human intestinal trefoil factor: goblet cell-specific expression of a peptide targeted for apical secretion. J Biol Chem. 1993;268:6694–702.
33. Theisinger B, Seitz G, Dooley S, Welter C. A second trefoil protein, ITF/hP1.B, is transcribed in human breast cancer. Breast Cancer Res Treat. 1995;38:145–51.
34. Tomasetto C, Rockel N, Mattei MG, Fujita R, Rio M-C. The gene encoding the human spasmolytic protein (SML1/hSP) is in 21q22.3, physically linked to the homologous breast cancer marker gene BCEI/pS2. Genomics. 1992;13:1328–30.
35. Schmitt H, Wundrack I, Beck S et al. A third P-domain peptide gene (TFF3), human intestinal trefoil factor, maps to 21q22.3. Cytogenet Cell Genet. 1996;72:299–302.
36. Chinery R, Williamson J, Poulsom R. The gene encoding human intestinal trefoil factor (TFF3) is located on chromosome 21q22.3 clustered with other members of the trefoil peptide family. Genomics. 1996;32:281–4.
37. Hauser F, Hoffman W. P-domains as shuffled cysteine-rich modules in integumentary mucin C.1 (FIM-C.1) from Xenopus laevis. J Biol Chem. 1992;267:24620–4.
38. Carr MD, Bauer CJ, Gradwell MJ, Feeney J. Solution structure of a trefoil-motif-containing cell growth factor, porcine spasmolytic protein. Proc Natl Acad Sci USA. 1994;91:2206–10.
39. De A, Brown DG, Gorman MA, Carr M, Sanderson MR, Freemont PS. Crystal structure of a disulfide-linked 'trefoil' motif found in a large family of putative growth factors. Proc Natl Acad Sci USA. 1994;91:1084–8.
40. Chadwick MP, May FEB, Westley BR. Production and comparison of mature single-domain 'trefoil' peptides pNR-2/pS2 Cys58 and pNR-2/pS2 Ser 58. Biochem J. 1995;308:1001–7.
41. Chinery R, Bates PA, De A, Freemont PS. Characterisation of the single copy trefoil peptides intestinal trefoil factor and pS2 and their ability to form covalent dimers. FEBS Lett. 1995;357:50–4.
42. Thim L, Woldike HF, Nielsen PF, Christensen M, Lynch-Devaney K, Podolsky DK. Characterization of human and rat intestinal trefoil factor produced in yeast. Biochemistry. 1995;34:4757–64.
43. Alison MR, Chinery R, Poulsom R, Ashwood P, Longcroft JM, Wright NA. Experimental ulceration leads to sequential expression of spasmolytic polypeptide, intestinal trefoil factor, epidermal growth factor, and transforming growth factor alpha mRNAs in rat stomach. J Pathol. 1995;175:405–14.
44. Wright NA, Poulsom R, Stamp G et al. Trefoil peptide gene expression in gastrointestinal epithelial cells in inflammatory bowel disease. Gastroenterology. 1993;104:12–20.
45. Wright NA, Poulsom R, Stamp GW et al. Epidermal growth factor (EGF/URO) induces expression

215

of regulatory peptides in damaged human gastrointestinal tissues. J Pathol. 1990;162:279–84.

46. Wright NA, Pike C, Elia G. Induction of a novel epidermal growth factor-secreting cell lineage by mucosal alteration in gastrointestinal stem cells. Nature. 1990;343:82–5.

47. Ahnen DA, Gullick W, Wright NA. Multiple growth factor production by the cell lineage induced by mucosal ulceration in Crohn's disease. Gastroenterology. 1991;100:A512.

48. Stamp GWH, Poulsom R, Chung LP et al. Lysozyme gene expression in inflammatory bowel disease. Gastroenterology. 1992;103:532–8.

49. Wright NA. Trefoil peptides and the gut. Gut. 1993;34:577–9.

50. Jørgensen KH, Thim L, Jacobsen HE. Pancreatic spasmolytic polypeptide (PSP): I. Preparation and initial chemical characterization of a new polypeptide from porcine pancreas. Reg Pept. 1982; 3:207–19.

51. Babyatsky MW, DeBeaumont M, Thim L, Podolsky DK. Oral trefoil peptides protect against ethanol- and indomethacin-induced gastric injury in rats. Gastroenterology. 1996;110:489–97.

52. Chinery R, Cox HM. Modulation of epidermal growth factor effects on epithelial ion transport by intestinal trefoil factor. Br J Pharmacol. 1995;115:77–80.

53. Williams R, Stamp GWH, Gilbert C, Pignatelli M, Lalani E-N. pS2 transfection of murine adenocarcinoma cell line 410.4 enhances dispersed growth pattern in a 3-D collagen gel. J Cell Sci. 1996;109:63–71.

54. Playford RJ, Marchbank T, Goodlad RA et al. Transgenic mice that overexpress the human trefoil peptide pS2 have an increased resistance to intestinal damage. Proc Natl Acad Sci USA. 1996; 93:2137–42.

55. Mashimo H, Wu D-C, Podolsky DK, Fishman MC. Impaired defense of intestinal mucosa in mice lacking intestinal trefoil factor. Science. 1996;274:262–5.

56. Lefebvre O, Chenard M-P, Masson R et al. Gastric mucosal abnormalities and tumorigenesis in mice lacking the pS2 trefoil protein. Science. 1996;274:259–62.

57. Marchbank T, Chinery R, Hanby AM, Poulsom R, Elia G, Playford RJ. Distribution and expression of pancreatic secretory trypsin inhibitor and its possible role in epithelial restitution. Am J Pathol. 1996;148:715–22.

58. Steinbakk M, Naess-Andresen C-F, Lingaas E, Dale I, Brandtzaeg P, Fagerhol MK. Antimicrobial actions of calcium binding leucocyte L1 protein, calprotectin. Lancet. 1990;336:763–5.

59. Schmid KW, Lügering N, Stoll R et al. Immunohistochemical demonstration of the calcium-binding proteins MRP8 and MRP14 and their heterodimer (27E10 antigen) in Crohn's disease. Hum Pathol. 1995;26:334–7.

60. Mahnke K, Bhardwaj R, Sorg C. Heterodimers of the calcium binding proteins MRP8 and MRP14 are expressed on the surface of human monocytes upon adherence to fibronectin and collagen. Relation to TNF alpha, IL-6 and superoxide production. J Leukocyte Biol. 1995;57:63–71.

61. Lügering N, Stoll R, Schmid KW et al. The myeloic related protein MRP8/14 (27E10 antigen) – usefulness as a potential marker for disease activity in ulcerative colitis and putative biological function. Eur J Clin Invest. 1995;25:659–64.

62. Jensen RA, Page DL, Holt JT. Identification of genes expressed in premalignant breast tissue by microscopy-directed cloning. Proc Natl Acad Sci USA. 1994;91:9257–61.

63. Brady G, Iscove NN. Construction of cDNA libraries from single cells. Methods Enzymol. 1993; 225:611–23.

19
Regulation of epithelial cell proliferation and differentiation in small bowel adaptation after resection and during ontogeny

D. C. RUBIN and M. S. LEVIN

INTRODUCTION

The mammalian small intestine contains a constantly proliferating and differentiating epithelium. Anchored stem cells in the crypts of Lieberkühn give rise to proliferating daughter cells that differentiate during migration onto the villus or to the base of the crypt[1]. The principal terminally differentiated cell types in the intestine include the absorptive enterocytes, goblet cells, enteroendocrine cells and Paneth cells. Despite perpetual renewal, a spatially complex epithelium is maintained from crypt to villus tip and from duodenum to colon.

One of the fundamental challenges in intestinal epithelial cell biology is to define the molecular mechanisms that regulate crypt cell proliferation and the switch to a well differentiated epithelium. Our laboratory has employed two approaches to address this problem. We have studied a rat model of small bowel adaptation after intestinal resection, in which there are dynamic alterations in the proliferation and differentiation of the epithelium. After 70% resection of the gut, the remaining adaptive crypt epithelium undergoes a marked proliferative response, resulting in crypt and villus cell hyperplasia and increased absorptive capacity to compensate for the loss of normal functional surface area[2-4]. We have used this model to begin to identify the molecules involved in regulating these processes, employing subtractive hybridization techniques to isolate genes that are transcriptionally regulated in adaptation[5]. The enterocytic response to loss of small bowel surface area has also been examined[6]. Specifically, the expression of a variety of enterocytic genes in control and adaptive tissues was quantitated by RNA blot hybridization, immunohistochemical and in situ hybridization techniques. In related studies, we have also attempted to identify factors that regulate the normal spatial differentiation of the gut, from crypt to villus tip and from duodenum to colon. Specifically, the role of luminal factors in regulating epithelial cell differentiation was examined using intestinal isograft implantation techniques[7-11]. We have employed the rodent model of intestinal development, focusing on fetal life, during crypt-villus morphogenesis and cytodifferentiation, and on postnatal ontogeny. Key aspects of this work will be reviewed.

THE INTESTINAL ADAPTIVE RESPONSE IS IMPORTANT FOR RECOVERY OF NORMAL FUNCTION FOLLOWING LOSS OF SMALL BOWEL SURFACE AREA

In the human, loss of functional small bowel surface area may occur following surgical resection for vascular injury, trauma, or Crohn's disease of the small bowel, or as a consequence of radiation injury or intestinal bypass for weight loss. In children, necrotizing enterocolitis and intestinal atresia are two other important causes of short bowel syndrome. After substantial intestinal resection, the magnitude of the adaptive response in the remnant normal intestine in part determines whether a patient may continue to be enterally nourished or whether short- or long-term total parenteral nutrition will be required for survival, due to severe short bowel syndrome. The medical and economic costs of long-term parenteral nutrition are substantial. Thus, an understanding of the molecular basis of the adaptive response is required to facilitate the design of new therapies to enhance small bowel surface area and prevent the adverse sequelae of short bowel syndrome.

THE ADAPTIVE EPITHELIUM RESPONDS RAPIDLY TO LOSS OF SMALL BOWEL SURFACE AREA BY INCREASING THE EXPRESSION OF SOME ENTEROCYTE-SPECIFIC GENE PRODUCTS

Enhanced crypt cell production rate resulting in crypt and villus hyperplasia is one of the cardinal features of the adaptive response. However, the individual contribution of the differentiated enterocyte to the adaptive process has been much less well described. The ability of this cellular population to respond to the loss of small bowel surface area is unclear. Although several studies have suggested that the adaptive enterocyte is functionally immature[12-14], others have shown a selective increase in enterocytic protein expression[15,16]. To begin to clarify and quantitate the enterocytic response to loss of small bowel surface area, we have used a rat model of small bowel adaptation after 70% intestinal resection[6]. Male Sprague–Dawley rats were randomly assigned to undergo control (sham) resection (small bowel transection and re-anastomosis) or 70% intestinal resection (Figure 1). A second control group consisted of sham-operated animals that underwent laparotomy without intestinal transection. The small intestines were harvested at various times after surgery, and segments of duodenum, jejunum and ileum were harvested for further analysis.

To assess the enterocytic response to loss of small bowel surface area, the expression of a variety of abundant, absorptive cell-specific genes was examined in the remnant ileum after small bowel resection. Apolipoprotein (apo) A-IV, apo

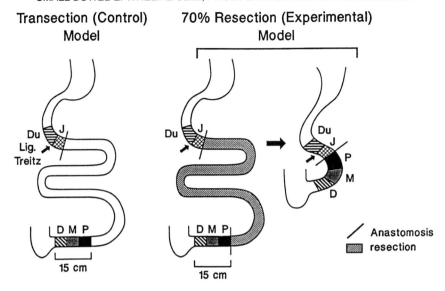

Figure 1 70% intestinal resection model. Left: transection or sham resection control model. The segments subjected to analysis as well as the site of transection and reanastomosis 5 cm distal to the ligament of Treitz are indicated. Right: resection model, with segment of intestine removed indicated. Du, duodenum; J, jejunum; P, proximal ileum; M, mid-ileum; D, distal ileum (reprinted from Ref. 5)

A-I, intestinal fatty acid binding protein (I-FABP) and liver fatty acid binding protein (L-FABP) mRNA levels were measured by RNA dot blot hybridization in sham, transfected, and experimental (adaptive) intestinal segments. These genes were chosen because they exhibit unique yet well-characterized regional and cell-specific patterns of expression in the developing and adult gut[17]. Adaptive ileal apo A-IV mRNA levels were markedly increased 48 h after resection compared with either control group (Figure 2A), and remained increased 1 week after resection (Figure 2B). To assess cell-specific expression of apo A-IV, in situ hybridization and immunohistochemical techniques were used. Apo A-IV mRNA and protein were expressed in villus-associated enterocytes but not in the crypt, in both adaptive and control intestine (Figure 3). However, apo A-IV mRNA and protein levels were increased in the adaptive compared with control enterocyte. Therefore, the changes in apo A-IV expression were not simply due to increased mucosal surface area. In contrast, no change in mRNA expression of a related gene, apo A-I, was found in any region of the adaptive gut 48 h after resection. The two cytoplasmic fatty acid binding proteins were also differentially regulated during adaptation (Figure 4). I-FABP mRNA levels were significantly increased in adaptive compared to control ileum 48 h after resection, but were no longer elevated by 1 week after surgery. In contrast, L-FABP levels were increased in proximal and mid ileum only compared with sham-operated animals 48 h after operation. The cell-specific expression of the FABPs (in villus-associated but not crypt enterocytes) remained unaltered during adaptation.

These results are in agreement with cytochemical findings and biochemical studies of other groups[15,16] who showed that expression of some enterocytic proteins

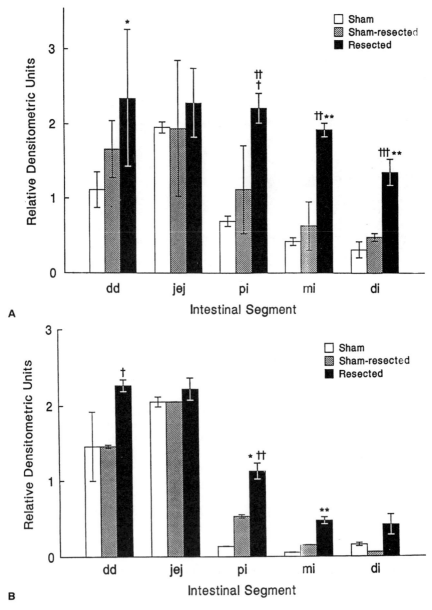

Figure 2 Apo A-IV mRNA expression is induced in adaptive ileum compared to sham or sham-resected intestine 48 h or 1 week after surgery. Segments of small intestine from duodenum to ileum were harvested from sham, sham-resected or resected animals 48 h (A) or 1 week (B) after surgery. Total RNA was prepared from individual segments and RNA dot blot hybridization analysis was performed using a ^{32}P-labelled apo A-IV rat cDNA probe that is specific for detecting apo A-IV mRNA. Data are means ± SEM. p values by Student's t-test for unpaired data: in (A) †$p < 0.01$ compared with sham-resected; **$p < 0.001$ compared with sham-resected; *$p < 0.05$ compared with sham; †††$p < 0.01$ compared with sham; ††$p < 0.001$ compared with sham. In (B) †$p < 0.02$ compared with sham-resected; *$p < 0.05$ compared with sham-resected; ††$p < 0.02$ compared with sham; **$p < 0.05$ compared with sham. dd, duodenum; jej, jejunum; pi, proximal ileum; mi, mid-ileum; di, distal ileum (reprinted from Ref. 6)

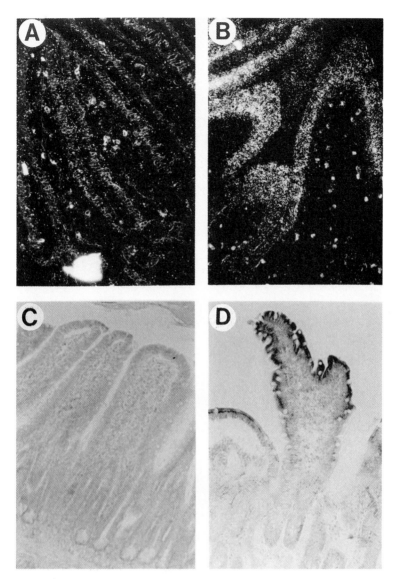

Figure 3 In situ hybridization (A,B) and immunohistochemical (C,D) analyses demonstrate adaptive enterocytic apo A-IV mRNA and protein levels are induced 48 h after surgery. Section of mid-ileum harvested 48 h after sham resection and hybridized to an [^{35}S]UTP-labelled apo A-IV cRNA (antisense) probe. Scattered white grains indicate low levels of cellular apo A-IV mRNA. (B) After 70% intestinal resection, there is a marked increase in enterocytic apo A-IV mRNA accumulation from the villus base to its tip in adaptive mid-ileum. Apo A-IV mRNA is not readily detectable in adaptive or control crypts. (C,D) Immunohistochemical analyses of control and adaptive proximal ileum. An anti-apo A-IV sera was used and antigen–antibody complexes were detected using immunogold–silver labelling techniques. Dark black staining indicates the presence of apo A-IV. (C) Section of control proximal ileum removed prior to resective surgery. Very light black staining is present on the tips of the villi. (D) Section of adaptive proximal ileum harvested 48 h after surgery. A marked increase in cellular apo A-IV accumulation is indicated by the dark black staining in villus enterocytes. There is a linear pattern of expression (arrow) consistent with apo A-IV localization in the Golgi apparatus. (A,B × 170; C, × 85; D, × 108.8; reprinted from Ref. 6)

221

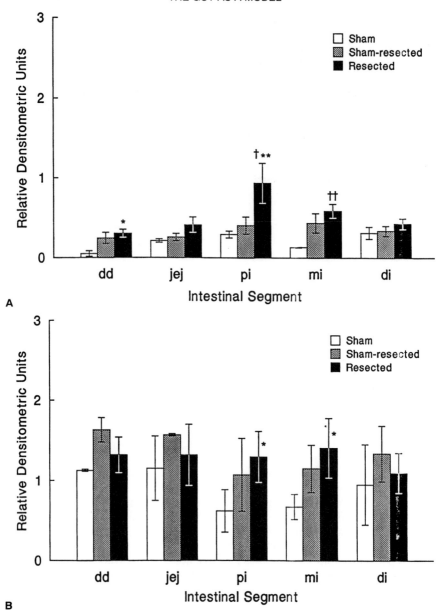

Figure 4 Differential regulation of the FABPs during intestinal adaptation. RNA dot blots were probed with ^{32}P-labelled I-FABP r L-FABP cDNA probes. Under the washing conditions specified only a single band representing the appropriate FABP could be detected by Northern blot hybridization. Quantitation of I-FABP mRNA expression in adaptive (resected) compared to sham or sham-resected intestine 48 h (A) or 1 week (C) after resection. Quantitation of L-FABP mRNA accumulation in adaptive, sham and sham-resected intestine at 48 h after resection (B). Abbreviations as per Figure 2. *$p < 0.05$ compared with sham; ††$p < 0.02$ compared with sham; †$p < 0.01$ compared with sham; **$p < 0.05$ compared with sham-resected (reprinted from Ref. 6).

is, in fact, selectively increased during the adaptive response. Thus, our data support the concept that the adaptive response is not limited to the crypt cell compartment, but includes the differentiated epithelium. The effects on enterocytic gene expression during adaptation are not likely to be mediated via the crypt (i.e. by inducing the appearance on the villus of a new lineage of adaptive enterocyte) since the response is too rapid. We and others[18,19] have shown that apo A-IV mRNA levels, for example, are up-regulated in villus tip adaptive ileal enterocytes as early as 16 h after surgery. Thus, the rodent enterocyte responds to loss of functional small bowel surface area by a selective increase in gene expression, at least in the short term. Further experiments are needed to clarify the molecular enterocytic response in long-term studies of adaptation, and to determine whether similar alterations in gene expression are found in humans.

INTESTINAL GENES ARE TRANSCRIPTIONALLY REGULATED IN RESPONSE TO LOSS OF SMALL BOWEL SURFACE AREA

Although the morphological features of the adaptive response have been clearly described, little is known about the underlying molecular and cellular mechanisms. It is clear that luminal nutrients are essential for full expression of the adaptive phenotype[20,21], yet the mechanism by which these substances affect the crypt cells is unknown. Polyamine synthesis is required for stimulating cellular pro-liferation[22]. Several likely humoral mediators of the adaptive proliferative response have been identified, including growth hormone, insulin-like growth factor-1 (IGF-1), glucagon, and related peptides[23], yet none has been shown to have an essential role in promoting the adaptive response.

As an approach to begin to define the molecular mechanisms underlying the adaptive intestinal response, we used subtractive hybridization techniques to identify genes that are differentially regulated in the adaptive intestine[5]. Isolation of genes that are transcriptionally regulated in the gut facilitates the identification of potential mediators and modulators of the adaptive response in a manner that is not biased by preconceptions about their identity. An adaptive cDNA library was constructed from ileum harvested 48 h postoperatively. This time point was chosen to eliminate non-specific changes in gene expression in response to the stress of surgery and to allow 24 h for the exposure of the gut to nutrients that are required for the maximal adaptive response. A subtracted experimental probe was prepared by hybridizing labelled adaptive ileal cDNA to biotinylated control ileal RNA to remove sequences in common[24]. This probe and a subtracted control probe were used to sequentially screen the cDNA library. Plaques that were positive after the screen with the experimental probe but negative when screened with the control probe were isolated and further analysed by sequence analysis and expression studies.

The cloned cDNAs that were isolated from the adaptive ileal library included known genes that were categorized as Group 1: enterocyte-specific genes involved in nutrient trafficking; Group 2: putative cell cycle regulators; and Group 3: genes involved in the regulation of protein synthesis and degradation (Table 1). Also cloned were 10 novel cDNAs (Group IV).

Table 1 Cloned cDNAs isolated from adaptive ileal library by subtractive hybridization

---

Group 1: Enterocyte specific genes involved in nutrient trafficking
    Cellular retinol binding protein II (CRBPII)
    Apolipoprotein A-IV
    Ileal lipid binding protein (ILBP)
    Liver fatty acid binding protein
Group II: Immediate early genes/putative cell cycle regulators
    PC4/TIS7
    Proteasome β-subunit
    Pancreatitis associated proteins I, II, III
    Protein phosphatase 1δ
Group 3: Genes involved in regulation of protein synthesis and degradation
    Glucose regulated protein (GRP) 78
    Proteasome β-subunit
    Ribosomal phosphoprotein 40S and 60S subunits
Group 4: Novel cDNAs ([10])

Group 1

The first group of cDNAs that encode enterocytic genes included apo A-IV and L-FABP, as would be predicted based on prior studies of the enterocytic response to small bowel surface area (Figure 2). Cellular retinol binding protein II (CRBPII), a cytoplasmic hydrophobic binding protein that facilitates intestinal vitamin A absorption and metabolism[25,26], and ileal lipid binding protein (ILBP), which is postulated to play a role in bile acid absorption in the ileum[27], were also cloned. Interestingly, these two proteins are also members of the FABP family. The expression of these genes may be increased in adaptation to enhance intestinal absorption of lipids and retinoids. Alternatively, their increased expression may indicate a specific role for their encoded proteins in mediating the adaptive response. For example, CRBPII could modulate intestinal vitamin A metabolism and subsequently the synthesis and trafficking of all-*trans* and 9-*cis* retinoic acids, ligands for nuclear retinoic acid and retinoid x receptors.

Group II

Of the putative cell cycle regulators, protein phosphatase 1 (PP1), a serine-threonine phosphatase, is of particular interest in adaptation. The protein phosphatase 1δ isoform of the catalytic subunit was cloned from the adaptive ileal library. Phosphorylation–dephosphorylation events are critical in the regulation of cellular growth and differentiation[28]. PP1 is required for completion of mitosis in yeast or *Drosophila*[28], and injection of anti-PP1 antibodies into mammalian cells arrests mitosis[29]. These studies suggested that PP1 may be important in early cellular proliferative events in adaptation.

The pancreatitis-associated proteins I, II and III are a group of proteins that demonstrate increased expression in experimental acute pancreatitis[30–32]. All three were cloned from the adaptive ileal cDNA library. These proteins are homologous with *reg*, another pancreatic protein that is a putative regulator of islet cell proliferation, as well as with the carbohydrate binding domain of Ca^{2+}-dependent lectins. PAP I, a secreted protein, is the best characterized of the three. Its expression appears to be regulated by tumour necrosis factor α, interferon γ, and IL-6 and glucocorticoids in combination[33]. The functions of PAP II and III are less well described, but all share significant sequence homology with each other. As secreted proteins with homology to *reg*, a potential role for these proteins as paracrine modulators of crypt cell proliferation can be hypothesized.

The β-subunit of the rat proteasome has also been cloned from the adaptive ileal library. Proteasomes are large multisubunit proteases important for nonlysosomal protein degradation. Both ubiquitin-dependent and ubiquitin-independent pathways of proteolysis have been described. Proteasomes appear to be important in antigen presentation and in the regulation of cellular proliferation, due to their role in degrading cyclins, p53, and *fos* as well as ornithine decarboxylase[34].

Group 3

The glucose-regulated peptide grp78 was included in the third group of cloned cDNAs. This member of the 70 kDa heat shock protein (hsp 70) family is known to facilitate correct folding of secretory proteins in the lumen of the endoplasmic reticulum[35], and may play a role in preventing cells from undergoing apoptotic death[36]. In conditions of stress such as cell injury and anoxia, grp78 accumulates in the endoplasmic reticulum and acts as a chaperone to rid the cell of abnormal proteins[37].

TEMPORAL AND CELL-SPECIFIC REGULATION OF CLONED cDNAs DURING GUT ADAPTATION

After these genes were identified and classified by sequence analysis and by comparison with known sequences in Genbank, we sought to define their role in adaptation. Our approach was to examine patterns of temporal, regional and cell-specific expression during adaptation, and to begin to identify regulators of their expression in the gut. Northern blot and in situ hybridization techniques were utilized. The temporal course of expression of these genes during adaptation was diverse. The expression of some of the cloned genes increased very early in the adaptive process. For example, PP1δ, grp78 and PAP I and III mRNA levels were increased in adaptive compared to control intestine at an early time after surgery (8 h; Figures 5, 6). On the other hand, PAP II expression was increased in adaptive intestine 48 h after surgery, but not at 8 h. PP1δ and grp78 mRNA levels were most increased in adaptive compared to control gut at 8 h, yet the increase in PAP III expression was highest at 48 h. There was also regional specificity in the intestinal response to loss of small bowel surface area (e.g. Figures 2, 4). In general, ileal segments and duodenum demonstrated the most marked changes in mRNA levels. In contrast, jejunal mRNA levels remained unchanged in the first 48 h after small bowel resection.

In situ hybridization and immunohistochemical analyses indicated that the cell-specific expression of the cloned genes was also quite diverse. Some genes, such as apo A-IV and L-FABP, were expressed only in villus-associated entero-

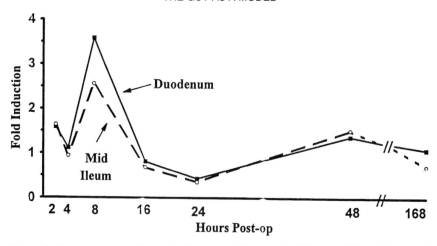

Figure 5 Temporal pattern of protein phosphatase 1δ expression following 70% small intestinal resection. At the indicated times following surgery, segments of the duodenum and mid-ileum were harvested from sham-resected control and resected experimental animals. Total RNA was extracted, RNA dot blots were prepared and hybridized with a radiolabelled PP1δ cDNA. Data are expressed as fold induction of the resected compared to the control animals (reprinted from Ref. 5)

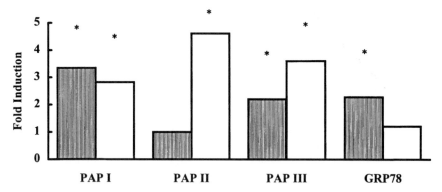

Figure 6 Increase in GRP78 and PAP I, II and III at 8 and 48 h after resection. RNA was harvested from the ileum 8 (shaded bars) and 48 h (open bars) following 70% intestinal resection or sham resection ($n = 7$–9 rats per surgical group). Northern blots were prepared and hybridized with radio-labelled GRP78 or PAP I, II or III cDNAs. Data are expressed as mean fold induction of the resected compared to the control animals. Fold induction is calculated by dividing the data from the experimental animals by the data from control animals. Thus values greater than 1 reflect an increase and values less than 1 reflect a decrease in transcript levels. $^*p < 0.05$ by Student's t-test (reprinted from Ref. 5)

cytes[6], whereas others, such as grp78, were expressed in crypts and villi[5]. However, the characteristic cellular localization of the respective mRNAs and proteins along the crypt-villus axis did not change in the adaptive compared to the control gut.

These results support the concept that the adaptive process consists of a complex series of temporally regulated events occurring in both crypt and villus cells. We have identified components of an 'early' transcriptional response that occurs in the first 48 h after surgery and includes the regulation of genes that may play a role in cellular proliferation/differentiation and protein synthesis and degradation. The complete description of these responses, as well as the identification of earlier and later events, provides much work for the future. However, we can suggest that the identification of genes that are transcriptionally regulated during adaptation provides a firm basis for further analysis of the underlying molecular pathways. The factors that regulate these genes can now be identified, and common regulatory pathways may subsequently be clarified.

REGULATION OF EPITHELIAL CELL DIFFERENTIATION DURING ONTOGENY: ROLE OF LUMINAL CONTENTS

Despite rapid proliferation, the gut epithelium maintains precise spatial differentiation in the crypt-villus and duodenal-colonic axes. As mentioned above, the four major differentiated cell types are produced from stem cells located near the base of the crypt. Absorptive enterocytes and goblet cells appear on the villus, Paneth cells differentiate during migration to the crypt base and enteroendocrine cells arise during ascent and descent from the proliferative zone. In addition to this complex pathway in the crypt-villus axis, spatial differentiation is also maintained from duodenum to colon. For example, there are regional differences in the expression of a variety of enterocytic genes such as those encoding the intestinal and liver fatty acid binding protein and apolipoprotein A-IV, with highest mRNA and protein concentrations in the proximal small bowel. At least 15 different enteroendocrine cell types can be defined by their principal neuroendocrine products, each having a distinctive distribution along this horizontal axis[38]. Finally, there are also regional differences in the number of goblet cells, and Paneth cells, as defined by lysozyme expression[8].

To determine whether these complex differentiation pathways could be established and maintained in the absence of a normal luminal environment, we examined the expression of a variety of enterocytic and enteroendocrine cell gene products in normal rodent intestine and in intestinal isografts[7-11]. We studied the mature intestine and also characterized spatial patterns of gene expression during ontogeny.

THE NORMAL CELLULAR AND SPATIAL DIFFERENTIATION OF THE GUT EPITHELIUM IS PRESERVED IN INTESTINAL ISOGRAFTS

In our initial studies, enterocytic differentiation was assessed by examining the expression of the fatty acid binding proteins. Enteroendocrine cell expression was characterized using serotonin, gastrin, CCK, GIP, secretin, neurotensin, PYY and substance P as neuroendocrine markers. Goblet cell distribution was assessed by periodic acid Schiff (PAS) stain, and Paneth cell differentiation was established by detecting lysozyme expression. Intestinal isograft implantation studies were performed by removing fetal intestines prior to cytodifferentiation and the formation of the villus, followed by implantation into the subcutaneous space of young adult host animals. The isografts were grown for 4–6 weeks, and differentiation

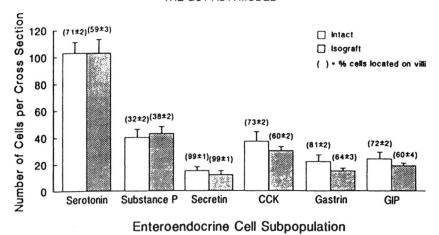

Figure 7 Enteroendocrine cell subpopulation frequency and distribution within intact jejunum and jejunal isografts. The number of immunoreactive enteroendocrine cells per cross-section and their distribution along the crypt-to-villus axis were determined. The average percentage of cells located on villi±SEM is given in parentheses (reprinted from Ref. 7)

pathways from crypt to villus tip[7] and duodenum to colon[8] were examined. Using immunohistochemical methods, we showed that the normal adult patterns of gene expression in enterocytic, enteroendocrine and Paneth cells were precisely recapitulated in the isografted intestine (Figures 7, 8). Goblet cell distribution from duodenum to colon was similarly unaltered. Thus the spatial differentiation programmes of the adult intestine appeared preserved despite the absence of luminal nutrients and pancreaticobiliary secretions.

LUMINAL CONTENTS MAY PLAY A MODULATORY ROLE IN SPATIAL DIFFERENTIATION ALONG THE CRYPT-VILLUS AXIS DURING ONTOGENY

We next wished to examine the influence of the luminal and hormonal environment on cellular differentiation during gut epithelial ontogeny, since there are marked alterations in the intestinal luminal environment during development (reviewed in Ref. 39). Amniotic fluid bathes the intestine during intrauterine life. At birth, mother's milk is ingested and during weaning, a solid diet is introduced. Gut maturation is also influenced by systemic hormonal changes, particularly thyroxine and glucocorticoid levels (reviewed in Ref. 39). During these stages, the rodent intestine also undergoes profound morphogenesis and cytodifferentiation. In fetal life, proliferation of undifferentiated endoderm and mesenchyme is followed by the formation of nascent villi[40]. Cellular proliferation becomes confined to the intervillus epithelium, the site of crypt formation. In the postnatal period, villus elongation and crypt fission are accompanied by further cytodifferentiation.

Do the profound luminal and hormonal changes that occur during gut ontogeny

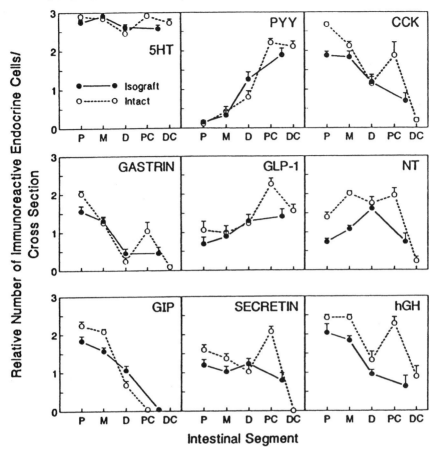

Figure 8 Regional distribution of enteroendocrine cell subpopulations along the duodenal to colonic axis of the intact intestine and intestinal isografts. The mean value for each enteroendocrine cell subpopulation (scored on a 0–3+ scale) is shown ±SE. Open circles, intact intestine; closed circles, values from isografts. P, M, D, proximal, mid and distal thirds of the small intestine; PC, proximal colon; DC, distal colon; 5HT, serotonin (reprinted from Ref. 8)

play a role in generating spatial differentiation in the gut? To answer this question, intestinal isografts were once again employed. We had previously shown that on gestation day 17–18 in the rat, L-FABP and CRBPII were initially expressed in a mosaic pattern in nascent enterocytes, coincident with villus formation[17,41]. To determine whether or not the normal fetal–maternal environment is required for the establishment of this pattern of cytodifferentiation, intestines were removed from fetuses on gestation day 12 and implanted in young adult host rats. Grafts were harvested 6–8 days later and examined for I-FABP expression by immunohistochemical means. The mosaic pattern of expression of L-FABP was preserved in these grafts despite the absence of a normal luminal and extraluminal environment from fetal day 12 (Figure 9)[10]. These results suggested that an intrinsic genetic differentiation programme is present in endoderm and mesenchyme which

229

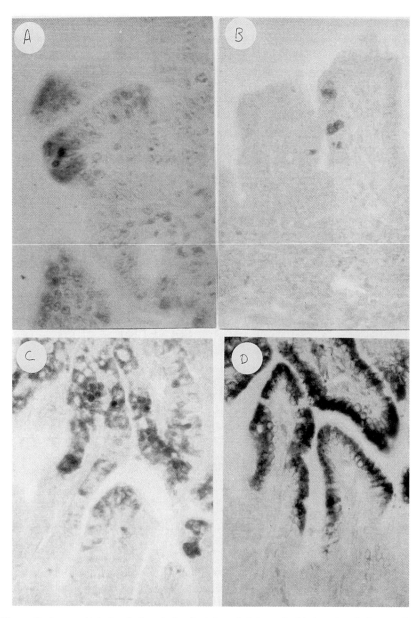

Figure 9 Immunohistochemical analysis of rat intestinal isografts implanted early in gestation. Sections were immunostained to detect L-FABP (A,C) or cellular retinol binding protein II (CRBPII), (B,D), using immunogold staining with silver enhancement. (A) Small intestinal isograft implanted on fetal day 12, grown in the subcutaneous space of an adult host rat for 6 days (equivalent to fetal day 17–18). A nascent, thumblike villus is seen with cells that either stain darkly for L-FABP (arrows) or are unstained, recapitulating the normal ontogenic pattern of FABP expression. (B) Immunostaining of an equivalent isograft as in (A), to detect CRBPII. (C) Intestinal isograft implanted on fetal day 12, harvested 9 days later (equivalent to fetal day 20–21). L-FABP is now expressed homogeneously in all villus enterocytes, as in the normal fetal intestine. (D) Similar isograft as in (C), stained to detect CRBPII (reprinted from Ref. 10)

is not dependent on systemic or luminal factors for its expression after day 12 of gestation.

We next wished to determine whether spatial patterns of enterocytic gene expression were altered in isografts during postnatal ontogeny[10]. In situ hybridization techniques showed a profound alteration in the pattern of expression of L-FABP and apo A-IV mRNA expression in isografts harvested at various times during development (Figure 10). In the normal postnatal week 1 or 2 rat intestine, L-FABP and apo A-IV mRNA expression appear to be predominantly localized to villus base enterocytes. However, the preferential accumulation of L-FABP or apo A-IV mRNA in villus base enterocytes was never observed in isografts (Figures 10, 11). Rather, a mature, adult pattern of mRNA distribution was seen. These results suggest that the gut lumen and/or its systemic environment modulate spatial patterns of gene expression from villus base to tip during ontogeny. We hypothesize that the dissimilar spatial patterns of gene expression may be due to altered epithelial cell migration rates in the isograft compared with normal developing intestine, secondary to differences in systemic hormone levels in the adult host compared with the normal suckling pup. Future studies will aim to reverse these differences by administration of systemic hormones that mimic the normal rise in glucocorticoids and thyroxine or by reintroduction of luminal contents.

CONCLUSIONS

We have used two model systems to begin to identify the mechanisms that regulate intestinal epithelial cell proliferation and differentiation. The intestinal adaptation model is a valuable tool for studying the pathways that control crypt cell proliferation and the switch to a differentiated state. Clarification of these molecular mechanisms also has relevance to the treatment of human bowel diseases, to facilitate the design of new therapies to enhance functional small bowel surface area after resection or following injury from a variety of intestinal illnesses. Intestinal isograft implantation experiments have established that the programme directing the differentiation of the gut epithelium is not dependent upon the presence of a normal intestinal luminal environment, yet during ontogeny a modulatory role for luminal and/or systemic factors has been identified. By altering the contents of the isograft lumen or by manipulating the systemic hormonal environment (via the host) the precise identity of these factors may be clarified. Since the differentiation of its epithelium is intact, the isograft may also be an excellent model to exploit for the study of epithelium−pathogen relationships that are toxic to the intact animal. In addition, transgenic isografts may be useful to study the consequences on the normal differentiation and organization of the gut of a specific targeted gene knockout, particularly one that would otherwise be lethal due to catastrophic effects on other organs.

References

1. Cheng H, Leblond CP. Origin, differentiation and renewal of the four main epithelial cell types in the mouse small intestine: unitarian theory of the origin of the four epithelial cell types. Am J Anat. 1979;41:537−62.

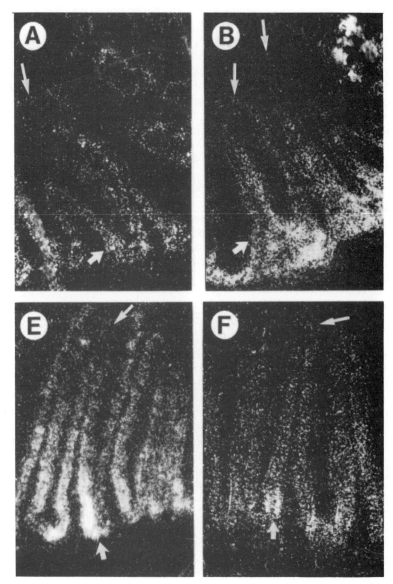

Figure 10 In situ hybridization analysis of the postnatal ontogeny of L-FABP and apo A-IV expression in normal intestine and intestinal isografts. Normal jejunum or jejunal isografts were hybridized to an L-FABP (A–D) or apo AIV (E–H) cRNA probe. Yellow grains indicate the presence of L-FABP or APO A-IV mRNA, viewed under darkfield microscopy. (A) Section of 1-week-old normal jejunum. Note decreased cellular L-FABP mRNA accumulation in the mid-villus and villus tip (long arrow) and increased yellow grains indicating L-FABP mRNA (short arrow). (B) Two-week-old normal jejunum. A marked gradient in expression of L-FABP mRNA from villus base to tip is still present at 2 weeks of gestation. (C) Section of 1-week-old jejunal isograft. The distinct spatial pattern of L-FABP mRNA expression from villus base to tip is altered in the isografted epithelium. Note the lack of L-FABP mRNA accumulation at the villus base (short arrow). In contrast, accumulation of grains is most abundant in the mid-villus and upper villus regions. (D) Two-week-old jejunal isograft. Cellular

232

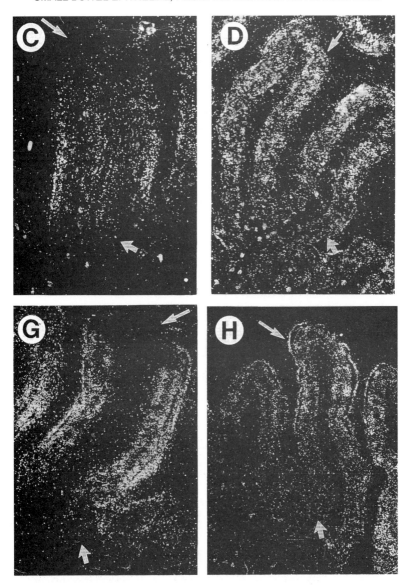

Figure 10 *Continued.* L-FABP mRNA expression is most prominent in mid and upper villus entero-cytes (long arrow) and decreases towards the villus base (short arrow). Slightly increased background signal is present on this section compared to the others in this series. (E) One-week-old intact jejunum hybridized with an anti-sense apo A-IV probe. Very high levels of apo A-IV mRNA are present in cells located at the villus base (short arrow) and decrease in the upper villus and villus tip (long arrow). (F) Two-week-old intact jejunum. Apo A-IV mRNA is still most abundantly expressed in enterocytes at the base of the villus. (G,H) Sections of 1- (G) and 2- (H) week-old jejunal isograft. As noted for L-FABP, apo A-IV expression is markedly altered in the crypt-villus axis of isografts. There is decreased cellular mRNA accumulation in villus base enterocytes (short arrow) with maximal expression in the mid and upper villus, and decreased expression at the villus tip in (G) (long arrow). (A,B,E,F × 130, C,D × 260, H × 104; reprinted from Ref. 10)

233

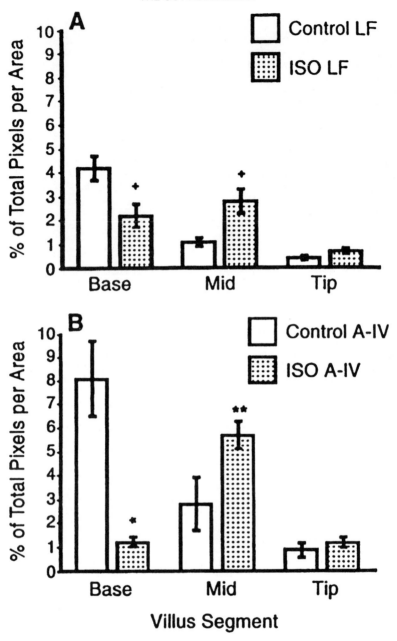

Figure 11 Quantitative assessment of enterocytic gene expression along the crypt-villus axis of 1-week-old jejunum compared to jejunal isografts. In situ hybridization analyses were performed as per Figure 10. Grain density was quantitated per unit area in three regions of the villus, including the base of the villus, the mid region and the villus tip. Grain density was measured in the villi of three different intact jejuna and three isografts. A total of six villi were counted per sample. (A) L-FABP, †$p < 0.001$. (B) Apo A-IV, *$p < 0.000001$, **$p < 0.02$ (reprinted from Ref. 10)

2. Cheng H, McCulloch C, Bjerknes M. Effect of 30% intestinal resection on whole population cell kinetics of mouse intestinal epithelium. Anat Rec. 1986;215:35–41.
3. Dowling RH, Booth CC. Structural and functional changes following small intestinal resection in the rat. Clin Sci Lond. 1967;32:139–49.
4. Williamson RCN, Buchholtz TW, Malt RA. Humoral stimulation of cell proliferation in small bowel after transection and resection in rats. Gastroenterology. 1978;75:249–54.
5. Dodson BD, Wang JL, Swietlicki EA, Rubin DC, Levin MS. Analysis of cloned cDNAs differentially expressed in adapting remnant small intestine after partial resection. Am J Physiol. 1996; 271:G347–56.
6. Rubin DC, Swietlicki EA, Wang JL, Dodson BD, Levin MS. Enterocytic gene expression in intestinal adaptation: evidence for a specific cellular response. Am J Physiol. 1996;270:G143–52.
7. Rubin DC, Roth KA, Birkenmeier EH, Gordon JI. Epithelial cell differentiation in normal and transgenic mouse intestinal isografts. J Cell Biol. 1991;113:1183–92.
8. Rubin DC, Swietlicki E, Roth KA, Gordon JI. Use of fetal intestinal isografts from normal and transgenic mice to study the programming of positional information along the duodenal-to-colonic axis. J Biol Chem. 1992;267:15122–33.
9. Rubin DC, Swietlicki E, Gordon JI. Use of isografts to study proliferation and differentiation programs of mouse stomach epithelia. Am J Physiol. 1994;267:G27–39.
10. Gutierrez ED, Grapperhaus KJ, Rubin DC. Ontogenic regulation of spatial differentiation in the gut epithelium in the crypt-villus axis of normal and isografted small intestine. Am J Physiol. 1995;269:G500–11.
11. Okuyama S, Rubin DC, Woodley MC, Peters MG. Regional expression of murine intestinal immune cells in normal and isografted intestine. Cell Immunol. 1995;163:198–205.
12. Buts JP, DeKeyser N, Dove C. Cellular adaptation of the rat small intestine after proximal enterectomy: changes in microvillus enzymes and in the secretory component of immunoglobulins. Pediatric Res. 1987;22:29–33.
13. Gleeson MD, Dowling RH, Peters TS. Biochemical changes in intestinal mucosa after experimental small bowel by-pass in the rat. Clin Sci. 1972;43:743–57.
14. Menge H, Robinson JWL. The relationship between functional and structural alterations in the rat small intestine following resection of varying extent. Res Exp Med. 1978;173:41–53.
15. Albert V, Young GP. Differentiation status of rat enterocytes after intestinal adaptation to jejunoileal bypass. Gut. 1992;33:1638–43.
16. Chaves M, Smith MW, Williamson RCN. Increased activity of digestive enzymes in ileal enterocytes adapting to proximal small bowel resection. Gut. 1987;28:981–7.
17. Rubin DC. Spatial analysis of transcriptional activation in fetal rat jejunal and ileal gut epithelium. Am J Physiol. 1992;263:G853–63.
18. Wang JL, Swietlicki E, Tudos R, Rubin DC, Levin MS. Analysis of rat intestinal apolipoprotein (apo) AIV HNF-4 gene expression in the early adaptive period following massive small bowel resection. Gastroenterology. 1995;108:A762.
19. Sonoyama K, Kiriyama S, Niki R. Adaptive response of apolipoprotein A-1 and A-IV mRNA in residual ileum after massive small bowel resection in rats. J Nutr Sci Vitaminol. 1995;41:253–64.
20. Bristol JB, Williamson RCN. Nutrition, operations and intestinal adaptation. J Parenter Enteral Nutr. 198;12:299–309.
21. Dowling RH. Cellular and molecular basis of intestinal and pancreatic adaptation. Scand J Gastroenterol. 1992;27(Suppl 193):64–7.
22. Luk GD, Baylin SB. Inhibition of intestinal epithelial DNA synthesis and adaptive hyperplasia after jejunectomy in the rat by suppression of polyamine biosynthesis. J Clin Invest. 1984;74: 698–704.
23. Taylor RG, Fuller PJ. Humoral regulation of intestinal adaptation. Bailliére's Clin Endocrinol Metab. 1994;8:165–83.
24. Sive HL, St John T. A simple subtractive hybridization technique employing photoactivatable biotin and phenol extraction. Nucleic Acids Res. 1988;16:10937.
25. Levin MS. Cellular retinol-binding proteins are determinants of retinol uptake and metabolism in stably transfected Caco-2 cells. J Biol Chem. 1993;268:8267–76.
26. Lissoos TW, Davis AE, Levin MS. Vitamin A trafficking in Caco-2 cells stably transfected with cellular retinol binding proteins. Am J Physiol. 1995;268:G224–31.
27. Kramer WF, Girbig F, Gutjahr U et al. Intestinal bile acid absorption. Na+ dependent bile acid transport activity in rabbit small intestine correlates with the coexpression of an integral 93 kDa

and a peripheral 14 kDa bile acid-binding membrane protein along the duodenum-ileum axis. J Biol Chem. 1993;268:18035–46.

28. Mumby MC, Walter G. Protein serine/threonine phosphatases: structure, regulation and functions in cell growth. Physiol Rev. 1993;73:673–99.

29. Fernandez A, Brautigan DI, Lamb NJ. Protein phosphatase type 1 in mammalian cell mitosis: chromosomal localization and involvement in mitotic exit. J Cell Biol. 1992;116:1421–30.

30. Iovanna JL, Orelle B, Keim V, Dagorn JC. Messenger RNA sequence and expression of rat pancreatitis-associated protein, a lectin-related protein overexpressed during acute experimental pancreatitis. J Biol Chem. 1991;266:24664–9.

31. Frigerio JM, Dusetti NJ, Keim V, Dagorn JC, Iovanna JL. Identification of a second rat pancreatitis-associated protein. Messenger RNA cloning, gene structure, and expression during acute pancreatitis. Biochemistry. 1993;32:9236–41.

32. Frigerio JM, Dusetti NJ, Garrido P, Dagorn JC, Iovanna JL. The pancreatitis associated protein III (PAP III), a new member of the PAP family. Biochim Biophys Acta. 1993;1216:329–31.

33. Dusetti NJ, Ortiz EM, Mallo GV, Dagorn JC, Iovanna JL. Pacreatitis-associated protein (PAP I), an acute phase protein induced by cytokines – identification of two functional interleukin-6 response elements in the rat PAP I promoter region. J Biol Chem. 1995;270:22417–21.

34. Ichihara AAU, Tanaka KTI. Roles of proteasomes in cell growth. Mol Biol Rep. 1995;21:49–52.

35. Lee AS. Mammalian stress response: induction of the glucose-regulated protein family. Curr Opin Cell Biol. 1992;4:267–73.

36. Sugawara S, Takeda K, Lee A, Dennert G. Suppression of stress protein grp78 induction in tumor B/C10ME eliminates resistance to cell mediated cytotoxicity. Cancer Res. 1993;53:5001–5.

37. Hartl FU, Hlodan R, Langer T. Molecular chaperones in protein folding: the art of avoiding sticky situations. Trends Biochem Sci. 1994;19:20–5.

38. Roth KA, Hertz JM, Gordon JI. Mapping enteroendocrine cell populations in transgenic mice reveals an unexpected degree of complexity in cellular differentiation within the gastrointestinal tract. J Cell Biol. 1990;110:1791–801.

39. Henning SJ, Rubin DC, Shulman RJ. Ontogeny of the intestinal mucosa. In: Johnson LR, editor. Physiology of the Gastrointestinal Tract, 3rd edn. New York: Raven Press. 1994:571–609.

40. Trier JS, Moxey PC. Morphogenesis of the small intestine during fetal development. In: Elliot K, Whelan J, editors. Development of Mammalian Absorptive Processes. New York: CIBA Foundation Symposium. 1979:3–29.

41. Rubin DC, Ong DE, Gordon JI. Cellular differentiation in the emerging fetal rat small intestinal epithelium: mosaic patterns of gene expression. Proc Natl Acad Sci USA. 1989;86:1278–82.

20
Protein synthesis and trafficking in polarized epithelia: the parietal cell model

J. M. CROTHERS JR, D.-C. CHOW and J. G. FORTE

INTRODUCTION

Most eukaryotic cells demonstrate some degree of spatial asymmetry, or polarization, arising early in development from the asymmetry of cell division. Epithelial cells are the simplest, and most definitive, types of polarized cells, demarcated by tight junctions with a basolateral surface communicating with body fluids and an apical surface facing an external compartment. In addition to their barrier function, epithelial cells must regulate a variety of asymmetrical transport processes that serve to maintain body fluid homeostasis. Because of the diversity of transporters, their asymmetrical location to apical or basolateral plasma membrane, and the ability to recruit and manipulate the activity of the transporter proteins, the cell can effect an infinite variety of translocation processes. The gastrointestinal epithelium provides an example of the variety and selectivity of secretory and absorptive processes designed for nutritional homeostasis[1,2].

One of the key questions in epithelial physiology concerns the mechanisms which establish and maintain the polarity of membranes and transporters within the cell[3,4]. Membrane proteins are synthesized in the endoplasmic reticulum (ER) and are directed through a series of cellular compartments to their ultimate target membrane. Highly selective trafficking processes ensure that a transporter resides in a given membrane for a given cell type. For example, with few exceptions, Na,K-ATPase operates in the basolateral membrane, whereas H,K-ATPase is targeted solely to the apical membrane. Targeting of other transport proteins, such as the Cl^-/HCO_3^- exchanger or the Na^+/H^+ exchanger, is definitive within a given cell type, but residence within a particular membrane varies depending on tissue function, as may be readily seen along the gastrointestinal tract[5,6].

There is a large volume of literature reporting on the phenomena of membrane synthesis, trafficking and sorting in epithelial cells[3,7–9]. Although useful, these studies have been largely confined to in vitro cell systems, in which there is the potential of change and adaptation. The gastric parietal cell contains two closely related cation transport pumps, Na,K-ATPase and H,K-ATPase, which are faithfully sorted to different plasma membranes (personal observation), thus representing a potentially useful model in which to study mechanisms of trafficking and targeting. Furthermore, parietal cells are relatively rich in these pump proteins so that they constitute a sizeable fraction of the cellular protein and commitment of physiological activity. Our immediate goal was to study in vivo synthesis and trafficking of H,K-ATPase in the parietal cell, with the hope of eventually distinguishing sorting criteria and pathways for the H,K- and Na,K-ATPases. Here we report on the trafficking and turnover of a membrane-bound pump protein, H,K-ATPase, identifying four pools of residence designated as a nascent pool within the ER, a pubescent pool (probably Golgi system), a mature pool of functioning pump protein, and a senescent pool. Using a transfected cell culture system we also show that the β-subunit of H,K-ATPase requires glycosylation to exit the ER.

MATERIALS AND METHODS

Pulse-labelling of animals with [^{35}S]methionine/[^{35}]cysteine

New Zealand White rabbits weighing 2–3 kg were treated with cimetidine (20 mg/kg, s.c.) to put parietal cells in a resting state. A pulse of 2 mCi of [^{35}S]methionine and [^{35}S]cysteine in an approximately 4:1 ratio ([^{35}S]met/cys, obtained from ICN, Costa Mesa, CA, or DuPont NEN, Boston, MA) was injected via an ear vein. Serum was sampled from the other ear and counted in a scintillation counter to assess isotope clearance time. Serum ^{35}S levels declined rapidly in the first 4 min, with $t_{1/2}$ of about 2 min, creating an effective pulse[10]. Labelling was terminated at various times after the pulse of [^{35}S]met/cys by a lethal dose of sodium pentobarbital (50 mg/ml, 1.5 ml, i.v.) and the stomach was immediately removed for further processing.

The gastric mucosa was processed as previously described[11] to obtain crude cell fractions, P0, P1, P2 and P3, and supernatant, S3. The microsomal fraction (P3), a high-speed (100 000g for 60 min) pellet from a 13 000g for 10 min supernatant, was resuspended in 300 mM sucrose in suspending buffer (SB: 5 mM Tris–Cl, pH 7.3, 0.4 mM EDTA), layered on top of continuous gradients of 10–40% sucrose (wt/vol) in SB, and centrifuged at 100 000g for 4 h. Membranes were recovered in 12–18 equal fractions with densities determined as previously described[11]. The gradient pellets were resuspended in 300 mM sucrose in SB.

LLC-PK cells transfected with H,K-ATPase β-subunit

We used an LLC-PK cell line stably transfected with H,K-ATPase β-subunit (H,K-β-subunit) by Gottardi and Caplan[12] and carried out cell culture as they described. Cells were also treated with tunicamycin (1 μg/ml medium) for various times, then scraped, washed in PBS, and solubilized in SDS–PAGE sample buffer. The samples were analysed by Western blot using monoclonal antibody 2G11 against the H,K-β-subunit. Cells were also plated on cover slips, grown for 1–2 days, and switched to tunicamycin-containing medium for 21 h. They were then immunoprobed with 2G11 as described by Gottardi and Caplan[40] and photographed with a Nikon microphot-FXA.

SDS–PAGE and Western blots

Protein assay and sodium dodecyl sulphate polyacrylamide gel electrophoresis (SDS–PAGE) were carried out as previously described[11]. Samples were solubilized in SDS–PAGE sample buffer and run through 4% acrylamide pH 6.8 stacking gels and 9% acrylamide pH 8.8 separating gels. Gels showing gradient distributions were loaded with a constant percentage of each recovered fraction. Western blotting, autoradiography, and the acquisition and analysis of digitized images were carried out as previously described[13].

RESULTS

The microsomal fraction is enriched in total and nascent H,K-ATPase

Fractions from differential centrifugation of gastric mucosal homogenate were analysed by SDS–PAGE. Autoradiography and total protein staining of sample gels are shown in Figure 1 for a stomach 12 min after [^{35}S]met/cys injection. Labelled and total 94 kDa bands, indicated by arrowheads, are seen to be enriched in P3, the microsomal fraction. We have previously shown[11,14] that the 94 kDa band in P3 is overwhelmingly the H,K-ATPase α-subunit. The β-subunit, because of its glycosylation and diffuse banding pattern, cannot be seen by autoradiography or protein staining in these fractions. The proteins with the highest ^{35}S specific activity, isoforms of the zymogen pepsinogen, ran in the region of 40 kDa and were recovered mainly in the lower-speed membrane fractions and supernatant (S3).

Subfractionation of microsomes reveals time course for movement of H,K-ATPase through multiple membrane domains

Microsomal fractions from stomachs taken 12–90 min after [^{35}S]met/cys injection, were subfractionated on continuous sucrose gradients, then analysed by SDS–PAGE, Western blot and autoradiography. Figure 2 shows autoradiographs for three such tests, clearly revealing the progress of labelled α-subunit from the densest subfractions at 12 min post-injection to the lighter subfractions after 90 min. Over the same time course, labelling of pepsinogen isoforms, in the region of 40 kDa, decreased in the microsomal fractions, probably reflecting movement into dense-core granules that sediment in lower speed primary fractions.

Western blots of these fractions from the 30-min test, probed for the α- and β-subunits, show the distribution of total mature H,K-ATPase (Figure 2, bottom). This distribution, a major low density peak (~1.06 g/ml) with a higher density shoulder (~1.11 g/ml), has been previously described[13,14] and is typical regardless of the distribution of labelled H,K-ATPase. The β-subunit probe, in addition to

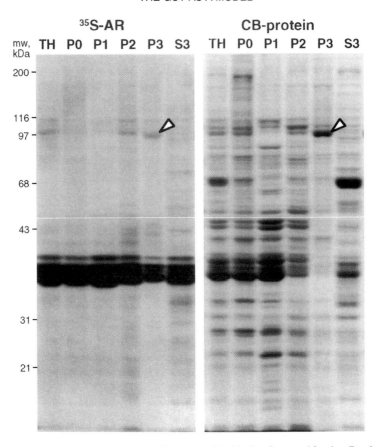

Figure 1 Pulse-labelled and total H,K-ATPase are enriched in the microsomal fraction. Fractions from differential centrifugation of resting gastric mucosal homogenate were analysed by SDS–PAGE. Autoradiography (left) and Coomassie Blue staining (right) of sample gels are shown for a stomach 12 min after [^{35}S]met/cys injection. Enrichment of the H,K-ATPase α-subunit (94 kDa band, open arrowheads) is seen in P3, the microsomal fraction. Heavily labelled pepsinogen isoforms, in the region of 40 kDa, were recovered mainly in the lower speed membrane fractions and the supernatant (S3)

identifying the 60–90 kDa mature β-subunit, also shows a narrow band, at ~52 kDa, which has been previously characterized[15,16] as the high-mannose precursor (ER form) of the β-subunit – sensitive to endoglycosidase H and recognized by GNA lectin, which is specific for terminal mannose. This precursor ('pre-β') is found in a single peak centred at ~1.14–1.15 g/ml (fraction 12), a peak which thus represents the distribution of parietal cell rough ER and which correlates well with the distribution of labelled α-subunit at the 12 min time point. Careful overlaying of a Western blot with the corresponding autoradiograph allowed identification of ^{35}S-labelled pre-β among closely positioned bands in the 45–55 kDa range. Labelling of this band was greatly diminished by 90 min, reflecting conversion of pre-β into the diffusely migrating mature β-subunit.

Tracing the movement of H,K-ATPase beyond the ER must rely on the labelled

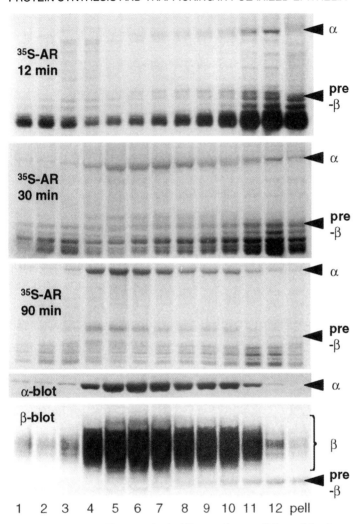

Figure 2 Pulse-labelled H,K-ATPase α-subunit shifts from denser to lighter subfractions on density gradients. Microsomes were separated on continuous sucrose gradients with fractions analysed by SDS–PAGE, autoradiography and Western blot. Gels are shown with high density to the right. Labelled α-subunit peaked in the densest fractions 12 min after [^{35}S]met/cys pulse (top panel), in fractions 7–8 after 30 min (2nd panel) and in fraction 5 after 90 min (3rd panel). The 4th and 5th panels show Western blots probed for total (unlabelled) α- and β-subunits of the H,K-ATPase. The latter (bottom panel) shows not only mature β-subunit (60–90 kDa), but also its ER precursor, 'pre-β' (52 kDa), which has the same distribution as 12 min labelled α-subunit. The unlabelled mature subunits peak mainly in fractions 5–6, with a secondary shoulder in fraction 10, a distribution that is typical of all normal resting microsomal preparations. The time course also shows a progressive loss of label from pre-β and from the pepsinogen recovered in P3.

α-subunit, which migrates in a similarly well focused band whether it is nascent or mature. Figure 3 shows the quantitation of ^{35}S-labelled α-subunit in the density gradient fractions measured at various time points after the pulse of [^{35}S]met/cys. Arrows identify approximate positions of four peaks, numbered according to the sequence in which labelled α-subunit appears in them. After 12 and 15 min most of the label was in a single dense peak (peak 1) matching the distribution of pre-β. However, a small shoulder at lower density appeared faintly by 12 min and became more obvious by 15 min. By 22 min this shoulder became a sharply distinct secondary peak, at ~1.09 g/ml (peak 2), and by 30 min became the dominant peak.

After 90 min, labelled α-subunit was almost entirely recovered at an even lower density (peak 3, centred at ~1.06–1.07 g/ml). The distribution of total α-subunit for the 90 min preparation (quantitated by Coomassie Blue staining of the 94 kDa band) is indicated by a dashed line, showing that the major labelled peak coincides with the large low density peak of total α-subunit, previously characterized as residing in mature tubulovesicles[11,13,14]. The 90 min results also show a small secondary peak of label, peak 4 (~1.11–1.12 g/ml), aligning with the secondary peak of total α-subunit rather than with peaks 1 or 2, and having much lower ^{35}S specific activity than peak 3.

β-Subunit glycosylation is required for transport beyond the ER

To study the influence of glycosylation on the trafficking of the β-subunit, we used an LLC-PK cell line that was stably transfected to express the H,K-β-subunit[12]. Under control conditions of growth, the β-subunit expressed in this cell line is N-glycosylated, with complex type glycans, and transported to the apical membrane. When the LLC-PK cells were treated with tunicamycin, an inhibitor of N-glycosylation, marked changes occurred in both glycosylation and transport of the H,K-β-subunit. The Western blot shown in Figure 4 demonstrates that tunicamycin effectively blocks N-glycosylation. Over the course of 3–10 h both complex glycosylation (~70 kDa) and high mannose core glycosylation (52 kDa) of H,K-β-subunit were eliminated and the non-glycosylated core β-subunit peptide (34 kDa) dominated the preparation. Comparison of cellular distribution of the H,K-β-subunit indicates that the normal trafficking pathway is dependent on glycosylation (Figure 5). In control LLC-PK cells immunofluorescent labelling of H,K-β-subunit occurred throughout the cells (Figure 5A), including transport to the apical plasma membrane. When glycosylation was blocked by tunicamycin, immunofluorescence was sequestered within the ER surrounding the

Figure 3 (Opposite) Quantitation of labelled α-subunit on density gradients shows migration through discrete peaks. Gradient subfractions were processed as described for Figure 2, and results were analysed by densitometry. Numbers at the top of the figure indicate approximate positions of peaks in which labelled α-subunit sequentially appeared: (1) the principal peak for the first 22 min after pulse, ~1.14–1.15 g/ml, (ER); (2) a peak that became distinct at 22 min and dominant by 30 min, ~1.09–1.10 g/ml, (Golgi); (3) a peak at ~1.07 g/ml that was dominant by 90 min, coinciding with the dominant peak of total (Coomassie Blue-stained) α-subunit in the same preparation, shown by dotted line (mature tubulovesicles); and (4) a peak at ~1.11–1.12 g/ml, coinciding with the secondary peak of total α-subunit, but with lower ^{35}S specific activity than peak 3 (senescent pool). See Discussion for more detailed characterization

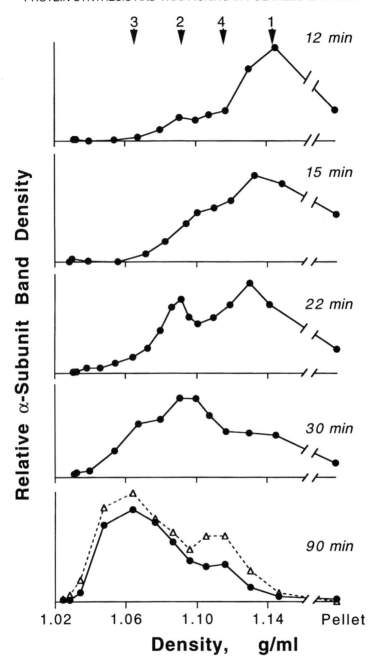

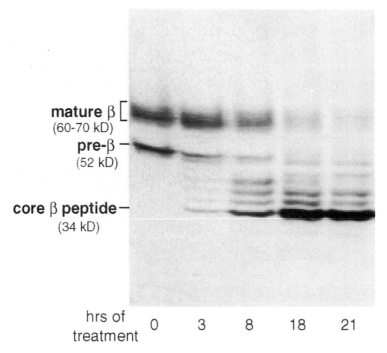

mature β [
(60-70 kD)
pre-β —
(52 kD)

core β peptide —
(34 kD)

hrs of treatment   0   3   8   18   21

Figure 4 Tunicamycin changes the pattern of glycosylation of H,K-ATPase β-subunit expressed in LLC-PK cells. LLC-PK cells transfected with β-subunit DNA were treated with 1 μg/ml tunicamycin and then harvested at the times indicated. The cells were lysed, developed by SDS-PAGE and blotted to nitrocellulose which was then probed for H,K-ATPase β-subunit. In untreated cells only mature β-subunit with complex N-glycosylation (60–70 kDa) and high mannose immature pre-β (52 kDa) were seen. These forms of β-subunit disappeared after tunicamycin treatment ($t_{1/2}$ ~8h), and they were replaced by the non-glycosylated core β-subunit peptide (34 kDa) which had about the same $t_{1/2}$ of appearance

nucleus (Figure 5B), thus demonstrating that N-glycans are important for transport of the β-subunit beyond the ER.

DISCUSSION

Using pulse-chase conditions to follow the amino acid incorporation and intra-cellular transport of H,K-ATPase we have been able to characterize the time course for synthesis and turnover of the enzyme in the in vivo parietal cell model. Shifts in the peak of radiolabelled α-subunit among density gradient subfractions of gastric microsomes were used to identify four sequential membrane compart-ments through which H,K-ATPase migrates, designated as peaks 1, 2, 3, and 4. Peaks 1 and 2 are discernible only by autoradiography, and contain less than 2% of the total enzyme. Western blotting, Coomassie Blue staining, and enzyme assay[11,13,14] reveal only peak 3, containing ~70% of total H,K-ATPase, and peak 4, containing ~30%.

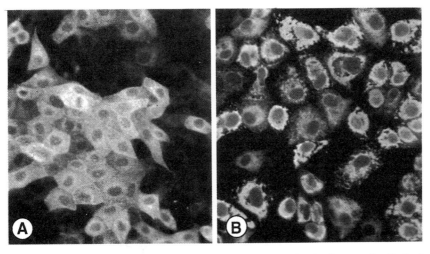

Figure 5 Glycosylation is necessary for β-subunit to exit the ER. LLC-PK cells expressing β-subunit were immunostained with and without treatment with tunicamycin to block N-glycosylation. (A) Control cells showed good expression of β-subunit with much of the label being present on the apical plasma membrane. (B) Tunicamycin-treated cells (1 μg/ml for 24 h) demonstrated an abundance of β-subunit, but the material was clumped in the perinuclear region of the ER and did not migrate to the plasma membrane. (Magnification ×56)

Peak 1 clearly represents H,K-ATPase in the rough ER. The coincident density gradient distribution of the earliest labelled pool of α-subunit with that of the core-glycosylated β-subunit, pre-β, provides support for characterizing peak 1 as nascent enzyme within the rough ER of parietal cells.

Peak 2 is a pubescent pool of enzyme proposed to be Golgi, but confirmation is complicated by the cellular heterogeneity of the gastric mucosa and the high level of zymogen synthesis in chief cells. Some galactosyltransferase was found in the peak 2 fractions, but as a shoulder on a large dense peak that might be mainly chief cell Golgi (not shown). Nevertheless, the dominance of peak 2 at 30 min is consistent with Golgi localization of the ^{35}S pulse[10], and the clear separation between peaks 1 and 2 after 22 min suggests that peak 2 represents the next major membrane compartment after the ER along the parietal cell synthetic pathway. In addition, the luminally acting H,K-ATPase inhibitor omeprazole (5 days in vivo) was previously shown to have no effect on the gradient distribution of 30 min labelled α-subunit, though it caused a marked shift of peak 3 into peak 4[11,13], suggesting that peak 2 membranes have not reached a pool that is affected by modification of apical membrane components.

The large, low density peak of total α-subunit (peak 3) has been characterized as mature tubulovesicles. These membranes are not seen in neonatal rabbit preparations, in which H,K-ATPase is recovered only in peak 4, but rapidly appear after the third postnatal week[14], concomitant with a large increase in acid secreting capability[17]. The peak 3 tubulovesicles have very low K$^+$ permeability, assayed by nigericin-dependent ATPase activity[14], and are proposed to sediment slowly in sucrose density gradients because of very low permeability to small solutes[11].

In fact, most H,K-ATPase could be recovered in peak 4 if microsomes were subjected either to hyposmotic lysis or to lengthy preincubation in high sucrose[11]. Thus, peak 3 is seen as functionally effective tubulovesicles having membrane properties critical for regulated recruitment to the apical membrane and establishment of a million-fold proton gradient during normal acid secretion.

The virtual congruence of labelled and total α-subunit in peak 3 after 90 min suggests that most newly synthesized H,K-ATPase reaches the mature tubulovesicle pool by this time. Since an H_2 blocker was used to maintain parietal cells in a resting state, the change in membrane properties causing peaks 2 and 3 to sediment differently may not require an apical membrane fusion step, but must involve lipid processing enzymes, beyond the Golgi compartment, that establish critical concentrations of particular lipids in tubulovesicles, or specific lipid 'flippase' enzymes that maintain a characteristic membrane asymmetry. Any such enzymes that reside in tubulovesicle membranes and move to and from the apical surface with each cycle of stimulation may be subject to inhibition by omeprazole. We previously reported that treatment of rabbits for 5 days with omeprazole resulted in a gradual alteration in tubulovesicle membrane properties, making them too leaky to maintain a large pH gradient and resulting in their recovery in peak 4 after gradient centrifugation, as with hyposmotically lysed vesicles[11].

Such membrane maintenance processes may also diminish with normal ageing of parietal cells. Both a decreased morphological response to stimulus[18] and a lower rate of H,K-ATPase synthesis[19] have been found in older parietal cells deep in the gastric gland, compared with younger cells near the neck of the gland. Furthermore, omeprazole treatment accelerated the morphological senescence of parietal cells, analysed by electron microscopy[20], even as it abolished the tubulovesicle properties that lead to recovery of peak 3. We previously showed[14] that stimulation shifts H,K-ATPase of peak 4 less completely (~70%) than that of peak 3 (~90%) to an apical membrane pool, consistent with peak 4 coming from less morphologically responsive cells. Although peak 4 might include a small pool of H,K-ATPase destined for degradation in the same cells that contain the 'tight' membranes of peak 3, the recruitability of much of peak 4 to the apical membrane and maintenance of distinctly different membrane properties between peaks 3 and 4 suggest that these two pools fuse with apical membranes in different cells. The low ^{35}S specific activity in peak 4 could reflect slower turnover than that occurring in cells yielding peak 3 membranes. An interpretation that peak 3 comes from the younger, more responsive cells, while older cells yield the 'senescent' vesicles of peak 4, seems to fit the preponderance of evidence thus far, an exception being made for neonatal cells, in which mature tubulovesicle properties have not yet appeared.

A schematic representation of the time course of H,K-ATPase synthesis and trafficking in parietal cells is shown in Figure 6. This time course, with an ER transit time of ~20 min, can be used in conjunction with the presence of a distinguishable ER form of the β-subunit for estimation of an H,K-ATPase half life. If the enzyme is at steady state, if α- and β-subunits are translated at equal rates, and if all nascent subunits are processed into mature H,K-ATPase, then pre-β as a fraction of total β-subunit represents the portion of total H,K-ATPase turned over in 20 min. In Western blots (as in Figure 2), pre-β averaged 0.6% of total β-subunit staining, and we have previously reported[13] that both subunits were

246

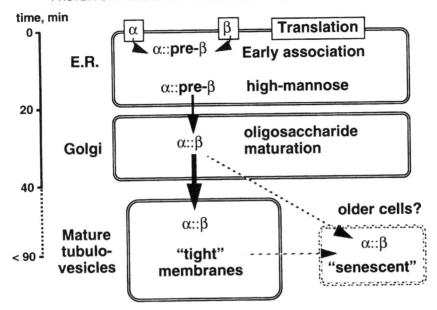

Figure 6 Diagram of H,K-ATPase synthesis and trafficking in parietal cells. Translated at equivalent rates, the α-subunit and pre-β quickly associate into dimers in the ER. Most of the nascent enzyme is undergoing oligosaccharide maturation to the complex type in the Golgi compartment by 30 min after translation and reaches the mature tubulovesicle pool by 90 min. Proposed secondary pathways are shown, with dotted lines, for movement of H,K-ATPase into leakier 'senescent' membranes, e.g. in omeprazole-treated stomachs, or in normally ageing adult parietal cells

translated at equivalent rates in vivo in the rabbit, quickly associating with each other in the ER with no detectable excesses of unassociated subunits subject to rapid breakdown. Thus, 0.6% of the enzyme is estimated to be turned over in 20 min or 1.8% per hour. Because the turnover rate is equivalent to the initial slope of the decay curve for loss of radioactivity in a pulse-labelled protein at steady state, and the derivative of the decay curve at $t = 0$ is $(\ln 0.5)/(\text{half life})$, we can estimate the half life of H,K-ATPase in the rabbit as $(\ln 0.5)/-0.018^{-h}$ – about 40 h. This method does not require sampling over several days to construct a decay curve and may prove useful for analysing acute changes in synthetic rate.

The H,K-β-subunit transfected into LLC-PK cells had a markedly shorter half life of ~8 h, as seen by the rate of loss of mature glycosylated form with tunicamycin treatment (Figure 4), suggesting instability of this subunit when it is not associated with the α-subunit. Both the ratio of pre-β to mature β-subunit (Figure 4) and the ratio of intracellular to plasma membrane immunostaining (Figure 5B) are consistent with low accumulation of mature β-subunit in the plasma membrane due to a high rate of breakdown. In transfected HEK cells, H,K-ATPase α-subunit was apparently stabilized only when cells were co-transfected with H,K-β-subunit[21]. Similar stabilization of Na,K-ATPase subunits in *Xenopus* oocytes was seen with co-injection of cRNa for the complementary subunit[22,23]. Even endogenous Na,K-ATPase β-subunits in LLC-PK cells, translated in excess over α-subunits, showed rapid breakdown of the unassociated excess, but stabilization of the dimeric form[24].

Transport of glycosylated but unassociated H,K-β-subunit to the plasma membrane in LLC-PK cells is in contrast to transport of Na,K-ATPase β-subunit in some cell systems. The latter was trapped in the ER of *Xenopus* oocytes unless associated with its α-subunit, regardless of N-glycosylation[22], but transported beyond the ER in α/β dimers even if glycosylation was inhibited[25]. However, rat Na,K-ATPase α- and β-subunits, separately expressed in different Sf-9 (insect) cells, were transported to the plasma membrane[26], suggesting caution in the interpretation of protein processing and trafficking patterns in various cell systems.

The possibility that glycosylation plays a role in protein transport or sorting is of special interest with regard to the parietal cell model, which has both H,K- and Na,K-ATPases, sorted to apical and basolateral domains respectively. Oligosaccharides of H,K-β-subunit have been found, in all species examined, to lack the common terminal sugar sialic acid[27], probably reflecting an adaptation to the very acidic conditions encountered by the luminal face of the enzyme. However, terminal sugars substituting for sialic acid vary among species. In the rabbit, this subunit has α-galactosyl termini on all its complex type branches[27], while all human samples we have analysed display mainly the Lewis Y antigen, a doubly fucosylated terminal tetrasaccharide[28,29].

The question of whether asialylation is characteristic of parietal cell apical glycoproteins, playing a role in sorting, or is a more general parietal cell adaptation characteristic of all its glycoproteins, remains to be answered. In some preliminary tests, lectin affinity chromatography with *Griffonia simplicifolia* I, which binds terminal α-galactose, has largely, though not completely, separated maturely glycosylated rabbit H,K-ATPase from Na,K-ATPase, implying differences in terminal glycosylation of their β-subunits and suggesting that such differences might be exploited in the parietal cell model to dissect the sorting pathways for these two highly homologous cation transporters.

Acknowledgements

We wish to thank Dr Adam Smolka for the antibody against the α-subunit of H,K-ATPase and Dr Michael Caplan for the gift of the transfected LLC-PK cells. This work was supported in part by a grant from the National Institutes of Health, DK38972.

References

1. Schultz SG. Cellular models of epithelial ion transport. In: Andreoli TE, *et al.*, editors. Physiology of Membrane Disorders. 2nd edn. New York: Plenum, 1986:135–50.
2. Powell D. Ion and water transport in the intestine. In: Andreoli TE, *et al.*, editors. Physiology of Membrane Disorders. 2nd edn. New York: Plenum, 1986:175–212.
3. Nelson WJ. Renal epithelial cell polarity. Curr Opin Nephrol Hyperten. 1992;1:59–67.
4. Bradbury NA, Bridges RJ. Role of membrane trafficking in plasma membrane solute transport. Am J Physiol. 1994;267:C1–24.
5. Tse M, Levine S, Yun C *et al.* Structure/function studies of the epithelial isoforms of the mammalian Na$^+$/H$^+$ exchanger gene family. J Membr Biol. 1993;135:93–108.
6. Sundaram U, Knickelbein RG, Dobbins JW. pH regulation in ileum: Na$^+$-H$^+$ and Cl$^-$-HCO$_3^-$ exchange in isolated crypt and villus cells. Am J Physiol. 1991;260:G440–9.
7. Mellman I, Yamamoto E, Whitney JA, Kim M, Hunziker W, Matter K. Molecular sorting in

polarized and non-polarized cells: common problems, common solutions. J Cell Sci. 1993;17 (Suppl):1–7.

8. Mostov K. Protein traffic in polarized epithelial cells: the polymeric immunoglobulin receptor as a model system. J Cell Sci. 1993;17(Suppl):21–6.

9. Le Gall AH, Yeaman C, Muesch A, Rodriguez-Boulan E. Epithelial cell polarity: new perspectives. Semin Nephrol. 1995;15:272–84.

10. Sztul ES, Howell KE, Palade GE. Intracellular and transcellular transport of secretory component and albumin in rat hepatocytes. J Cell Biol. 1983;97:1582–91.

11. Crothers JM Jr, Chow DC, Forte JG. Omeprazole decreases H⁺-K⁺-ATPase protein and increases permeability of oxyntic secretory membranes in rabbits. Am J Physiol. 1993;265:G3231–41.

12. Gottardi CJ, Caplan MJ. An ion-transporting ATPase encodes multiple apical localization signals. J Cell Biol. 1993;121:283–93.

13. Crothers JM Jr, Chow DC, Scalley ML, Forte JG. In vivo trafficking of nascent H⁺-K⁺-ATPase in rabbit parietal cells. Am J Physiol. 1995;269:G883–91.

14. Crothers JM Jr, Reenstra WW, Forte JG. Ontogeny of gastric H⁺-K⁺-ATPase in suckling rabbits. Am J Physiol. 1990;259:G913–21.

15. Chow DC, Forte JG. Characterization of the β-subunit of the H⁺-K⁺-ATPase using an inhibitory monoclonal antibody. Am J Physiol. 1993;265:C1562–70.

16. Horisberger JD, Jaunin P, Reuben MA et al. The H,K-ATPase β-subunit can act as a surrogate for the β-subunit of Na,K-pumps. J Biol Chem. 1991;266:19131–4.

17. Mulvihill SJ, Garcia R, Fonkalsrud EW, Debas HT. Ontogeny of basal and stimulated acid secretion in the rabbit. Gastroenterology. 1985;88:1511.

18. Karam SM, Yao X, Forte JG. Functional heterogeneity of parietal cells along the pit-gland axis. Am J Physiol. 1996;272:G161–71.

19. Bamberg K, Nylander S, Helander KG, Lundberg LG, Sachs G, Helander HF. In situ hybridization of mRNA for the gastric H⁺,K⁺-ATPase in rat oxyntic mucosa. Biochim Biophys Acta. 1994; 1190:355–9.

20. Karam SM, Forte JG. Inhibiting gastric H⁺-K⁺-ATPase activity by omeprazole promotes degeneration and production of parietal cells. Am J Physiol. 1994;266:G745–58.

21. Asano S, Tega Y, Konishi K, Fujioka M. Functional expression of gastric H,K-ATPase and site-directed mutagenesis of the putative cation binding site and the catalytic center. J Biol Chem. 1996;271:2740–5.

22. Ackermann U, Geering K. β₁- and β₃-subunits can associate with presynthesized α-subunits of Xenopus oocyte Na,K-ATPase. J Biol Chem. 1992;267:12911–15.

23. Ackerman U, Geering K. Mutual dependence of Na,K-ATPase α- and β-subunits for correct posttranslational processing and intracellular transport. FEBS Lett. 1990;269:105–8.

24. Lescale-Matys L, Putnam DS, McDonough AA. Na⁺-K⁺-ATPase α₁- and β₁-subunit degradation, evidence for multiple subunit-specific rates. Am J Physiol. 1993;264:C583–90.

25. Geering K. Subunit assembly and functional maturation of Na,K-ATPase. J Membr Bol. 1990; 115:109–21.

26. DeTomaso AW, Blanco G, Mercer RW. The α and β subunits of the Na,K-ATPase can assemble at the plasma membrane into functional enzyme. J Cell Biol. 1994;127:55–69.

27. Tyagarajan K, Townsend RR, Forte JG. The β-subunit of the rabbit H,K-ATPase – A glycoprotein with all terminal lactosamine units capped with α-linked galactose residues. Biochemistry. 1996;35:3238–46

28. Appelmelk BJ, Simoons-Smit I, Negrini R et al. Potential role of molecular mimicry between Helicobacter pylori lipopolysaccharide and host Lewis blood group antigens in autoimmunity. Infect Immun. 1996;64:2031–40.

29. Crothers JM Jr, Appelmelk BJ, Tyagarajan KT, Townsend RR, Forte JG. Lewis Y (Leʸ) antigen is prominently expressed on the β-subunit of human gastric H,K-ATPase. Gastroenterology. 1996;110:A85.

Section IV
Cell differentiation

21
Mechanisms of sucrase-isomaltase gene transcription: implications for intestinal development

P. G. TRABER

INTRODUCTION

The function of the mammalian intestinal mucosa is defined by the sets of genes expressed in differentiated epithelial cell phenotypes. The expression of individual proteins in the intestine may be regulated at multiple control points, including synthesis and degradation of mRNA, translation of mRNA into protein, and processing or modification of synthesized proteins. Control of RNA synthesis, or gene transcription, is one critical regulatory control point, particularly for tissue-specific, differentiation-dependent and developmental expression. An understanding of the mechanisms that regulate transcription of gene sets that define specific cellular phenotypes often leads to an understanding of the underlying mechanisms of tissue development and differentiation. Many classes of transcription factors have been shown to be involved in directing developmental processes in multiple organisms and tissues. Specific information regarding intestinal development and differentiation has resulted from an understanding of the transcriptional regulation of the sucrase-isomaltase (SI) gene. This brief review updates the subset of information on transcriptional regulation of the SI gene that was originally discussed in a previous review on intestinal gene transcription[1].

SI GENE EXPRESSION WITHIN THE COMPLEX ARCHITECTURE OF THE INTESTINAL EPITHELIUM

An understanding of intestinal gene transcription must be placed in the context of the architecture of the intestinal epithelium, a structure with an exquisitely regulated spatial organization. The epithelium of the adult intestine is continually replaced from committed stem cells that are fixed approximately four cell positions above the base of the crypt[2-4]. Stem cells give rise to four highly specialized

253

epithelial phenotypes including absorptive enterocytes, mucus-secreting goblet cells, a variety of enteroendocrine cells that secrete specific hormones, and Paneth cells that synthesize antibacterial peptides and enzymes[5]. Crypt cells undergo several rounds of cell division while they reside in the crypt compartment. Enterocytes, oligomucous cells and enteroendocrine cells migrate towards the villus tip, whereas Paneth cells reside in the base of the crypt. Because ultrastructural features of specific phenotypes are clearly identifiable in crypts, it appears that the commitment to a particular lineage occurs early after the initial stem cell division. The preponderance of absorptive enterocytes on villi suggests that immature enterocytes in crypts are the most abundant proliferating cells. Proliferation ceases in the upper third of the crypt and cell division does not occur once the cells migrate onto the villus.

Most gene products that are characteristic of the differentiated enterocyte are first expressed in the upper crypt region near the crypt-villus junction. Many mRNAs, proteins and enzymatic activities that define important enterocyte functions have been shown to be expressed first at this critical junction. This discussion focuses on SI, which is first expressed in the upper third of the crypt and crypt-villus junction, is expressed at high levels to the mid-villus and then decreases at the villus tips[6-8]. Although direct measurement of transcription is not feasible in the intestinal epithelium, the abrupt increase in mRNA levels at the crypt-villus junction and evidence from transgenic mouse studies (outlined below) suggest that transcriptional induction of the SI gene is intimately associated with the cessation of proliferation of cells in the upper third of the crypt.

The intricate structure of the adult epithelium arises as a result of multiple developmental transitions beginning in the mouse embryo and culminating after weaning which occurs during the third week of life. The primitive gut tube, comprised of endoderm surrounded by mesenchyme, is established by completion of embryo turning at approximately embryonic day 9 (E9). At E15 the stratified endoderm undergoes a cranial to caudal transition into a simple columnar epithelium with nascent villi. Simultaneous with this important morphological change, the expression of certain intestine-specific genes is first detected[9,10]. The SI gene is expressed at very low levels beginning at this transition[11]. From immediately before birth (at E19) to the second week of life, crypts develop from the intervillus epithelium and villi lengthen. Near the end of the third week of life the transition from suckling to weaning occurs, another major change in the developing mouse intestine[12,13]. This transition is marked by a cranial to caudal wave of cytodifferentiation and induction of gene expression, including marked induction of SI gene expression. Although this transition occurs at the time of weaning and may occur precociously by forced weaning or administration of corticosteroids or thyroid hormones, the occurrence of this transition appears to be genetically predetermined. Thus, by the middle of the fourth postnatal week, the mouse small intestine has attained its adult form with high level SI gene expression in differentiated enterocytes.

Within the complex architecture and developmental transitions of the intestinal epithelium, therefore, expression of the SI gene mirrors a number of important developmental and differentiation events. We have used this gene to explore regulatory mechanisms that underlie its pattern of expression and ultimately intestinal developmental mechanisms.

REGULATION OF INTESTINAL PATTERNS OF SI GENE TRANSCRIPTION

Transitions in cell phenotypes are directed by the combinatorial effects of ubiquitous, tissue-restricted and tissue-specific transcription factors. Although the regulation of developmental transitions occurs through multiple mechanisms, including cell–matrix and cell–cell interactions and growth factors, it is the regulation of transcription that ultimately controls major phenotypic changes in cells. The use of transgenic mice to examine patterns of intestinal gene transcription, pioneered by Gordon and colleagues[14,15], has provided multiple insights into transcriptional mechanisms. Regulation of gene transcription in transgenic mice has been studied for several enterocyte genes, including members of the fatty acid binding protein gene family and disaccharidases, as well as a few genes expressed in non-enterocytic cell lineages. The discussion is restricted to a description of the SI gene.

The regulation of both the human and mouse SI genes has been investigated in transgenic mice[8,16]. Initially, long segments of both the human (-3524 to $+54$)[8] and mouse (-8500 to $+54$)[16] genes were shown to direct transcription specifically to intestinal epithelial cells. More recently, a short evolutionarily conserved promoter region (-201 to $+54$ in the mouse gene) has been shown to direct transcription specifically to the intestinal epithelium in most transgenic lines, similar to the longer constructs[11]. Examination of the patterns of expression of these transgenes has defined a variety of functional DNA regulatory regions in the SI gene 5'-flanking region that fall into three general areas: the promoter, nucleotides -8500 to -201, and outside of -8500 to $+54$ (Figure 1).

The evolutionarily conserved promoter region has the regulatory elements necessary for directing development- and differentiation-dependent expression in small intestinal enterocytes in the same pattern as the endogenous gene[11]. Expression of the transgene is first seen in enterocytes at postnatal day 17 and expression is limited to differentiated enterocytes located at the crypt-villus junction and on the villus. Additionally, the promoter construct drives expression ectopically in a subset of enteroendocrine cells.

Results of the transgenic experiments suggest that there may be several functional DNA regulatory elements within the area bounded by nucleotides -8500 to -201 (Figure 1). Transgenic mice containing a construct linking bases -8500 to $+54$ of the mouse SI gene to the human growth hormone gene demonstrated intestine-specific expression, but high levels of GH were detected in each of the four phenotypes, including enterocytes, enteroendocrine cells, goblet cells and Paneth cells[16]. These data suggest that all intestinal epithelial cells contain the cellular machinery to direct transcription of the SI gene in the adult mouse epithelium. In addition, the expression in various transgenic lines was independent of insertion site in the genome and expression was transgene copy number dependent. These findings suggest that DNA elements between nucleotides -8500 and -201 may be required to insulate the promoter from surrounding chromatin effects determined by the site of insertion of the transgene. These types of regulatory elements have been described for numerous genes and may be important standard components of gene structure[17-19]. The developmental expression of the transgene in these animals suggested that there was a sequential activation of the transgene in different cell lineages (including goblet and Paneth

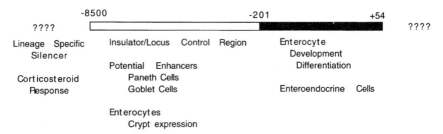

Figure 1 Functional regulatory elements of the SI gene as defined by experiments in transgenic mice. The promoter region of the SI gene (−201 to +54) is capable of directing expression of transgenes to enterocytes in a pattern that recapitulates the pattern of the endogenous gene expression. The transgene is expressed first at the suckling–weaning transition and limited in expression to villus-associated enterocytes. The promoter also directs expression to some enteroendocrine cells. The region located between nucleotides −8500 and −201 contains a number of putative regulatory regions. When this region is added to the promoter transgenes are expressed in an insertion site-independent, copy number-dependent fashion, whereas the expression of promoter constructs is dependent on the insertion site. These data suggest the presence of an insulator, matrix attachment region or locus control region in the area bounded by −8500 to −201. Because transgene expression is noted in Paneth and goblet cells when −8500 to −201 are added to the promoter, this region may contain an enhancer(s) for expression in these cells. Expression of the transgene extends into the crypt enterocytes with the long construct. This may be due to higher levels of expression in general in comparison to the promoter, or the presence of an enhancer element. The question marks on the figure indicate putative elements that are postulated to exist outside of nucleotides −8500 to +54, including a silencer of transcription for non-enterocyte lineages and response elements that mediate precocious expression in response to corticosteroids

cells) with full expression in all epithelial cells attained by 33 days after birth[16]. One possible explanation for this finding would be a developmentally regulated enhancer for these lineages. Finally, there is some ectopic expression of hGH in crypt associated enterocytes in the long construct lines which may be due to an enhancer for expression in these cells or simply the result of higher levels of expression in the animals harbouring the long construct versus the short promoter construct.

What does the pattern of expression of the transgene in all epithelial cells imply for the regulation of the endogenous SI gene? One possibility is that the SI gene is transcribed in all epithelial cells, but that there is differential regulation of SI mRNA stability which results in stable expression of SI mRNA only in enterocytes. A second possibility is that transcription of the SI gene may be normally repressed in non-enterocytic cells via DNA elements that are not contained in the −8500 to +54 construct (Figure 1). We favour the hypothesis of a transcriptional silencer since data from enterocytic and enteroendocrine cell lines are consistent with such a hypothesis[16].

It is well known that stress, via corticosteroid secretion, induces precocious maturation of the suckling rodent intestine (reviewed in Ref. 13). Recent evidence suggested that this precocious maturation may be mediated through a pathway separate from that which directs the normal developmental process[20]. Our data in transgenic mice provide molecular evidence that indeed normal and precocious expression are mediated via different pathways. In support of this hypothesis, we found that both long and short transgenic constructs lacked the ability to respond

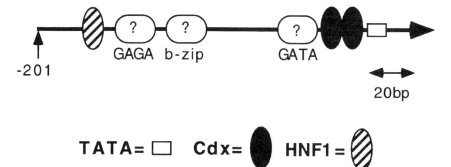

Figure 2 Confirmed and potential regulatory elements in the SI gene promoter. Well described regulatory elements and their cognate DNA binding proteins are indicated by the defined symbols (Cdx = binding site for caudal-related homeodomain proteins; HNF1 = binding site for hepatocyte nuclear factor 1 proteins). Potential regulatory elements are indicated by an oval DNA element and a question mark to indicate that the functional significance is still to be determined. GATA indicates a sequence that appears to be important for SI promoter transcription and interacts with GATA type zinc finger proteins, but the role of GATA factors is still uncertain. b-zip is a sequence that is capable of interacting with basic-leucine zipper type transcriptional proteins, but its function in the SI promoter remains unclear. GAGA is a region that is conserved between mouse and human promoters that has yet to be experimentally examined

to corticosteroid treatment with precocious expression of the transgene. Thus, elements responsible for this response must be located outside of nucleotides -8500 to -201 (Figure 1).

THE SUCRASE-ISOMALTASE PROMOTER

The promoter region of the SI gene (-201 to $+54$) has been mapped in cell lines for nuclear protein binding sites and transcriptionally functional elements[21-24]. A summary of the confirmed and possible regulatory sites is shown in Figure 2. Most analysis of these regulatory elements has been performed in cell lines derived from carcinomas, although some of the DNA–protein interactions have been evaluated using intestinal epithelial cell nuclear extracts. The primary cell line used in these studies was Caco-2 which was derived from a colonic adeno-carcinoma and, in some respects, models a differentiated enterocyte in cell culture, particularly in the post-confluent state[25]. For the analysis of the SI promoter it is important to note that Caco-2 cells express significant amounts of SI mRNA and protein.

SIF1 binding proteins and the caudal-related family of transcription factors

Sequence analysis of the SI promoter revealed a 22bp region immediately upstream of the putative TATA box that was identical between mouse[22] and human[21] genes. Studies on the interaction of nuclear proteins with the promoter region confirmed that this evolutionarily conserved DNA sequence may be important for SI gene transcription. DNAase I footprint analysis showed that nuclear proteins from Caco-2 cells protected this 22 base region whereas nuclear extracts from HepG2 cells, a liver cancer cell line, or HeLa cells, a cervical cancer cell line, did not contain nuclear proteins that interacted with this site (the site was named SIF1 for *Sucrase Isomaltase Footprint 1*). Additional analysis showed that this site interacted with nuclear proteins in some intestinal cell lines and intestinal epithelial cells, but not with nuclear extracts from multiple other cell types[22]. Transfection of chimeric SI promoter–luciferase plasmids into Caco-2, HepG2, and HeLa cells demonstrated that the human SI promoter (– 183 to + 54) directed transcription specifically in Caco-2 cells and that this activity was in large part dependent on the SIF1 sequence[22]. Thus, the SIF1 element was found to be a functional activator of SI promoter transcription which binds nuclear proteins only found in intestinal cell lines.

SIF1 interacting proteins were cloned by screening a mouse small intestinal λgt11 expression library utilizing the molecular interaction between the SIF1 DNA sequence and fusion proteins expressed by the phage vector[24]. One cDNA isolated in this fashion encoded a protein in the caudal family of homeodomain containing proteins. Caudal is a homeobox gene (*cad*) that is involved in early axial pattern formation in *Drosophila melanogaster*[26–29]. Using the sequence of the *cad* gene, other caudal family members have been cloned from multiple animal species[30–37]. In mouse, there have been three independent caudal related genes cloned, designated *Cdx1*[38], *Cdx2*[24,30,39] and *Cdx4*[40]. The cloned cDNA that interacted with the SIF1 element was found to contain the full coding sequence of *Cdx2*[24]. Studies have confirmed that Cdx2 protein interacts specifically with the SIF1 element and that it serves to activate transcription of the SI promoter[24]. Antibodies generated to Cdx2 protein were used to show that the predominant, if not the exclusive, SIF1 binding protein in intestinal cell lines is the Cdx2 protein[24]. Therefore, Cdx2 is an excellent candidate as a critical transcriptional factor for regulation of the SI gene in the intestine.

The current information regarding the function of the SIF1 element and Cdx2 does not definitively confirm their importance for SI gene transcription in vivo. Function of the SIF1 element has been demonstrated in cell lines which must be confirmed by site directed mutants of the promoter expressed in transgenic mice. The most direct assessment of the importance of Cdx2 on expression of SI would be to eliminate expression of the Cdx2 protein in Caco-2 cells and determine whether SI expression is effected. This approach is feasible since Cdx2 seems to be the only SIF1 binding protein expressed in Caco-2 cells. Despite these caveats, the evidence is strong that the Cdx2 protein is involved in transactivation of the SI promoter.

Other potential SI promoter DNA regulatory elements

A number of other sites in the SI promoter have been identified that may be important for regulation of intestinal gene transcription. In the human SI promoter two DNA binding elements were identified that interact with hepatocyte nuclear factor 1 (HNF1)[23]. Subsequently, we have shown that HNF1 only interacts with the SIF3 site in the mouse promoter, the site with the most activity (Zhu and Traber, unpublished data). HNF1 is a member of a class of transcription proteins that contain a DNA binding domain which is distantly related to the homeodomain and which bind to DNA as dimers (for review see Ref. 41). The two members of this family that have been described are HNF1α[42–46], which is expressed in liver, kidney, stomach, and small and large intestine[46–48], and HNFIβ[42,49–51], which is expressed in liver, stomach, large and small intestine, kidney, ovary and lung[42]. Because of the wide tissue distribution of both HNF1α and HNF1β, it is clear that these proteins are not sufficient for intestinal transcription of the SI gene. However, they may interact with other proteins, such as Cdx2 or others, resulting in augmentation of transcription.

A consensus GATA site is present in the SI promoter (TGATG) and there is preliminary evidence that intestinal cell lines express GATA binding proteins, that known GATA binding proteins interact with the SI promoter GATA site, and that mutation of the GATA site significantly impairs SI promoter transcription (Silberg DG, Long S, Chen L and Traber PG, unpublished data). Additional work will be required to characterize regulation of the SI promoter via this element and to determine which GATA factors may be involved in this regulation, or whether other proteins bind to this site.

One element in the SI promoter that is evolutionarily conserved contains an inverted repeat of TTTA separated by two bases. Although there is a weak footprint in this region using Caco-2 nuclear extracts[22], there is a strong footprint using liver nuclear extract[52]. Screening a liver cDNA expression library with a double-stranded oligonucleotide probe for SIF4 resulted in identification of the mouse orthologue of human E4BP4[52], a transcription factor of the basic-leucine zipper class that has been shown to be a transcriptional repressor protein[53]. The mRNA for this protein seems to be ubiquitously expressed in the mouse and it is unclear what function it may play in the regulation of the SI gene. However, it is likely that other members of the basic leucine zipper class of transcription factors are able to bind to this site. Thus, the element remains a potentially important region of the SI gene for regulation of the promoter, either by the ubiquitous factor we cloned or other unidentified proteins.

Another potentially interesting site is a conserved (GA)$_3$. There is a nuclear protein that binds to the pentamer GAGAG which is of functional importance in other genes. The GAGA protein binds to GA/CT rich promoter regions in multiple *Drosophila* genes[54], the human CD11a gene[55], and the rat serine protease inhibitor 2.1 gene[56], creating DNase I hypersensitivity sites in DNA. The binding of the GAGA protein appears to disrupt the arrangement of nucleosomes allowing access to the DNA for the initiation of transcription[56–59]. In *Drosophila*, the GAGA protein is bound constitutively to the promoter region of the uninduced *hsp70* and *hsp26* genes. After heat shock the GAGA protein binds to the DNA in a 5' to 3' progression during transcription. The recruitment of GAGA protein to the induced *hsp70* and *hsp26* gene has kinetics similar to that found previously for RNA polymerase II. The distribution of the GAGA protein and its pattern of binding to genes during transcription, suggests that the protein may be necessary for transcription by opening the nucleosome structure allowing RNA polymerase II binding and transcription[60]. Experimental evidence of a role for this protein in the SI promoter is not available.

Function of the SI promoter

It is clear that no one transcriptional protein that has been identified to date is sufficient to direct the pattern of developmental and spatial expression found in the −201 to +54 mSI transgene. The *Cdx* genes are clearly insufficient since they are expressed in both small intestine and colon in adult animals and are expressed at the time of the endoderm−intestinal epithelial junction, when there is little SI gene expression. The patterns of SI gene transcription are, therefore, probably modulated by the combined effects of multiple transcription factors. In addition, protein modifications such as phosphorylation during development and in various cell lineages may be important for stage- or cell-specific function. Most importantly, there are probably protein co-factors that interact with the DNA binding proteins to functionally link them to the basal transcriptional apparatus. Such co-factors could be envisioned to act by binding to a single DNA binding protein, such as Cdx2, or to a complex of interacting proteins simultaneously bound to the SI promoter. It is clear that once the majority of the DNA binding proteins that interact with specific elements are identified and functionally characterized, a great deal of work will remain to properly fit the pieces of the transcription factor puzzle together on the SI promoter.

FUNCTION OF TRANSCRIPTION PROTEINS IN DEVELOPMENT

A remarkable outgrowth of the characterization of transcription factors that direct tissue-specific gene transcription is that, in many cases, these same factors have important regulatory roles in development of the complete tissue or organ. Examples include the function of GATA proteins in haematopoietic development[61,62], myoD and others in muscle development[63], and Pit1 in development of the anterior pituitary[64]. The discovery that Cdx2 is an important transcriptional protein for the SI promoter raises the issue of whether the caudal-related genes may have a more general function in intestinal development. Although caudal-related genes are found in many animal species and the patterns of expression have been carefully explored in some of these species, their function and gene targets have not been well described. In *Drosophila*, knockout of *cad* leads to impaired formation of posterior structures, including the proctodeum and hindgut and portions of the distal midgut[28]. These and other data suggest that the *cad* gene plays a role in axial pattern formation in early *Drosophila* development. An important gene target for *cad* in *Drosophila* is the segmentation gene fuzi tarazu (*ftz*) which has a number of functional *cad* binding sites in its promoter[65].

Developmental patterns of *Cdx* gene expression in mice suggest important roles in early embryonic development. *Cdx1* mRNA and protein are first expressed in mouse embryos at day 7.5 in the region of the primitive streak, predominantly in nuclei of ectoderm and mesoderm and some in visceral endoderm[66]. At day 7.75 expression extends to the entire posterior area, but there is no expression in definitive endoderm. Between embryonic day 8.25 and 12 there is variable expression of *Cdx1* in a number of tissues including the neural tube, somites, the mesoderm and limb buds. By day 12 there is marked reduction in expression which correlates with undetectable levels of mRNA between days 11 and 14[38].

At approximately day 14 *Cdx1* mRNA is expressed in embryonic intestine[38], which is the time when the pseudostratified endoderm undergoes a transition to a columnar epithelium organized in nascent villi. *Cdx2* is also expressed in early embryonic tissues, including preimplantation time points, with decreasing levels in most tissues in mid-gestation[39]. Cdx2 protein expression appears to increase in the endoderm just before the time of the endoderm–intestinal epithelial transition and continues to be expressed in adult mice along the entire crypt-villus axis of the small intestine and in crypts of the colon[39] (unpublished data). *Cdx4* is expressed in posterior structures early in embryogenesis, but is not expressed in the intestinal epithelium[40]. Therefore, the currently available data on the pattern of expression of *Cdx* genes in mice suggest a role in early developmental events and later during morphogenesis of the visceral endoderm into intestinal epithelium.

Gene knockout experiments have yet to reveal sufficient information to understand the function of *Cdx1* and *Cdx2* in development and maintenance of the intestinal epithelium. Mice null for *Cdx1* have been reported to have skeletal abnormalities, but the effects on the intestinal epithelium have not yet been published[67]. Preliminary data on mice null for *Cdx2* indicate that the homozygous state is associated with preimplantation lethality[68]. Thus, more directed approaches to the intestine will be required to assess function in the intestinal epithelium.

Another approach to understanding the function of Cdx proteins is to use cell lines to perform gain of function and loss of function studies. Using gain of function in intestinal cell lines, we have recently shown that *Cdx2* has effects on proliferation, morphogenesis and gene expression in intestinal cell lines[69]. The expression of *Cdx2* in undifferentiated intestinal cell line, IEC-6, was shown to have a profound effect on cellular proliferation and morphogenesis[69]. Induced expression of *Cdx2* in IEC-6 cells resulted in cessation of cellular pro-liferation that lasted for several days, followed by cellular growth to confluency. After confluency, the cultures expressing high levels of *Cdx2* formed a well-differentiated intestinal type epithelium in the context of a complex architecture of cells with different morphologies. The epithelium consisted of columnar cells with tight junctions, a basement membrane, lateral membrane interdigitations characteristic of the intestinal epithelium, and well formed microvilli. Neither the parental IEC-6 cells, nor cells expressing very low levels of *Cdx2* attained a differentiated morphology. Based on these data we proposed that Cdx2 is a critical regulatory protein in the network of regulatory factors that direct intestinal epithelial differentiation. Recently, we have obtained preliminary evidence that Cdx1 has similar effects on proliferation, but lacks the ability to induce morphogenesis in IEC-6 cells (Suh ER and Traber PG, unpublished).

Thus, the circumstantial data on the temporal pattern of expression in endoderm combined with these functional data in undifferentiated intestinal epithelial cells make caudal-related genes an important target for study to elucidate the mechanisms of intestinal development.

SUMMARY

Accumulating evidence shows that multiple regulatory regions in the SI gene act in complex patterns during intestinal development and maintenance of the intestinal phenotype. An understanding of the transcription factors that interact with these DNA regulatory elements and how they interact with each other will be necessary for building a model of SI gene transcription. Moreover, a complete model will involve a second layer of regulatory mechanisms that will be dependent on transcriptional co-adaptor proteins that link the DNA binding proteins with the basal transcriptional apparatus. Thus, after the characterization of all DNA elements and cognate binding proteins of the SI gene, the even more involved task of the integration of transcription factor complexes, identification of functional post-translational modifications, and the cloning of transcriptional cofactors must be tackled.

The process of completely characterizing the transcriptional regulatory mechanisms that direct the complex patterns of expression of even one gene, such as SI, will provide insight into developmental mechanisms. The first example of this is the discovery that Cdx proteins regulate SI promoter function and have a broader role in the regulation of intestinal epithelial cell proliferation and morphogenesis. As additional transcriptional mechanisms are uncovered, such as co-adaptor proteins, it is likely that these will also play important roles in the overall developmental processes of intestinal epithelial cell development and differentiation.

References

1. Traber PG, Silberg DG. Intestine-specific gene transcription. Annu Rev Physiol. 1996;58:275–97.
2. Cheng H, Leblond CP. Origin, differentiation and renewal of the four main epithelial cell types in the mouse small intestine. I. Columnar cell. Am J Anat. 1974;141:461–80.
3. Gordon HI, Schmidt GH, Roth KA. Studies of intestinal stem cells using normal, chimeric, and transgenic mice. FASEB J. 1992;6:3039–50.
4. Gordon JI. Understanding gastrointestinal epithelial cell biology: Lessons from mice with help from worms and flies. Gastroenterology. 1993;104:315–24.
5. Cheng H, Leblond CP. Origin, differentiation and renewal of the four main epithelial cell types in the mouse small intestine. V. Unitarian theory of the origin of the four epithelial cell types. Am J Anat. 1974;141:537–62.
6. Traber PG. Regulation of sucrase-isomaltase gene expression along the crypt-villus axis of rat small intestine. Biochem Biophys Res Commun. 1990;173:765–73.
7. Traber PG, Yu L, Wu G, Judge T. Sucrase-isomaltase gene expression along the crypt-villus axis of human small intestine is regulated at the level of mRNA abundance. Am J Physiol. 1992;262:G123–30.
8. Markowitz AJ, Wu GD, Birkenmeier EH, Traber PG. The human sucrase-isomaltase gene directs complex patterns of gene expression in transgenic mice. Am J Physiol. 1993;265:G526–39.
9. Rubin DC, Ong DE, Gordon JI. Cellular differentiation in the emerging fetal rat small intestinal epithelium: Mosaic patterns of gene expression. Proc Natl Acad Sci USA. 1989;86:1278–82.
10. Rings EHHM, DeBoar PAJ, Moorman AFM et al. Lactase gene expression during early development of rat small intestine. Gastroenterology. 1992;103:1154–61.
11. Tung J, Markowitz AJ, Silberg DG, Traber PG. Developmental expression of the sucrase-isomaltase gene in transgenic mice is regulated by an evolutionarily conserved promoter. Am J Physiol. 1997; in press.
12. Henning SJ. Ontogeny of enzymes in the small intestine. Annu Rev Physiol. 1985;47:231–45.
13. Henning SJ. Functional development of the gastrointestinal tract. In: Johnson LR, editor. Physiology of the Gastrointestinal Tract. New York: Raven Press, 1987:285–300.
14. Sweetser DA, Hauft SM, Hoppe PC, Birkenmeier EH, Gordon JI. Transgenic mice containing intestinal fatty acid-binding protein-human growth hormone fusion genes exhibit correct regional and cell-specific expression of the reporter gene in their small intestine. Proc Natl Acad Sci USA. 1988;85:9611–15.

15. Sweetser DA, Birkenmeier EH, Hoppe PC, McKeel DW, Gordon JI. Mechanisms underlying generation of gradients in gene expression within the intestine: an analysis using transgenic mice containing fatty acid binding protein-human growth hormone fusion genes. Genes Dev. 1988;2: 1318–32.
16. Markowitz AJ, Wu GD, Bader A, Cui Z, Chen L, Traber PG. Regulation of lineage-specific transcription of the sucrase-isomaltase gene in transgenic mice and cell lines. Am J Physiol. 1995; 269:G925–39.
17. Wilson C, Bellen HJ, Gehring WJ. Position effects on eukaryotic gene expression. Annu Rev Cell Biol. 1990;6:679–714.
18. Forrester WC, vanGenderen C, Jenuwein T, Grosschedl R. Dependence of enhancer-mediated transcription of the immunoglobulin μ gene on nuclear matrix attachment regions. Science. 1994; 265:1121–5.
19. Festenstein R, Tolaini M, Corbella P et al. Locus control region function and heterochromatin-induced position effect variegation. Science. 1996;271:1123–5.
20. Nanthakumar NN, Henning SJ. Distinguishing normal and glucocorticoid-induced maturation of intestine using bromodeoxyuridine. Am J Physiol. 1995;268:G139–45.
21. Wu GD, Wang W, Traber PG. Isolation and characterization of the human sucrase-isomaltase gene and demonstration of intestine-specific transcriptional element. J Biol Chem. 1992;267:7863–70.
22. Traber PG, Wu GD, Wang W. Novel DNA-binding proteins regulate intestine-specific transcription of the sucrase-isomaltase gene. Mol Cell Biol. 1992;12:3614–27.
23. Wu GD, Chen L, Forslund K, Traber PG. Hepatocyte nuclear factor 1α (HNF-1α) and HNF-1β regulate transcription via two elements in an intestine-specific promoter. J Biol Chem. 1994;26: 17080–5.
24. Suh E-R, Chen L, Taylor J, Traber PG. A homeodomain protein related to caudal regulates intestine-specific gene transcription. Mol Cell Biol. 1994;14:7340–51.
25. Pinto M, Robine-Leon S, Appay M-D et al. Enterocyte-like differentiation and polarization of the human colon carcinoma cell line Caco-2 in culture. Biol Cell. 1983;47:323–30.
26. Mlodzik M, Fjose A, Gehring WJ. Isolation of caudal, a Drosophila homeo box-containing gene with maternal expression, whose transcripts for a concentration gradient at the pre-blastoderm stage. EMBO J. 1985;4:2961–9.
27. Mlodzik M, Gehring WJ. Expression of the caudal gene in the germ line of Drosophila: formation of an RNA and protein gradient during early embryogenesis. Cell. 1987;48:465–78.
28. Macdonald PM, Struhl G. A molecular gradient in early Drosophila embryos and its role in specifying the body pattern. Nature. 1986;324:537–45.
29. Mlodzik M, Gibson G, Gehring WJ. Effects of ectopic expression of caudal during Drosophila development. Development. 1990;109:271–7.
30. James R, Kazenwadel J. Homeobox gene expression in intestinal epithelium of adult mice. J Biol Chem. 1991;266:3246–51.
31. Freund J-N, Boukamel R, Benazzouz A. Gradient expression of cdx along the rat intestine throughout postnatal development. FEBS Lett. 1992;314:163–6.
32. Burglin TR, Finney M, Coulson A, Ruvkun G. Caenorhabditis elegans has scores of homeobox-containing genes. Nature. 1989;341:239–43.
33. Frumkin A, Rangini Z, En-Yehuda A, Gruenbaum Y, Fainsod A. A chicken caudal homologue, CHox-cad, is expressed in the epiblast with posterior localization and in the early endodermal lineage. Development. 1991;112:207–19.
34. Serrano J, Scavo L, Roth J, de la Rosa EJ, de Pablo F. A novel chicken homeobox-containing gene expressed in neurulating embryos. Biochem Biophys Res Commun. 1993;190:270–6.
35. German MS, Wang J, Chadwick RB, Rutter WJ. Synergistic activation of the insulin gene by a LIM-homeo domain protein and a basic helix-loop-helix protein: building a functional insulin minienhancer complex. Genes Dev. 1992;6:2165–76.
36. Joly J-S, Maury M, Joly C, Duprey P, Boulekbache H, Condamine H. Expression of a zebrafish caudal homeobox gene correlates with the establishment of posterior cell lineages at gastulation. Differentiation. 1992;50:75–87.
37. Blumberg B, Wright CVE, DeRobertis EM, Cho KWY. Organizer-specific homeobox genes in Xenopus laevis embryos. Science. 1991;253:194–253.
38. Duprey P, Chowdhury K, Dressler GR et al. A mouse gene homologous to the Drosophila gene caudel is expressed in epithelial cells from the embryonic intestine. Genes Dev. 1988;2:1647–54.
39. James R, Erler T, Kazenwadel J. Structure of the murine homeobox gene cdx-2: Expression in embryonic and adult intestinal epithelium. J Biol Chem. 1994;269:15229–37.

40. Gamer LW, Wright CVW. Murine *Cdx-4* bears striking similarities to the *Drosophila* caudal gene in its homeodomain sequence and early expression pattern. Mech Dev. 1993;43:71–81.
41. Mendel DB, Crabtree GR. HNF-1, a member of a novel class of dimerizing homeodomain proteins. J Biol Chem. 1991;266:677–80.
42. Mendel DB, Hansen LP, Graves MK, Conley PB, Crabtree GR. HNF-1α and HNF-1β (vHNF-1) share dimerization and homeo domains, but not activation domains, and form heterodimers in vitro. Genes Dev. 1991;10:1042–56.
43. Kuo CJ, Conley PB, Hsieh C-L, Francke U, Crabtree GR. Molecular cloning, functional expression, and chromosomal localization of mouse hepatocyte nuclear factor 1. Proc Natl Acad Sci USA. 1990;87:9838–42.
44. Frain M, Swart G, Monaci P *et al.* The liver-specific transcription factor LF-B1 contains a highly diverged homeobox DNA binding domain. Cell. 1989;59:145–57.
45. Lichtsteiner S, Schibler U. A glycosylated liver-specific transcription factor stimulates transcription of the albumin gene. Cell. 1989;57:1179–87.
46. Baumhueter S, Mendel DB, Conley PB *et al.* HNF-1 shares three sequence motifs with the POU domain proteins and is identical to LF-B1 and APF. Genes Dev. 1990;4:372–9.
47. Evans RM. The steroid and thyroid hormone receptor superfamily. Science. 1988;240:889–95.
48. Lipson KE, Baserga R. Transcriptional activity of the human thymidine kinase gene determined by a method using the polymerase chain reaction and an intron-specific probe. Proc Natl Acad Sci USA. 1989;86:9774–7.
49. Baumhueter S, Courtois G, Crabtree GR. A variant nuclear protein in dedifferentiated hepatoma cells binds to the same functional sequences in the β fibrinogen gene promoter as HNF-1. EMBO J. 1988;7:2485–93.
50. De Simone V, De Magistris L, Lazzaro D, Gerstner J, Monaci P, Cortese R. LFB3, a heterodimer-forming homeodomain of the LFB1 family, is expressed in specialized epithelia. EMBO J. 1991;10:1435–43.
51. Rey-Campos J, Chouard T, Yaniv M, Cereghini S. vHNF1 is a homeoprotein that activates transcription and forms heterodimers with HNF1. EMBO J. 1991;10:1445–57.
52. Wu GD, Wang W, Traber PG. Molecular cloning of a transcriptional repressor protein (SIRP-1) which binds to the intestine-specific promoter region of the sucrase-isomaltase gene. Gastroenterology. 1993;104:A290.
53. Cowell IG, Skinner A, Hurst HC. Transcriptional repression by a novel member of the bZIP family of transcription factors. Mol Cell Biol. 1992;12:3070–7.
54. Soeller WC, Oh CE, Kornberg TB. Isolation of cDNAs encoding the Drosophila GAGA transcription factor. Mol Cell Biol. 1993;13:7961–70.
55. Shelley CS, Farokhzad OC, Arnaout MA. Identification of cell-specific and developmentally regulated nuclear factors that direct myeloid and lymphoid expression of the *CD11a* gene. Proc Natl Acad Sci USA. 1993;90:5364–8.
56. LeCam A, Pantescu V, Paquereau L, Legraverend C, Fauconnier G, Asins G. *Cis*-acting elements controlling transcription from rat serine protease inhibitor 2.1 gene promoter. J Biol Chem. 1994;269:21532–9.
57. Tsukiyama T, Becker PB. ATP-dependent nucleosome disruption at a heat-shock promoter mediated by binding of GAGA transcription factor. Nature. 1994;267:525–31.
58. Lu Q, Wallrath LL, Granok H, Elgin SCR. (CT)n (GA)n repeats and heat shock elements have distinct roles in chromatin structure and transcriptional activation of the *Drosophila hsp26* gene. Mol Cell Biol. 1993;13:2802–14.
59. Farkas G, Gausz J, Galloni M, Reuter G, Gyurkovics H, Karch R. The trithorax-like gene encodes the drosophila GAGA factor. Nature. 1994;371:806–8.
60. O'Brien T, Wilkins RC, Giardina C, Lis JT. Distribution of GAGA protein on *Drosophila* genes in vivo. Genes Dev. 1995;9:1098–110.
61. Pevny L, Simon MC, Robertson E *et al.* Erythroid differentiation in chimeric mice blocked by a targeted mutation in the gene for transcription factor GATA-1. Nature. 1991;349:257–60.
62. Tsai F-Y, Keller G, Kuo FC *et al.* An early haematopoietic defect in mice lacking the transcription factor GATA-2. Nature. 1994;371:221–6.
63. Weintraub H. The myoD family and myogenesis: Redundancy, networks, and thresholds. Cell. 1993;75:1241–4.
64. Vossa JW, Rosenfeld MG. Anterior pituitary development: Short tales from dwarf mice. Cell. 1992;70:527–30.

65. Dearolf CR, Topol J, Parker CS. The caudal gene product is a direct activator of fushi tarazu transcription during *Drosophila* embryogenesis. Nature. 1989;341:340–3.
66. Meyer BI, Gruss P. Mouse *cdx-1* expression during gastrulation. Development. 1995;117:191–203.
67. Subramanian V, Meyer BI, Gruss P. Disruption of the murine homeobox gene *Cdx1* affects axial skeletal identities by altering the mesodermal expression domains of *Hox* genes. Cell. 1995;83: 641–53.
68. Chawengsaksophak K, Hammond V, James R, Kontgen F, Beck F. Investigation of the functional role of Cdx2 during embryogenesis. Mol Biol Cell. 1996;7:3727.
69. Suh E-R, Traber PG. An intestine-specific homeobox gene regulates proliferation and differentiation. Mol Cell Biol. 1996;16:619–25.

22
Intestinal mucin gene expression

J. R. GUM JR, J. W. HICKS and Y. S. KIM

THE STRUCTURE AND PROPERTIES OF INTESTINAL MUCINS

The mucosal surfaces of the gastrointestinal tract represent a highly selective barrier between an organism and its environment. Nutrients must be able to pass through this barrier but pathogens and toxins must be repelled. The mucosa is lubricated, moistened, and protected by a thick layer of mucus which is secreted by the cells of the epithelium and underlying glands. Mucus gels are hydrophilic, viscous, and sticky: these properties are confirmed by their content of mucin glyco-proteins, large macromolecules containing approximately 80% carbohydrate and 20% protein. Mucin glycoprotein monomers can polymerize to form multimers with $Mr > 10\,000\,000$[1-3]. In the large and small intestine, at least three different forms of mucin, encoded by different genes, are expressed. These genes are designated *MUC2*, *MUC3*, and *MUC4*, numbered according to their order of discovery[4-6]. The complete protein sequence of the product of only one of these genes, *MUC2*, is known[7-9].

MUC2 monomers have a well defined domain structure. The central portion of the molecule is occupied by two distinct repetitive domains highly enriched in potential O-glycosylation sites, Thr and Ser residues. The larger of these two domains consists of tandem repeats of 23 residues each with an average threonine content of 55%[7,9]. Different alleles of *MUC2* have different numbers of tandem repeats although most alleles have slightly greater than 100 repeat units. Thus, in most alleles of *MUC2*, this domain codes for more than 2300 amino acid residues. The central portion of MUC2 also contains a second repetitive region of 347 residues containing repeats of irregular length, between 7 and 24 residues each. This domain, which is not polymorphic within the human population, is enriched in both Thr and Ser residues[7]. The central repetitive regions of MUC2 are flanked by Cys-rich domains with structural similarity to the D-domains of von Willebrand factor. There are three of these D-domains in the amino terminus portion of the molecule and one in the carboxyl terminus. In von Willebrand factor, the first two domains constitute a propeptide but whether this occurs in MUC2 is not known[9]. Details of the processing of large secretory mucins are only recently beginning to be elucidated[10,11].

MUC3 is a second major mucin expressed in the intestine. *MUC3* contains 51 bp

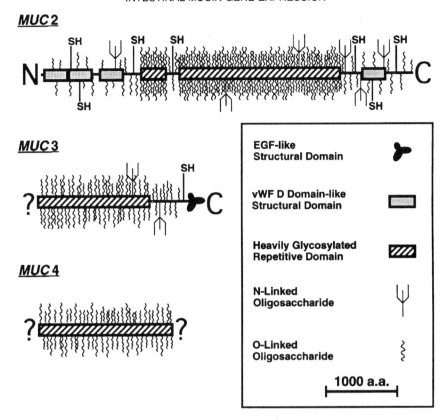

Figure 1 Models depicting the known structures of intestinal mucins. Note that the entire sequence of MUC2 is known, that only the carboxyl terminus sequence is known for MUC3, and that nothing is known of the unique sequences of MUC4

tandem repeats that encode a 17 residue amino acid sequence enriched in both Thr and Ser[5]. Much less is known however, about the remainder of the MUC3 protein. Only the carboxyl terminus domain has been cloned and this region has no sequence similarity to MUC2 (J.R. Gum, J.L.L. Ho, J.W. Hicks, A. Hill, D.M. Swallow and Y.S. Kim, unpublished). Instead, the carboxyl terminus of MUC3 contains a domain with sequence similarity to the epidermal growth factor-like structural motif. MUC4 contains 48 bp tandem repeats but nothing else is known about its structure[6]. *MUC2, MUC3*, and *MUC4* are clearly different genes, encoded on different chromosomes[12,13]. Figure 1 shows model structures for these three mucins.

CELL TYPE-SPECIFIC EXPRESSION OF INTESTINAL MUCINS

Mucin gene expression is exquisitely regulated with expression limited to just a few cell types in select epithelia. *MUC2* gene expression is especially selective.

267

Copious quantities of MUC2 message are produced in the goblet cells of the small intestine and colon as visualized by both in situ hybridization and immuno-histochemistry using antibodies to the deglycosylated peptide backbone[14,15]. Intestinal enterocytes express little if any *MUC2*. The expression of *MUC2* in the airways has also been noted and appears to be considerable, at least in certain pathological conditions, although systematic studies are lacking[16,17]. *MUC3* is expressed in the small intestine and colon in both goblet cells and enterocytes[14,15]. Significant expression of *MUC3* by the gall bladder epithelium is also evident[18]. *MUC4* was originally obtained in a screening of a human tracheo-bronchial cDNA library but is also expressed in both goblet cells and enterocytes of the small intestine and colon as well as in the epithelium of the breast, cervix, and stomach[15].

Because mucin gene expression is so tightly regulated, if offers an excellent opportunity for detailed analysis of gene expression in epithelia. We have recently succeeded in cloning the 5'-flanking region of the *MUC2* gene[19]. This has enabled us to begin analysis of the regulation of *MUC2* gene expression as outlined in the next section.

THE *MUC2* GENE 5'-FLANKING REGION

As part of our continuing effort to characterize intestinal mucins we isolated a number of genomic DNA clones including GMUC 46 (Figure 2A). A region of this lambda phage clone stretching over 11 000 bp was sequenced[19]. This region of the clone contained three introns and four exons, including the first exon. The clone also contained more than 8000 bases of 5'-flanking sequence. Immediately upstream of the first exon, a consensus TATA box was found. Several consensus binding sites for the ubiquitous transcription factor Sp1 were also identified, although these are all very far upstream, making their role in regulating tran-scription questionable. A repetitive motif of over 1000 bp was found far upstream here, and not pictured, a repetitive motif was also found in the second intron. We noted, in fact, that repetitive motifs were found in several *MUC2* introns. Thus, the *MUC2* gene contains repetitive motifs in both expressed and non-expressed regions.

Comparison of human and rodent sequences may provide clues as to regions that may be important in gene function. Accordingly, following our identification of the human *MUC2* 5'-flanking region we sought to extend these studies to rats[20]. Figure 3 shows a sequence similarity matrix comparing human and rodent *MUC2* 5'-flanking sequence. When the 5'-flanking regions of mouse *MUC2* are compared with those of rat *MUC2* a high degree of similarity is present throughout the entire 700 bp common region, as is evident from the solid line stretching the entire length of the similarity matrix. When mouse is compared with human, however, only a few regions of high similarity are evident. These regions include the first exon, a stretch of 31 nucleotides surrounding the TATA box, a stretch of approximately 200 nucleotides beginning 60 bases upstream of the start of tran-scription, and a smaller stretch located further upstream. These sequences, con-served over evolution, may be important for the initiation and regulation of *MUC2* gene transcription.

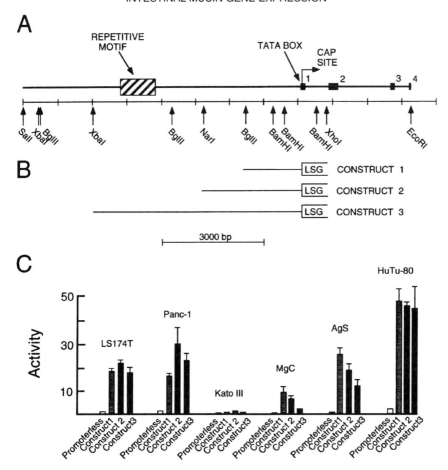

Figure 2 The MUC2 gene promoter. Part A shows the overall structure of the MUC2 gene near the transcription start site. The first four exons are shown as filled boxes and the cap site is shown. The locations of the TATA box and a repetitive motif located in the 5'-flanking region are also shown. Part B shows the relative lengths of the pGL2-Basic promoter/reporter constructs used for transfection. LSG denotes the luciferase structural gene. Part C shows the relative luciferase activity observed following transfection of the various constructs into gastrointestinal cancer cell lines. Cells were transfected with lipofectin (Gibco BRL) and harvested for assay 2 days later. Results are expressed as percentage of that obtained using the pGL2-Control vector, which employs the SV-40 promoter and enhancer to drive transcription of the luciferase structural gene

PROMOTER ACTIVITY OF THE *MUC2* 5'-FLANKING SEQUENCE IN CULTURED CELLS

We next wanted to determine whether the 5'-flanking region of the *MUC2* gene has functional promoter activity in vitro. Accordingly, lengths of the *MUC2* 5'-upstream sequence totalling 1742 bp, 2912 bp and 6115 bp were cloned upstream of a firefly luciferase gene using the pGL2-Basic vector (Promega). These promoter/reporter constructs were then transfected into a variety of cell types

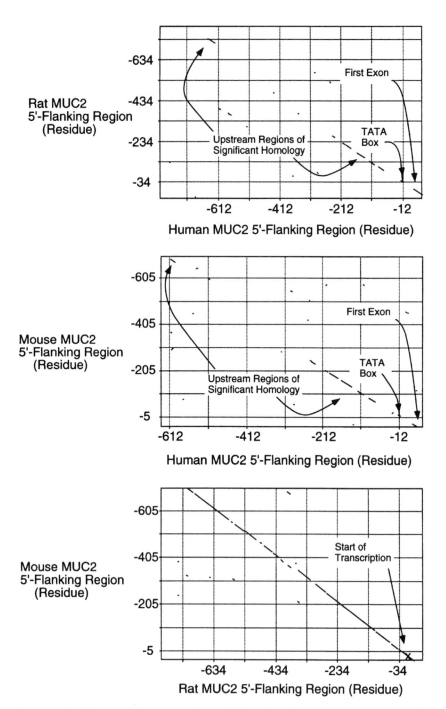

Figure 3 Similarity matrices depicting regions of high similarity between rodent and human *MUC2*. The Pustell DNA similarity matrix routine of MacVector 5.0 was used with a window of 15 residues and a cutoff of 65% similarity. Strings and dots which join together to form lines indicate regions of significant similarity

using lipofectin (Gibco/BRL) and luciferase activity was measured after 2 days. All of these constructs exhibited high levels of activity (Figures 2B, C). Interestingly, activity was observed in almost all cell lines tested, whether they expressed the *MUC2* message or not. Thus, cell type specificity was not observed with these constructs. This could be due to several factors including the possibilities that transcription of luciferase message actually initiates from an upstream sequence not utilized in vivo or that regulatory sequences are found in introns. We then prepared shorter promoter constructs to determine which sequences are absolutely required for activity. In these experiments we used four cell lines that produced varying amounts of *MUC2* message[19]. We determined that the region between base – 91 and base – 73 with respect to the start of transcription is important for a basal level of activity in all tested cell lines. This suggests the presence of an element in this region important for promoter activity. Another increase in activity was observed going from bases – 228 to – 171. This increase was considerably more pronounced in a high *MUC2*-producing cell line than in the other cell lines however, suggesting that this region may be important in conferring specificity[19]. DNase footprinting experiments demonstrated nuclear protein binding to these regions as well.

WORKING MODEL OF THE *MUC2* PROMOTER

Our initial experiments with cultured cells define some important characteristics of the *MUC2* promoter. Like many tissue specific promoters, the *MUC2* promoter contains a TATA box immediately upstream of its transcription start site. The region between bases – 73 and – 91 is important for transcriptional activity as shown by transient transfection experiments. Computer analysis of this region indicates that it contains a CACCC box, previously shown to be important in the activity of several promoters. This motif, which is also known as the β-globin consensus sequence, appears to bind different nuclear factors in different cell types. The nine nucleotide sequence 5'-GCCACACCC has a degree of similarity to the Sp1 recognition site and has been shown to bind this transcription factor in several cell types[21-23]. Other cell types, however, appear to utilize a factor shown to be clearly different from Sp1[24,25]. It will be important to determine which factor is utilized in goblet cells. The region between bases – 171 and – 228 is important for transcription activity in C1a cells and may be important for conferring specificity. A model depicting these features of the *MUC2* promoter is depicted in Figure 4. The mechanisms responsible for the exquisite specificity of expression remains unproven however, and a subject for further study. It is possible that elements important for *MUC2* specificity lie in introns or even in the 3'-region of the gene.

TRANSCRIPTION OF *MUC2* IN VITRO

In order to attempt to gain insight into the relative rates of transcription of the *MUC2* gene in cultured cells we conducted nuclear run on assays using standard protocols[26,27]. Despite repeated attempts with different probes representing different

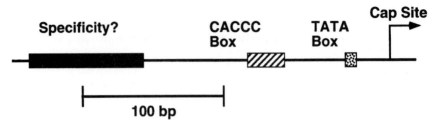

Figure 4 Proximal portion of the *MUC2* promoter. The cap site demarcates the start of transcription. The location of a cognate TATA box is given as a CACCC box. Deletion of this latter site results in a dramatic decrease in promoter activity in all cell lines tested. An upstream region that may be important for specific expression is also depicted

portions of the *MUC2* message, we failed to achieve high enough signals compared with background to be able to assess relative *MUC2* transcription rates confidently (data not shown). This occurred despite obtaining robust signals for β-actin, used as a positive control in these experiments. We interpret these results as indicating that the rate of *MUC2* transcription in cultured cells is very low. We next studied the rate of degradation of the *MUC2* message using actinomycin D to inhibit message biosynthesis, following the rate of message degradation with RNA blot analysis[19]. Here we found a very long half-life for the *MUC2* message, much longer than the 12 h window allowed by the experimental technique used because of adverse effects of actinomycin D on cell viability. This experiment revealed no evidence for a shorter half-life in cell lines with low levels of *MUC2* message, although this could not be ruled out. Thus, *MUC2* message levels in cultured cells are likely to be achieved by low degradation rates in spite of low transcription rates.

MUC2 EXPRESSION IN VIVO

RNA blot analysis indicates that the intestinal mucosa contains considerably higher levels of *MUC2* message than is observed even in the highest producing cell lines[4,5,28]. Moreover, only a fraction of epithelial cells are goblet cells. Therefore, it is clear that the *MUC2* message is expressed at very much higher levels in goblet cells in vivo than in any cultured cell model. Accordingly, cultured cells may lack features of *MUC2* regulation found in vivo. This implies that any experimentation that depends heavily upon cultured cell models may well fail to detect elements that are important for the regulation of *MUC2* in tissues. Thus, it will be important for future studies of *MUC2* and other mucin gene expression to utilize animal models and techniques that can be applied to tissues. Experimentation along these lines may be necessary to elucidate factors important for the expression of mucin and other epithelium-specific genes.

Acknowledgements

This work was supported by the Department of Veterans Affairs Medical Research Service and by grant CA 24321 from the United States National Cancer Institute.

References

1. Allen DC, Connolly NS, Biggart JD. Mucin profiles in ulcerative colitis with dysplasia and carcinoma. Histopathology. 1988;13:413–24.
2. Gum JR. Mucin genes and the proteins they encode: Structure, diversity, and regulation. Am J Resp Cell Mol Biol. 1992;7:557–64.
3. Gum JR. Human mucin glycoproteins: varied structures predict diverse properties and specific functions. Biochem Soc Trans. 1995;23:795–9.
4. Gum JR, Byrd JC, Hicks JW, Toribara NW, Lamport DTA, Kim YS. Molecular cloning of human intestinal mucin cDNAs. Sequence analysis and evidence for genetic polymorphism. J Biol Chem. 1989;264:6480–7.
5. Gum JR, Hicks JW, Swallow DM et al. Molecular cloning of cDNAs derived from a novel human intestinal mucin gene. Biochem Biophys Res Commun. 1990;171:407–15.
6. Porchet N, Van Cong N, Dufosse J et al. Molecular cloning and chromosomal localization of a novel human tracheo-bronchial mucin cDNA containing tandemly repeated sequences of 48 base pairs. Biochem Biophys Res Commun. 1991;175:414–22.
7. Toribara NW, Gum JR, Culhane PJ et al. MUC-2 human small intestinal mucin gene structure. Repeated arrays and polymorphism. J Clin Invest. 1991;88:1005–13.
8. Gum JR, Hicks JW, Toribara NW, Rothe EM, Lagace RE, Kim YS. The human MUC2 intestinal mucin has cysteine-rich subdomains located both upstream and downstream of its central repetitive region. J Biol Chem. 1992;267:21375–83.
9. Gum JR, Hicks JW, Toribara NW, Siddiki B, Kim YS. Molecular cloning of human intestinal mucin (MUC2) cDNA: Identification of the amino terminus and overall sequence similarity to pre-pro-von Willebrand factor. J Biol Chem. 1994;269:2440–6.
10. Asker N, Baeckstrom D, Axelsson MAB, Carlstedt I, Hansson GC. The human MUC2 mucin apoprotein appears to dimerize before O-glycosylation and shares epitopes with the insoluble mucin of rat small intestine. Biochem J. 1995;380:873–80.
11. Perez-Vilar J, Eckhardt AE, Hill RL. Porcine submaxillary mucin forms Disulfide-bonded dimers between its carboxyl-terminal domains. J Biol Chem. 1996;271:9845–50.
12. Griffiths B, Matthews DJ, West L et al. Assignment of the polymorphic intestinal mucin gene (MUC2) to chromosome 11p15. Ann Hum Genet. 1990;54:277–85.
13. Fox MF, Lahbib F, Pratt W et al. Regional localization of the intestinal mucin gene MUC3 to chromosome 7q22. Ann Hum Genet. 1992;56:281–7.
14. Chang SK, Dohrman AF, Basbaum CB et al. Localization of mucin (MUC2 and MUC3) messenger RNA and peptide expression in human normal intestine and colon cancer. Gastroenterology. 1994;107:28–36.
15. Audie JP, Janin A, Porchet N, Copin MC, Gosselin B, Aubert JP. Expression of human mucin genes in respiratory, digestive, and reproductive tracts ascertained by in situ hybridization. J Histochem Cytochem. 1993;43:1479–85.
16. Dohrman A, Young C, Gallup M et al. MUC2 mucin gene expression is upregulated in human airways by products of Pseudomonas Aeruginosa. Am J Res Crit Care Med. 1995;151:A160.
17. Gerard C, Eddy RL, Shows TB. The core polypeptide of cystic fibrosis tracheal mucin contains a tandem repeat structure. Evidence for a common mucin in airway and gastrointestinal tissue. J Clin Invest. 1990;86:1921–7.
18. Baeckstrom D, Karlsson N, Hansson GC. Purification and characterization of sialyl-Le(a)-carrying mucins of human bile; evidence for the presence of MUC1 and MUC3 apoproteins. J Biol Chem. 1994;269:14430–7.
19. Gum JR, Hicks JW, Kim YS. Identification and characterization of the MUC2 (human intestinal mucin) gene 5'-flanking region: Promoter activity in cultured cells. Biochem J. 1997; in press.
20. Nogami H, Ohmori H, Li J et al. Sp1 protein contributes to airway-specific rate MUC2 mucin gene transcription. Submitted 1996;
21. Dittmer J, Gegonne A, Gitlin SD, Ghysdael J, Brady JN. Regulation of parathyroid hormone-related protein (PTHrP) gene expression. Sp1 binds through an inverted CACCC motif and regulates promoter activity in cooperation with Ets1. J Biol Chem. 1994;269:21428–34.
22. Gegonne A, Bosselut R, Bailly RA, Ghysdael J. Synergistic activation of the HTLV1 LTR Ets-responsive region by transcription factors Ets1 and Sp1. EMBO J. 1993;12:1169–78.
23. Fischer KD, Hease A, Nowock J. Cooperation of GATA-1 and Sp1 can result in synergistic transcriptional activation or interference. J Biol Chem. 1993;268:23915–23.

24. DeVack C, Lupp B, Nichols M, Kowenz-Leutz E, Schmid W, Schutz G. Characterization of the nuclear proteins binding the CACCC element of a glucocorticoid-responsive enhancer in the tyrosine aminotransferase gene. Eur J Biochem. 1993;211:459–65.

25. Hartzog GA, Myers RM. Discrimination among potential activators of the beta-globin CACCC element by correlation of binding and transcriptional properties. Mol Cell Biol. 1993;13:44–56.

26. Greenberg ME, Ziff EB. Stimulation of 3T3 cells induces transcription of the c-*fos* proto-oncogene. Nature. 1984;311:433–8.

27. Celano P, Berchtold C, Casero RA. A simplification of the nuclear run-off transcription assay. Biotechniques. 1989;7:942–4.

28. Ho SB, Niehans GA, Lyftogt C *et al*. Heterogeneity of mucin gene expression in normal and neoplastic tissues. Cancer Res. 1993;53:641–51.

23
Gastrointestinal cell lines as a model for differentiation

R. H. WHITEHEAD and N. K. WATSON

INTRODUCTION

The intestinal mucosa comprises millions of discrete units, the crypts, in which proliferation and differentiation continually occur. The stem cells located in each crypt differentiate into at least five phenotypically distinct cell lineages: four cell types are common to all parts of the intestine (columnar or absorptive, goblet, caveolated and endocrine) while the fifth cell type, the Paneth cell, is restricted to the small intestine in the healthy bowel[1]. The complexity becomes greater when one examines the type of peptide granules being produced by endocrine cells, with specific peptides being produced in different regions of the intestine[2]. Similarly the type of mucin produced by the goblet cell varies in different regions of the colon[3]. The localization and differentiation signals acting on the stem cells or their uncommitted daughter cells in the crypt are still unknown.

The ideal system for identifying the factors controlling the differentiation pathways defined by the Unitarian hypothesis would be an in vitro culture system where cells can be induced to differentiate along specific lineages. This has been achieved in the haemopoietic system, where a culture method was devised for the bone marrow precursor cells[4]. Using this system, a whole family of growth and differentiation factors has been discovered. These factors have been shown to control the proliferation of the bone marrow stem cells and induce differentiation of the daughter cells along specific lineages[5]. No such system is possible for the intestinal mucosa, as normal mucosal epithelial cells have proved very difficult to culture in vitro. Because culturing normal intestinal mucosal cells has proved so difficult, many of the studies that have confirmed the Unitarian theory by demonstrating the ability of cells to differentiate into mature phenotypes have utilized colonic carcinoma cell lines.

Columnar and goblet cell differentiation

In his excellent review, Laboisse[6] nominated three markers of intestinal differentiation: VIP receptors, as a marker of basolateral membrane function; sucrase-

Table 1 Factors which induce differentiation in 'normal' and malignant intestinal epithelial cell lines

Treatment	Cell line	Reference
Spontaneous	LIM1863	17
Confluent growth and time	Caco-2, LIM1899, T84, HT-29Cl.16E	6, 17, 18
Sodium butyrate	Many	6, 25, 26, 28
Glucose-deprivation	HT-29, HCT-Geo, HCT-EB	18, 21
Forskolin	HT-29	38
IGF autocrine loop	HT-29	66
Xenograft growth	HRA-19, Caco-2	41, 44
Association with basement membrane proteins	HRA-19, NCI-H719, SW1222, IEC-17, IEC-6	33, 40, 42, 53, 54
Ras	Caco-2, IMCE	43, 44, 45
Cdx-2 (homeobox gene)	IEC-6	57

isomaltase, a brush border hydrolase, as a measure of brush border-related function, and mucus production as a measure of goblet cell differentiation. VIP receptors will not be considered further in this review as Laboisse gave a comprehensive introduction to this topic in his review[6].

Columnar cells are defined both by morphology and function in vivo. Morphology of cells in culture is best defined by electron microscopy as it is difficult, if not impossible, to identify brush border structures at the light microscope level in cultured cells. The functional aspects of the cells that are readily tested are the presence of brush border proteins such as villin[7] and brush border-associated enzymes such as alkaline phosphatase, dipeptidases and disaccharidases[8,9]. Goblet cells are defined by morphology and the presence of large mucus inclusions which can be demonstrated either histochemically using stains such as periodic acid–Schiff or Alcian blue or using mucin-specific antibodies.

Endocrine cell differentiation

Endocrine cells are defined either by ultrastructure where the presence of dense core granules is indicative or by immunohistochemistry. An antibody to chromogranin A, an acidic protein present in neurosecretory granules[10], is usually used, although antibodies to specific endocrine peptides have occasionally been used[11].

STUDIES USING COLON CARCINOMA CELL LINES

It is one of the interesting properties of colon carcinoma cell lines that many of them can be induced to differentiate along one or many of the known colonic differentiation pathways. Some examples of these findings are summarized in Table 1 and described below.

Absorptive cell differentiation

Many colon carcinoma cell lines spontaneously secrete brush border enzymes and some also show a columnar morphology e.g. post-confluent[12], T84[13–15], LIM1215[16], LIM1899[16] and LIM1863[17].

Although spontaneous differentiation does occur in colon carcinoma cell lines it is uncommon. Chantret et al.[18] studied 20 colonic carcinoma cell lines for evidence of enterocytic differentiation. These workers used the presence of villin and brush border hydrolases (both dipeptidases and disaccharidases) as markers of enterocytic differentiation. Other properties such as the ability to form a polarized monolayer were considered to be markers of partial differentiation. Of the 20 lines studied, only Caco-2 differentiated spontaneously with a polarized brush border expressing brush border-related enzymes. Three cell lines (HT-29, HCT-EB and HCT-GEO) could be induced to differentiate when grown in glucose-free medium but only the HT-29 cell line was considered to have differentiated completely with expression of a range of brush border enzymes. Eight cell lines formed a polarized monolayer but did not produce a brush border or any of the brush border-related peptides and the remainder remained undifferentiated under all culture conditions.

We have analysed eight colon carcinoma cell lines which we have developed and characterized in our laboratory for evidence of a differentiated phenotype[16]. Some of these cell lines have retained the ability to form a polarized monolayer with a well-developed brush border which stains positively for the known brush border enzymes[16]. One cell line, LIM1863[17], grows as non-adherent organoids. When these organoids were sectioned it was found that the cells were highly organized and that each organoid contained a central lumen lined with a well-developed brush border. The majority of the cells were columnar and the nuclei were displaced to the base of the cell as in the crypt (Figure 1). In addition to the columnar cells, these organoids also contain about 5% of morphologically mature goblet cells[19] and a small percentage of caveolated (tuft) cells[20].

As mentioned above, HT-29 cells undergo enterocytic differentiation when grown in medium in which glucose has been replaced by either galactose or inosine (reviewed in Ref. 6). Although Chantret et al.[18] found that two of 15 other cell lines could be partially differentiated in glucose-free medium, we were unable to influence the differentiation state of any of our lines following growth in glucose-free medium. These findings indicate that this is not a universal mechanism and its physiological relevance is unknown. It may be a property of the HT 29 cell line that, although the parental line is undifferentiated, it can be induced to differentiate using a number of different treatments[21,22].

Of possibly more physiological relevance have been the findings that addition of sodium butyrate to the growth medium can alter the differentiation status of a number of colon carcinoma cell lines. Sodium butyrate is found in the colonic lumen at high concentration[23] and is a preferred energy source for colonic enterocytes[24]. It has been shown that when some colon carcinoma cell lines are cultured in the presence of 1 mM sodium butyrate for 5–7 days, the growth rate decreases and the levels of alkaline phosphatase and dipeptidases produced by the cells increase markedly[25,26]. Although butyrate is only one of a number of short chain fatty acids produced in the colon as a result of fermentation of fibre[27], we found that it was the most efficient of the short chain fatty acids tested for inducing the up-regulation of alkaline phosphatase and dipeptidase in the LIM1215 cell line[28].

Although sodium butyrate has been the most widely used compound in differentiation induction studies, a number of other compounds and culture conditions have also been shown to induce differentiation of colon carcinoma cell lines. One

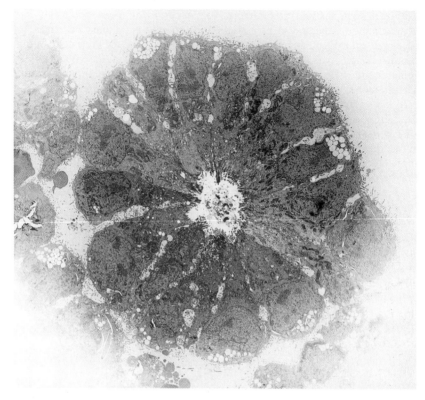

Figure 1 Electron micrograph of a section through an organoid formed by LIM1863 cells in culture. The organoids contain a central lumen which is lined with a brush border. The nuclei are polarized to the base of the cells (× 1600)

interesting finding was that glandular differentiation could be induced in the SW1222 cell line by culture in a collagen gel[29]. In a further study which investigated the role of the interaction of cell lines with basement membrane-related proteins in the induction of differentiation, del Buono et al.[30] found that culture on either fetal mesenchymal cells or on a basement membrane extract (Matrigel) induced morphological differentiation in two of the five cell lines tested. The differentiation induced in this system could be inhibited by an RGD-containing peptide, suggesting that integrin binding is involved.

Although the studies described above demonstrate that the phenotype of at least some colon carcinoma cell lines can be altered using the appropriate culture conditions, not all cell lines are responsive. We have not been successful in altering the proportion of the various cell types found in the LIM1863 cell line despite using most of the methods used in previous studies. As described above, the LIM1863 cell line is possibly the most differentiated of all the readily available cell lines. The presence of three of the four colonic mucosal cell phenotypes in the organoids suggested that the tumour from which the cell line was derived had arisen in a very primitive multipotential cell in the crypt. In spite of the multipotential nature of the cells, all attempts to alter the proportion of each cell type in the organoids of this cell line have failed. In one experiment, the LIM1863 organoids were disaggregated to single cells by culturing the organoids in Ca^{2+} free medium for 48 h. The single cell suspension was cloned in semisolid agar and 32 individual clones were picked and cultured. Comprehensive morphological, ultrastructural and immunohistochemical studies on each of these clones failed to demonstrate any difference in phenotype from the parental culture (Hayward and Whitehead, unpublished results).

Goblet cell differentiation

Colon cancer cell lines vary in the degree to which they can be induced to differentiate into a goblet cell phenotype. Some cell lines spontaneously form goblet cells. Sectioning of LIM1863 organoids reveals that approximately 5% of the cells in the organoid are mature goblet cells full of mucin[17]. Similarly LS174T[31], a human adenoma line PC/AA[32], HRA-19[33], LIM1215[34], LIM2463[35] and Caco-2[36] all spontaneously form goblet cells or secrete mucin in culture. Treatment of HT-29 cells for 23 days with sodium butyrate followed by cloning of those cells in the treated culture that had developed a distinctive morphology led to the development of a stable clone (Cl.16 E) with a goblet cell phenotype[37]. The HT-29 Cl.16E line has been shown to respond to cell contact inhibition by expressing a fully differentiated goblet cell phenotype[38]. In another study, treatment of the parental HT-29 line with forskolin induced expression of both *MUC2* AND *MUC3* genes whereas sodium butyrate treatment induced only the *MUC3* gene[38].

Endocrine cell differentiation

Very few colon carcinoma cell lines spontaneously differentiate into endocrine cells in vitro. The NCI-H716 cell line was described by Park et al.[39] as showing evidence of endocrine differentiation with cells containing electron-dense granules characteristic of endocrine cells. Recently, endocrine differentiation in this line was shown to be significantly enhanced when the cells were grown in contact with basement membrane proteins. A number of membrane-associated proteins were equally active. Culture on fibroblast feeder layers or in the presence of extracellular matrix or on a collagen IV/heparan sulphate proteoglycan mix or on a collagen IV coated surface in defined medium supplemented with fibroblast growth factor all induced significant differentiation. In these studies, endocrine cells were defined by chromogranin staining and by electron microscopy[11,40]. Recently Kirkland and Henderson[33] have reported that the HRA-19 cell line, which previously only differentiated into endocrine cells when grown as a xenograft in nude mice[41], could be induced to differentiate into mucous and endocrine cells if post-confluent cultures were grown in medium containing 1% fetal calf serum. In the case of both HRA-19 and NCI-H716 cells, interaction with the stroma when the cells are grown as xenografts appears to be required for induction of endocrine cell differentiation. Apart from stromal cell or basement membrane protein interaction, little is known about the factors that determine differentiation along the endocrine pathway. Kirkland and Henderson[33] found that transforming growth factor-β (TGF-β) inhibited formation of both endocrine and mucous cells in HRA-19 cells; however, Pignatelli and Bodmer[42] found that addition of TGF-β greatly enhanced glandular formation by SW1222 cells when the cells were grown in a collagen gel.

Effects of transformation with oncogenes

One surprising finding is that transfection of cell lines with an activated *Ras* oncogene can lead to the induction of differentiation-related properties. *Ras* is generally considered to be a transforming oncogene and the differentiation-related features appear in these transformed cells in addition to the properties associated with transformation such as rapid growth and tumour formation in animals. Celano et al.[43] expressed an activated v-*Ha-Ras* oncogene in Caco-2 cells and found that over-expression of this oncogene led to the expression of multiple markers characteristic of intestinal brush border differentiation. Sucrase-isomaltase and alkaline phosphatase activities were increased markedly compared to the parental line. Although the authors commented that the morphology of the Caco-2/Ras cell line changed, no ultrastructural studies were reported. In a similar study, de Bruine et al.[44] transfected Caco-2 cells with a point-mutated *Ha-Ras* gene. They found that although the tumorigenicity of the transfected Caco-2 cells was apparently increased, the tumours which formed contained cells representative of all the intestinal lineages. They demonstrated brush border staining for sucrase isomaltase, mucin presence by PAS/diastase and Alcian blue staining and the presence of endocrine cells using chromogranin A, chromogranin A/B and synaptophysin antibodies. Dense core granules were also seen by electron microscopy. In addition Paneth cells were demonstrated by staining for lysozyme. Ras proteins have also been shown to induce differentiation in phaeochromocytoma (PC12) cells, F9 teratoma cells and human medullary thyroid carcinoma cells (see Ref. 43).

We have recently found that transfection of a phenotypically normal, conditionally immortalized mouse colonic cell line which was derived from an SV40 large T/MIN hybrid transgenic mouse with *Ha-Ras* oncogene led to both transformation of the cells[45] and the expression of morphological characteristics associated with a differentiated phenotype. These studies are described below.

STUDIES USING 'NORMAL' INTESTINAL EPITHELIAL CELLS

Very few cell lines derived from normal intestinal mucosal cells have been widely used in differentiation studies. The most commonly used 'normal' intestinal cell lines have been the IEC series derived by Quaroni et al.[46] These lines and the RIE-1 line[47] were derived from the small intestinal mucosa of newly weaned rats. Other cell lines have been derived from fetal rat small intestine[48], suckling rat colon[49]; fetal human colonic mucosa[50] and adult rabbit colonic mucosa[51]. None of these cell lines has been widely used outside the laboratory of origin. We have recently derived conditionally immortalized 'normal' epithelial cell lines from the small intestinal and colonic mucosa of adult SV40 large T (ts mutant) transgenic mice[52].

Although the IEC lines have an undifferentiated phenotype, interaction of the cells with either mesenchyme or basement membrane proteins is able to induce differentiation. Kedinger et al.[53] packaged a sheet of IEC-17 cells between two sheets of cultured fetal rat gut mesenchymal cells and placed the cell packages under the kidney capsule of adult rats. When the tissue was harvested 9–10 days later, a small number of the IEC-17 implants showed full morphological differentiation with columnar (absorptive), goblet, endocrine and Paneth cells present. In their studies, the parental IEC-17 cells were devoid of alkaline phosphatase or disaccharidase activity; however, all these enzymes could be demonstrated on the IEC-17 cells after implantation. Carroll et al.[54] cultured IEC-6 cells on basement membrane protein (Matrigel) and found that the cells cultured on Matrigel developed microvilli, a markedly increased rough endoplasmic reticulum and showed staining for alkaline phosphatase and sucrase. Addition of nucleotides to the medium has recently been shown to increase alkaline phosphatase and sucrase activity of IEC-6 cells grown on Matrigel[55].

The importance of epithelial–mesenchyme interactions in directing epithelial cell differentiation has been emphasized by the recent report of the growth of fetal human small intestinal epithelial cells on either a standard plastic surface or on an extracellular matrix preparation. Cells growing on plastic were dedifferentiated whereas when the cells were grown on extracellular matrix, the level of alkaline phosphatase produced by the cells increased. Formation of microvilli was also described[56]. Sucrase activity could be demonstrated in primary intestinal sheets grown on a fibroblast feeder layer and the level of sucrase activity was increased by the addition of sodium butyrate to the culture medium[56].

All of the experiments described to date describe external influences that can act on mucosal epithelial cells to induce differentiation. The recent finding by Suh and Traber[57] that transfection of IEC-6 cells with a homeobox gene, *Cdx-2*, led to full morphological differentiation of the cells indicates possible gene control mechanisms for this process. They found that conditional expression of *Cdx-2* led to arrest of proliferation for several days followed by a period of growth which resulted in multicellular structures. These structures contained a layer of cells which was composed of columnar cells with well organized microvilli and tight junctions. Goblet cells were also present. The *Cdx-2* gene is a member of the homeobox family of genes and it was originally cloned by James and Kazenwadel[58] using RNA derived from purified colonic crypts using a PCR strategy. It is intestine-specific in the adult animal with greatest expression in the proximal colon. This gene was subsequently isolated by Traber's group[59] while they were attempting to isolate factors controlling the transcription of the sucrase-isomaltase gene. They found that transcription of this gene was dependent on the binding of Cdx-2 protein to a promoter element in the sucrase-isomaltase gene.

RECENT STUDIES

As mentioned earlier, we have derived conditionally immortalized cell lines from the small intestine (designated MSIE) and colon (YAMC) of adult SV40 large T transgenic mice[52,60]. These cells proliferate at the permissive temperature (33°C) in medium containing murine interferon-γ but die within 7 days at the non-

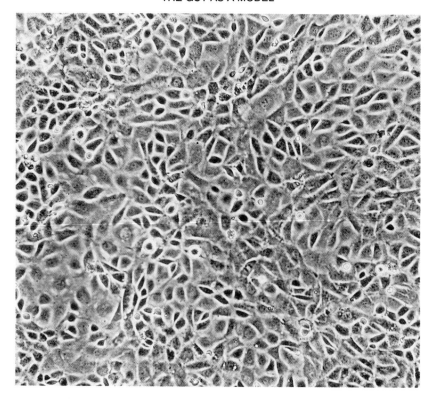

Figure 2 Phase contrast photograph of YAMC cells in monolayer culture. The cells are uniform and have an undifferentiated phenotype (× 125)

permissive temperature (39°C). These cells do not form colonies in agar or grow as xenografts in nude mice. By all standard criteria these cells still have a normal phenotype. Morphologically, the cells are very undifferentiated (Figure 2) and extensive ultrastructural studies indicate that the cells do not form tight junctions or microvilli. Cultures have been grown both as monolayers and on filter inserts with a range of growth factors and many hundreds of cells have been examined for the presence of tight junctions and microvilli without success. The cells stain poorly with antibodies to keratin 18 but staining can be induced by the addition of 10^{-7} M phorbol 12-myristate 13-acetate (PMA) to the cultures for 7 days. Epidermal growth factor and fibroblast growth factor are mitogenic for these cells and growth is inhibited by TGF-β[52].

As part of an attempt to develop in vitro models of colon cancer, these SV40 large T transgenic mice[60] were crossed with the Min mouse which carries a mutation of the murine *APC* gene[61]. The progeny of these matings were typed by PCR for the presence of both the SV40 large T gene and the mutant murine *APC* gene. Cell lines (designated IMCE) were derived from the colonic mucosa of adult mice carrying both genes[62]. The presence of a mutant murine *APC* gene was demonstrated in these cell lines; however the phenotype of the cell lines was

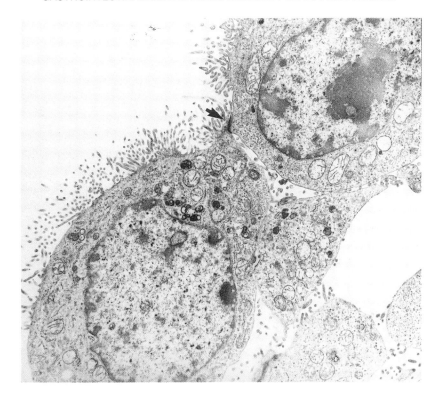

Figure 3   Electron micrograph of cells in a culture of *Ras*-transfected IMCE cells. In contrast to the parental IMCE cell line, there are a large number of microvilli present on the apical surface of the cells and the cells are joined at the apical surface by a well-formed tight junction (arrow) (× 7600)

almost identical to the parental YAMC cell line phenotype. The cells were still only conditionally immortalized, would not form colonies in agar and did not form tumours when injected into nude mice. Ultrastructurally, the cells were undifferentiated with no evidence of tight junctions or desmosomes and no microvilli. The only difference found between the two cell lines was that the IMCE cells stained more strongly for the presence of keratin fibres.

Both the YAMC and the IMCE cell lines have now been transfected with an activated Ha-Ras virus[45]. The phenotype of the YAMC/Ras cell line was almost unchanged from the parental YAMC phenotype. The IMCE cells transfected with Ras were, however, fully malignant and formed tumours in nude mice and could be grown clonally in soft agar at the non-permissive temperature. The IMCE/Ras cells grew as a loosely adherent monolayer with many floating cells which grew into aggregates of cells[45]. These cells stained much more strongly for keratin fibres than either the YAMC or IMCE cell lines. When the ultrastructure of these cell clumps was examined we were surprised to find well formed tight junctions between the cells and evidence of microvilli formation (Figure 3).

The mechanism by which over-expression of an activated Ras protein might

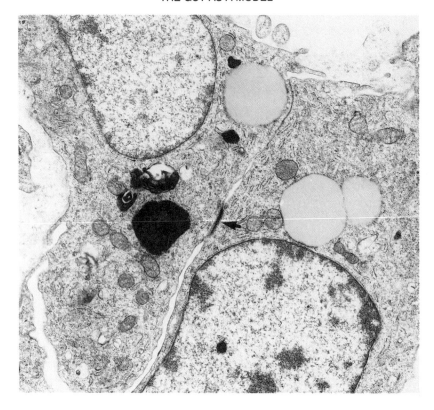

Figure 4 Electron micrograph of parental IMCE cells cultured in agar-coated flasks for 7 days. The cells grow unattached and form spheroids. Under these growth conditions, desmosomes form (arrow) (× 12 600)

induce differentiation in these cell lines is unknown. Ras proteins are involved in many intracellular signalling pathways[63,64] and an activated/over-expressed Ras protein would be expected to activate many, if not all, of these pathways.

We have begun to explore the mechanisms by which the transfection of the IMCE cell line by an activated Ras gene could lead to both malignant transformation and morphological differentiation changes. Initially, we cultured the parental IMCE line in medium containing combinations of factors known to stimulate different intracellular signalling pathways. Combinations of EGF, FGF, keratinocyte growth factor (KGF), hepatocyte growth factor (HGF), TGF-β and PMA were used. The cells were cultured both as monolayers and over agar-coated surfaces. Agar coating prevents cell adherence thus forcing the cells to grow in suspension and form spheroids. The cells were cultured for 5 days, harvested and examined by electron microscopy. As mentioned earlier we were unable to detect any tight junctions in parental IMCE monolayer cultures. However all the cultures grown in suspension including the parental line formed good desmosomal structures (Figure 4). Culture in a combination of TGF-α

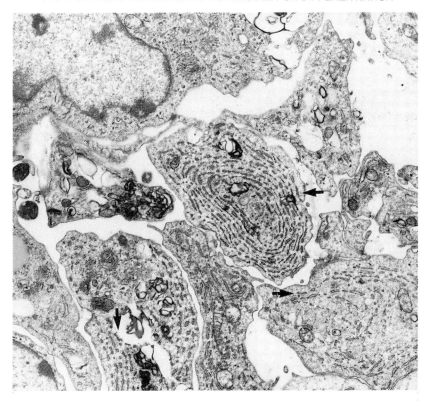

Figure 5 Electron micrograph of IMCE cells cultured in agar-coated flasks in medium containing TGF-α and KGF. Many of the cells developed extensive arrays of rough endoplasmic reticulum (arrows) ($\times 10\ 000$)

+ HGF + PMA or TGF-α + KGF + PMA increased the percentage of cells joined by tight junctions markedly (Table 2). Not only did the number of cells joined by tight junctions increase, the number of tight junctions per cell increased also.

In addition to tight junction formation there was a marked increase in the amount of endoplasmic reticulum present in the cells grown in suspension. The combination of TGF-α plus KGF induced the most cells containing large arrays of endoplasmic reticulum (Figure 5; Table 2). The nature of these cells is unknown. The endoplasmic reticulum arrays seen in these cells are common to many cell types synthesizing large amounts of protein. In the intestinal tract, the cell which the cells most resemble is the chief cell of the gastric mucosa.

The undifferentiated nature of the conditionally immortalized cell lines is also shown by the low levels of disaccharidase, dipeptidase and alkaline phosphatase expressed by the cells. We have attempted to increase the levels of activity of these enzymes by growing the cells in the presence of growth and differentiation factors such as sodium butyrate and phorbol 12-myristate 13-acetate (PMA). Disaccharidase levels (measured by the method of Dahlqvist[65]) were more than

Table 2 Morphological differentiation of IMCE cells grown in suspension culture in agar-coated flasks

Culture	Tight junctions (%)	Microvilli	Endoplasmic reticulum (%)
Monolayer	0[a]	–	<5[b]
Control on agar	37	+	11
TGF-α+KGF	43[c]	+	30
TGF-α+HGF	43[c]	+	25
HGF+KGF	42[c]	++	12
TGF-α+KGF+PMA	50[c]	+	23
TGF-α+HGF+PMA	50[c]	+	22

[a]Percentage of cells joined to an adjacent cell by at least one tight junction
[b]Percentage of cells containing arrays of endoplasmic reticulum in the cytoplasm
[c]More than one tight junction per cell

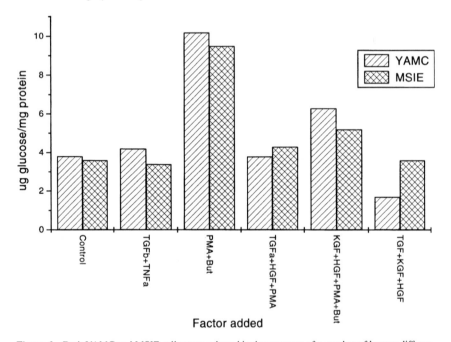

Figure 6 Both YAMC and MSIE cells were cultured in the presence of a number of known differentiating agents for 5 days. The cells were harvested by scraping, sonicated in lysis buffer and the supernate assayed for disaccharidase activity by the method of Dahlquist[65]. Protein content of the extract was determined using a BCA Protein Assay Kit (Pierce Chemical Co., Illinois). Addition of a combination of 1 mM sodium butyrate and 10^{-6} M PMA increased the level of disaccharidase activity in the cells significantly

doubled in both YAMC and MSIE cultures following growth for 5 days in the presence of 1 mM sodium butyrate and 10^{-6} M PMA (Figure 6).

Because culture of the IMCE cell line in suspension led to an increase in morphological differentiation of these cells, disaccharidase levels of the cell lines after suspension culture were determined. MSIE cells grown in agar coated plates

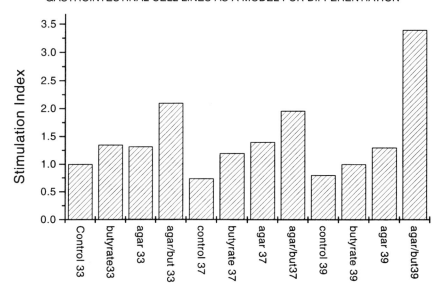

Figure 7 MSIE cells were cultured both as a monolayer and in suspension in agar-coated flasks. Disaccharidase activity was assayed after either 5 days at 33°C, 2 days at 33°C, 2 days at 33°C and 3 days at 37°C or 2 days at 33°C and 3 days at 39°C. In control cultures both addition of 1 mM sodium butyrate or culture over agar increased disaccharidase levels. The greatest increase in disaccharidase levels was obtained when cells were cultured at the non-permissive temperature for 3 days in medium containing 1 mM sodium butyrate. Results are expressed as a stimulation index being the increase in disaccharidase levels in test cultures compared with the control culture

expressed more disaccharidase activity than control monolayer cultures (Figure 7). Addition of 1 mM sodium butyrate to these cultures led to a doubling of disaccharidase levels. These cells are only conditionally immortalized: they stop proliferating within 48 h and die within 7 days at the non-permissive temperature (39°C). Cells cultured for 2 days at the permissive temperature followed by 3 days at 39°C showed a 3.5-fold increase in disaccharidase activity when grown over agar with 1 mM sodium butyrate (Figure 7).

These ongoing studies indicate that these very undifferentiated cell lines can be induced to develop both biochemical (increased brush border-related enzyme production) and morphological changes consistent with a more differentiated phenotype (keratin expression, tight junction formation, microvilli and large arrays of endoplasmic reticulum) when grown in conditions shown by others to induce differentiation in colon carcinoma cell lines.

SUMMARY

Studies with both colon carcinoma cell lines and cell lines derived from normal intestinal mucosa demonstrate that a range of factors can induce 'differentiation'.

In most cases the differentiation seen is, at best, partial. In only very few instances has differentiation into the mature cellular phenotypes characteristic of the intestinal mucosa been achieved. In most cases interactions between the epithelial cell and stromal elements have been essential for differentiation to occur. One assumes that the differentiation seen is being induced either by factors secreted by the mesenchyme or by cellular pathways induced by integrin-dependent binding between the two cell types. The finding by Suh and Traber[57] that over-expression of a homeobox gene (*Cdx-2*) can induce apparently complete phenotypic differentiation in the undifferentiated IEC-6 cell line may lead us to both the intracellular pathways and the factors involved in differentiation.

Acknowledgements

The authors wish to thank Dr I.P. Hayward for his contribution to the LIM1863 studies and Ms K. Demmler for her excellent technical assistance.

References

1. Cheng H, Leblond CP. Origin, differentiation and renewal of the four main epithelial cell types in the mouse small intestine. V. Unitarian theory of the origin of the four epithelial cell types. Am J Anat. 1974;41:537–62.
2. Sjolund K, Sanden G, Hakanson R, Sundler F. Endocrine cells in human intestine. An immuno-cytochemical study. Gastroenterology. 1983;85:1120–30.
3. Shamsuddin AM. Normal and pathological anatomy of the large intestine. In: Moyer MP, Poste GH, editors. Colon Cancer Cells. San Diego: Academic Press, 1990:15–40.
4. Bradley TR, Metcalf D. The growth of mouse bone marrow cells *in vitro*. Aust J Exp Biol Med Sci. 1966;44:287–300.
5. Metcalf D. The molecular control of cell division, differentiation commitment and maturation in haemopoietic cells. Nature. 1989;339:27–30.
6. Laboisse CL. Differentiation of colon cells in culture. In: Augenlicht L, editor. Cell and Molecular Biology of Colon Cancer. Boca Raton: CRC Press, 1989:27–43.
7. Bretscher A, Weber K. Villin: the major microfilament-associated protein of the intestinal micro-villus. Proc Natl Acad Sci USA. 1979;76:2321–5.
8. Hauri HP, Quaroni A, Isselbacher KJ. Biogenesis of intestinal plasma membrane: post-translational route and cleavage of sucrase-isomaltase. Proc Natl Acad Sci USA. 1979;76:5183–6.
9. Kenny AJ, Maroux S. Topology of microvillar membrane hydrolases of kidney and intestine. Physiol Rev. 1982;62:91–128.
10. Wiedenmann B, Huttner WB. Synaptophysin and chromogranins/secretogranins – widespread constituents of distinct types of neuroendocrine vesicles and new tools in tumor diagnosis. Virchows Archiv B Cell Pathol. 1989;58:95–121.
11. DeBruine AP, Dinjens WNM, Pijls MMJ *et al*. NCI-H716 cells as a model for endocrine differentiation in colorectal cancer. Virchows Archiv B Cell Pathol. 1992;62:311–20.
12. Fogh J, Fogh JM, Orfeo T. One hundred and twenty-seven cultured human tumor cell lines producing tumors in nude mice. J Natl Cancer Inst. 1977;59:221–5.
13. Murakami H, Masui H. Hormonal control of human colon carcinoma cell growth in serum-free medium. Proc Natl Acad Sci USA. 1980;77:3464–8.
14. Dharmsathaphorn K, Mandel KG, Masui H, McRoberts JA. Vasoactive intestinal polypeptide-induced chloride secretion by a colonic epithelial cell line. J Clin Invest. 1985;75:462–71.
15. Madara JL, Stafford J, Dharmsathaphorn K, Carlson S. Structural analysis of a human intestinal epithelial cell line. Gastroenterology. 1987;92:1133–45.
16. Whitehead RH, Zhang HH, Hayward IP. Retention of tissue-specific phenotype in a panel of colon carcinoma cell lines: Relationship to clinical correlates. Immunol Cell Biol. 1992;70:227–36.
17. Whitehead RH, Jones JK, Gabriel A, Lukeis RE. A new colon carcinoma cell line (LIM1863)

that grows as organoids with spontaneous differentiation into crypt-like structures in vitro. Cancer Res. 1987;47:2683–9.

18. Chantret I, Barbat A, Dussaulx E, Brattain MG, Zweibaum A. Epithelial polarity, villin expression, and enterocytic differentiation of cultured human colon carcinoma cells: a survey of twenty cell lines. Cancer Res. 1988;48:1936–42.

19. Hayward IP, Whitehead RH. Patterns of growth and differentiation in the colon carcinoma cell line LIM 1863. Int J Cancer. 1992;50:752–9.

20. Barkla DH, Whitehead RH, Foster H, Tutton PJM. Tuft (caveolated) cells in a new human colon carcinoma cell line. Am J Pathol. 1988;132:521–5.

21. Pinto M, Appay MD, Simon-Assmann P et al. Enterocytic differentiation of cultured human colon cancer cells by replacement of glucose by galactose in the medium. Biol Cell. 1982;44:193–6.

22. Lesuffleur T, Porchet N, Aubert JP et al. Differential expression of human mucin genes MUC1 to MUC5 in relation to growth and differentiation of different mucus-secreting HT29 cell subpopulations. J Cell Sci. 1993;106:771–83.

23. Rombeau JL, Kripke SA. Metabolic and intestinal effects of short chain fatty acids. J Parent Ent Nutr. 1990;14:181s–5s.

24. Roediger WEW. Utilization of nutrients by isolated epithelial cells of the rat colon. Gastroenterology. 1982;83:424–9.

25. Kim YS, Tsao D, Siddiqui B et al. Effects of sodium butyrate and dimethyl sulfoxide on biochemical properties of human colon cancer cells. Cancer. 1980;45:1185–92.

26. Tsao D, Morita A, Bella A, Luu P, Kim YS. Differential effects of sodium butyrate, dimethyl sulfoxide, and retinoic acid on membrane-associated antigen, enzymes, and glycoproteins of human rectal adenocarcinoma cells. Cancer Res. 1982;42:1052–8.

27. Cummings JH. Short chain fatty acids in the human colon. Gut. 1981;22:763–79.

28. Whitehead RH, Young GP, Bhathal PS. The effects of short chain fatty acids on a new human colon carcinoma cell line (LIM1215). Gut. 1986;27:1457–63.

29. Richman PI, Bodmer WF. Control of differentiation in human colorectal carcinoma cell lines. Epithelial–mesenchyme interactions. J Pathol. 1988;156:197–211.

30. Del Buono R, Pignatelli M, Bodmer WF, Wright NA. The role of arginine-glycine-aspartic acid-directed cellular binding to type I collagen and rat mesenchymal cells in colorectal tumour differentiation. Differentiation. 1991;46:97–103.

31. Tom BH, Rutzky LP, Jakstys MM, Oyasu R, Kaye CI, Kahan BD. Human colon adenocarcinoma cells. 1. Establishment and description of a new line. In Vitro. 1976;12:180–91.

32. Paraskeva C, Buckle BG, Sheer D, Wigley CB. The isolation and characterization of colorectal epithelial cell lines at different stages in malignant transformation from familial polyposis coli patients. Int J Cancer. 1984;34:49–56.

33. Kirkland SC, Henderson K. Endocrine and mucous differentiation by a cloned human rectal adenocarcinoma cell line (HRA-19) in vitro: Inhibition by TGFβ. J Cell Sci. 1994;107:1041–6.

34. Whitehead RH, Macrae FA, St John DJB, Ma J. A colon cancer cell line (LIM1215) derived from a patient with inherited nonpolyposis colorectal cancer. J Natl Cancer Inst. 1985;74:759–65.

35. Whitehead RH, Van Eeden P, Lukeis RE. A cell line (LIM2463) derived from a tubulovillous adenoma of the rectum. Int J Cancer. 1991;48:693–6.

36. Niv Y, Byrd JC, Dahiya R, Kim YS. Mucin synthesis and secretion in relation to spontaneous differentiation of colon cancer cells in vitro. Int J Cancer. 1992;50:147–52.

37. Augeron C, Laboisse CL. Emergence of permanently differentiated cell clones in a human colonic cancer cell line in culture after treatment with sodium butyrate. Cancer Res. 1984;44:3961–9.

38. Velcich A, Palumbo L, Jarry A, Laboisse C, Racevskis J, Augenlicht L. Patterns of expression of lineage-specific markers during the in vitro-induced differentiation of HT29 colon carcinoma cells. Cell Growth Diff. 1995;6:749–57.

39. Park J-G, Oie HK, Sugarbaker PH et al. Characteristics of cell lines established from human colorectal carcinoma. Cancer Res. 1987;47:6710–18.

40. De Bruine AP, Dinjens WNM, v.d. Linden EPM, Pijls MMJ, Moerkerk PT, Bosman FT. Extracellular matrix components induce endocrine differentiation in vitro in NCl-H716 cells. Am J Pathol. 1993;142:773–82.

41. Kirkland SC. Endocrine differentiation by a human rectal adenocarcinoma cell line (HRA-19). Differentiation. 1986;33:148–55.

42. Pignatelli M, Bodmer WF. Integrin-receptor mediated differentiation and growth inhibition are enhanced by transforming growth factor-beta in colorectal tumour cells grown in collagen gel. Int J Cancer. 1989;44:518–23.

43. Celano P, Berchtold CM, Mabry M *et al*. Induction of markers of normal differentiation in human colon carcinoma cells by v-*ras*^{H} oncogene. Cell Growth Diff. 1993;4:341–7.

44. De Bruine AP, de Vries JE, Dinjens WNM *et al*. Human Caco-2 cells transfected with c-*Ha-Ras* as a model for endocrine differentiation in the large intestine. Differentiation. 1993;53:51–60.

45. D'Abaco G, Whitehead RH, Burgess AW. Synergy between *Apc* and an activated *ras* mutation is sufficient to induce colon carcinomas. Mol Cell Biol. 1996;16:884–91.

46. Quaroni A, Wands J, Trelstad RL, Isselbacher KJ. Epithelioid cell cultures from rat small intestine: Characterization by morphologic and immunologic criteria. J Cell Biol. 1979;80:248–65.

47. Blay J, Brown KD. Characterization of an epithelioid cell line derived from rat small intestine: Demonstration of cytokeratin filaments. Cell Biol Int Rep. 1984;8:551–60.

48. Negrel R, Rampal P, Nano J-L, Cavenal C, Ailhaud G. Establishment and characterization of an epithelial intestinal cell line from rat fetus. Exp Cell Res. 1983;143:427–37.

49. Yeh K-Y, Chopra DP. Epithelial cell cultures from the colon of the suckling rat. In Vitro. 1980; 16:876–86.

50. Siddiqui KM, Chopra DP. Primary and long term epithelial cell cultures from human fetal normal colonic mucosa. In Vitro. 1984;20:859–68.

51. Vidrich A, Ravindranath R, Farsi K, Targan S. A method for the rapid establishment of normal adult mammalian colonic epithelial cell cultures. In Vitro Cell Dev Biol. 1988;24:188–94.

52. Whitehead RH, VanEeden PE, Noble MD, Ataliotis P, Jat PS. The establishment of conditionally immortalized epithelial cell lines from both colon and small intestine of adult H-2K^b-tsA58 transgenic mice. Proc Natl Acad Sci USA. 1993;90:587–91.

53. Kedinger M, Simon-Assman PM, Lacroix B, Marxer A, Hauri HP, Haffen K. Fetal gut mesenchyme induces differentiation of cultured intestinal endodermal and crypt cells. Dev Biol. 1986;113: 474–83.

54. Carroll KM, Wong TT, Drabik DL, Chang EB. Differentiation of rat small intestinal epithelial cells by extracellular matrix. Am J Physiol. 1988;254:G355–60.

55. He Y, Chu S-HW, Walker A. Nucleotide supplements after proliferation and differentiation of cultured human (Caco-2) and rat (IEC-6) intestinal epithelial cells. J Nutr. 1993;123:1017–27.

56. Sanderson IR, Ezzell RM, Kedinger M *et al*. Human fetal enterocytes in vitro: Modulation of the phenotype by extracellular matrix. Proc Natl Acad Sci USA. 1996;93:7717–21.

57. Suh E, Traber PG. An intestine-specific homeobox gene regulates proliferation and differentiation. Mol Cell Biol. 1996;16:619–25.

58. James R, Kazenwadel J. Homeobox gene expression in the intestinal epithelium of adult mice. J Biol Chem. 1991;266:3246–51.

59. Suh E, Chen L, Taylor J, Traber PG. A homeodomain protein related to caudal regulates intestine-specific gene transcription. Mol Cell Biol. 1994;14:7340–51.

60. Jat PS, Noble MD, Ataliotis P *et al*. Direct derivation of conditionally immortal cell lines from an H-2K^b-tsA58 transgenic mouse. Proc Natl Acad Sci USA. 1991;88:5096–100.

61. Moser AR, Pitot HC, Dove WF. A dominant mutation that predisposes to multiple intestinal neoplasia in the mouse. Science. 1990;47:322–4.

62. Whitehead RH, Joseph JL. Derivation of conditionally immortalized cell lines containing the Min mutation from the normal colonic mucosa and other tissues of an 'Immortomouse'/Min hybrid. Epithelial Cell Biol. 1994;3:119–25.

63. Burgering BMT, Pronk GJ, Medema JP *et al*. Role of p21^{ras} in growth factor signal transduction. Biochem Soc Trans. 1993;21:888–94.

64. Marshall MS. Ras target proteins in eukaryotic cells. FASEB J. 1995;9:1311–18.

65. Dahlqvist A. Assay of intestinal disaccharidases. Anal Biochem. 1968;22:99–107.

66. Remacle-Bonnet M, Garrouste F, el-Atiq F, Roccabianca M, Marvaldi J, Pommier G. des-(1-3)-IGF-1, an insulin-like growth factor analog used to mimic a potential IGF-II autocrine loop, promotes the differentiation of human colon-carcinoma cells. Int J Cancer. 1992;52:910–17.

24
Growth, differentiation and apoptosis: mechanisms of control and deregulation during colorectal tumorigenesis

A. HAGUE, D. J. E. ELDER, A. J. BUTT and C. PARASKEVA

INTRODUCTION

In the human colonic crypt, tissue homeostasis is maintained by a precise balance between an increase in cell number due to mitosis at the base of the crypt and a decrease in cell number as a result of cell death at the luminal surface. As colonic epithelial cells migrate towards the upper half of the colonic crypt they cease proliferation and undergo differentiation. The two main differentiated cell types of the colon are the mucus-producing goblet cells and the absorptive columnar cells. Towards the top of the crypt, the majority of cells are of the columnar type. Although there is still some debate as to the precise mechanism of cell shedding at the luminal surface, there is increasing evidence that the differentiated cells die by programmed cell death (apoptosis), completing the final step in a terminal differentiation pathway[1,2]. Further evidence to support this has come from in vitro studies which have shown that the differentiation agent butyrate is able to induce apoptosis in colorectal tumour cell lines[3,4] and that the apoptotic cells exhibit high levels of alkaline phosphatase activity, a marker of colonic columnar cell differentiation[4].

Genetic factors in the control of apoptosis

Despite its clear importance, relatively little is known about the relationship between growth control, differentiation and apoptosis in the colon or the factors which regulate these processes. The regulation of cell survival and apoptosis involves members of the Bcl-2 family of proteins. The differential distribution of Bcl-2 and homologous proteins (Bcl-x, Bax, Bak, Mcl-1) within the colonic crypt is further evidence that apoptosis is important in controlling cell numbers in the colon[5–11].

There are a number of possible different pathways to apoptosis in response to different cell death signals. For example, programmed cell death, which is thought to regulate cell shedding at the luminal surface[2], may be activated by a different mechanism to the rapid p53-dependent apoptosis which occurs in response to cell damage deeper within the colonic crypt, within the proliferation zone[12,13]. The death of cells at the luminal surface must be independent of p53, since p53-null mice have a histologically normal colon[14]. In genetically altered premalignant or malignant cells further apoptosis pathways have been identified. For example, cells with a deregulated c-*myc* gene, in which a growth arrest signal provides conflicting information for the cells, undergo apoptosis, eliminating potential precancerous cells[15]. This response of cells with a deregulated c-*myc* gene in growth restrictive conditions explains the oncogene co-operation between c-*myc*, which drives both proliferation and apoptosis, and *Bcl-2*, which protects against cell death.

Defects in the *fas*-mediated cell death pathway protect tumour cells from cyto-toxic T cell-mediated cell killing. For example, it has recently been shown that most colon carcinomas overexpress FAP-1, a negative regulator of the fas/APO1/CD95 death receptor (Kataoka S, personal communication). Thus, tumour cells may evade cell death signals by defects in different pathways to apoptosis. Many of the early genetic changes which occur during colon carcinogenesis may result in a breakdown of the normal regulation of cell numbers, such that the extent of apoptosis is no longer sufficient to balance the levels of proliferation and cell death in the epithelium. Relevant to this report, Bcl-2, an oncoprotein which promotes cell survival, may reduce the incidence of cell death during adenoma formation by inappropriate or high level expression[6].

Transforming growth factor-β and the control of cell number within the colonic epithelium

Transforming growth factor-$\beta 1$ (TGF-$\beta 1$) is endogenous to the colon. Immuno-staining for TGF-$\beta 1$ protein in the normal colonic mucosa has shown it to be differentially expressed within the crypt, with enhanced immunoreactivity in the non-proliferating, more differentiated cells in the upper parts of the crypt and an absence of expression in the lower proliferating cell compartment[16]. This autocrine growth inhibitor has been demonstrated to negatively regulate intestinal epithelial cell growth in vitro[17-21]. These observations suggest a role for TGF-$\beta 1$ in the regulation of colonic epithelial cell growth and/or differentiation. A breakdown in the regulation of this fine balance, for example through loss of responsiveness to growth regulatory signals, is thought to be an important step toward the deregulated growth which is characteristic of colonic neoplasia[22]. Carcinoma cells are frequently resistant to the growth inhibitory effects of TGF-$\beta 1$[19] and some carcinomas may actually acquire a growth-stimulatory response to TGF-$\beta 1$[23,24].

Dietary factors modulating proliferation, differentiation and apoptosis

In addition to endogenous growth regulators, evidence is accumulating to suggest that dietary factors may also play an important role in growth control in the colonic epithelium. Epidemiological studies have suggested that a diet low in fat and high in fibre could be protective against colorectal cancer[25,26]. In addition, Sandler et al.[27] have demonstrated that diets high in fat and low in fibre, typical of those found in industrialized countries, increase the risk of development of colon cancer. In the colonic lumen, dietary fibre is fermented by symbiotic bacteria producing the short-chain fatty acids butyrate, propionate and acetate, as major by-products in millimolar amounts[28]. A putative role for sodium butyrate in the negative regulation of growth in the colon has been suggested by several studies that have demonstrated its antiproliferative effects on colon carcinoma cells in vitro[29–31], and its ability to induce apoptosis in colonic tumour cells[3]. There is evidence that butyrate induces apoptosis via the induction of differentiation[4,32]. Therefore, the concentration of butyrate within the colonic lumen may affect the extent of apoptosis within the colonic epithelium.

Survival signals for colonic epithelial cells

Further factors may regulate apoptosis within the colonic epithelium. It has been proposed that cells will undergo apoptosis unless continually signalled not to do so[33]. Such survival signals may be in the form of cell–cell contact, cytokines or extracellular matrix components. The reduced availability of survival factors may initiate the death program in colonic epithelial cells. The development of autonomous growth factor signalling pathways is a well established mechanism by which tumour cells become able to grow in unusual cellular environments. It is becoming clear that, in many cases, such pathways also permit cell survival. Tumour cells may also become capable of survival in the absence of cell–cell contacts, a situation in which the normal epithelial cell would initiate the death program.

Therapeutic goals

There are, therefore, a number of different routes by which apoptosis is regulated in the colonic epithelium, and tumour cells may have defects in the molecular pathways which transduce apoptosis signals. It is therefore important to determine apoptosis signals to which colorectal carcinoma cells are still sensitive. Our recent studies have indicated that colon carcinoma cells are more sensitive to the induction of apoptosis by salicylate than are premalignant adenoma cells[34]. These results suggest that with appropriate understanding of the molecular basis for this differential sensitivity salicylate-like drugs could be used in the treatment of colorectal cancer, as well as in its prevention.

In this chapter we review our recent work demonstrating the different modes of action of butyrate and TGF-β1, providing evidence for differentiation-dependent and -independent pathways to apoptosis in colonic epithelial cells. We address the molecular mechanisms by which these agents are able to induce apoptosis. We also review our work showing that adenoma cells retain dependence on several factors for their survival, including cell–cell contact and cytokines such as the insulin-like growth factors. Finally, we review recent work showing that the aspirin metabolite salicylate induces apoptosis in colorectal tumour cell lines and discuss this in the context of the mechanisms by which non-steroidal anti-inflammatory drugs (NSAIDs) appear to be chemopreventive. Research in this area, as well as being important for the development of new strategies to prevent and treat colorectal cancer, has given new insights into the molecular mechanisms controlling epithelial growth, differentiation and apoptosis.

APOPTOSIS INDUCED BY DIFFERENTIATION-DEPENDENT AND -INDEPENDENT PATHWAYS: DIFFERENT MECHANISMS FOR INDUCTION BY SODIUM BUTYRATE AND TGF-β1

Both sodium butyrate and TGF-β1 have growth inhibitory effects on colonic adenoma-derived cell lines[19,22]. However, in two adenoma cell lines (S/RG/C2 and PC/AA/C1), butyrate treatment induced apoptosis whereas TGF-β1 did not, suggesting that these factors may act through different growth-inhibitory pathways[3]. The ability of butyrate to induce apoptosis in colorectal tumour cell lines has been hypothesized to be one of the reasons why dietary fibre could be protective against large bowel cancer[3]. Recently, we have found that TGF-β1 can induce apoptosis in two other adenoma-derived cell lines, PC/BH/C1 and S/RR/C1 (A. Hague and C. Paraskeva, unpublished results). This is consistent with a recent report by Wang et al.[35], showing that TGF-β1 can induce apoptosis in the human colon adenoma cell line VACO-330. TGF-β1 is, therefore, growth inhibitory to colonic epithelial cells and, in addition, TGF-β1 induces apoptosis in some colorectal tumour cell lines, but not in others. Whether a colonic epithelial cell line undergoes apoptosis in response to TGF-β1 may depend on the genetic background of the cell line or on the degree of sensitivity to TGF-β1-induced growth inhibition[35]. It should be noted that apoptosis in response to TGF-β1 is not an immediate response. Although growth inhibition was apparent at 48 h of treatment, apoptosis was not detected until 72 h (A. Hague and C. Paraskeva, manuscript in preparation).

Having shown that TGF-β1 can induce apoptosis in the adenoma cell lines PC/BH/C1 and S/RR/C1, the next question we addressed was whether this is via a terminal differentiation pathway (as is apparent for butyrate[4,32]) or by a differentiation-independent pathway, for example due to conflicting growth signals[15]. Adenoma cells that are growth inhibited by TGF-β1 without the induction of apoptosis (AA/C1 and S/RG/C2), and adenoma cells that are sensitive to TGF-β1-induced apoptosis (PC/BH/C1 and S/RR/C1) were treated with a range of TGF-β1 concentrations known to cause growth inhibition/apoptosis to determine whether this led to an increase in the differentiation markers alkaline phosphatase (ALP) activity and E-cadherin expression. There was no increase in expression of ALP or E-cadherin whether TGF-β1 induced apoptosis or not, suggesting that TGF-β1 can induce a growth arrest in response to colonic epithelial cells without the induction of differentiation and that additional signals from other growth and/or dietary factors (e.g. sodium butyrate) may be required for cells to become further differentiated. The failure of TGF-β1 to induce differentiation in the cell lines sensitive to TGF-β1-induced apoptosis suggests that the cells are undergoing apoptosis independent of differentiation. Our in vitro data therefore indicate that both differentiation-dependent and differentiation-independent pathways

294

to apoptosis may be induced in colonic epithelial cells. Sodium butyrate induces apoptosis as the end point of a differentiation pathway, whereas TGF-β1 induces apoptosis via a differentiation-independent pathway.

The presence of TGF-β1 protein expression in the non-proliferating region of the human colonic crypt[16] may suggest a role for this growth factor in mediating a stable growth arrest which is a prerequisite for differentiation. Differentiating agents such as hexamethylene bisacetamide (HMBA), retinoic acid and sodium butyrate can also induce TGF-β1 expression[31,36,37], suggesting a role for TGF-β1 in the maintenance of a differentiated phenotype. The function of TGF-β1 in the human colonic crypt may be in the maintenance of a non-proliferative state, to allow subsequent induction and stabilization of a differentiated phenotype by additional growth and/or dietary factors and through interactions with extracellular matrix (ECM). TGF-β1 may induce an apoptotic response in PC/BH/C1 and S/RR/C1 cells by eliciting conflicting growth signals in these cells, for example by an inability to down-regulate Myc expression, as has been suggested by studies in fibroblast[15], myeloid[38] and T cells[39]. Indeed, following treatment of the cells with TGF-β1, Myc protein expression declined slowly (apparent at 48 h) in PC/BH/C1 cells, but rapidly (apparent at 4 h) in PC/AA/C1 and S/RG/C2 cells – which do not apoptose in response to TGF-β1. There is, therefore, deregulation of Myc in the PC/BH/C1 cells. The apoptotic response to TGF-β1 observed in PC/BH/C1 and S/RR/C1 appears to be along a pathway that is distinct from a terminal differentiation pathway and may be due to conflicting growth signals.

The alternative hypothesis is that apoptosis is a normal response to TGF-β1. In this case, it could be argued that the delayed apoptosis which occurs in response to TGF-β1 would give the normal colonic epithelial cells time to reach the top of the crypt before undergoing apoptosis. Previous studies have reported that a reduced response or loss of response to the growth inhibitory effects of TGF-β1 may be an important event during colorectal carcinogenesis[19]. Recently, it has also been suggested that an escape from TGF-β1-induced apoptosis may be important in colorectal cancer development[35]. The failure of RG/C2 and AA/C1 cells to undergo apoptosis in response to TGF-β1 may reflect one stage in the development of TGF-β1 resistance. Thus, resistance to TGF-β1-induced apoptosis and resistance to TGF-β1-induced growth inhibition may be involved in tumour progression.

There is a further possibility that TGF-β1 could have a dual role in maintaining normal cell numbers in the normal colon, first, as a growth inhibitor mediating a stable growth arrest (G_1/G_0) which is a prerequisite for differentiation, and second, to eliminate any defective cells which may have acquired gene mutations leading to conflicting signals in a part of the normal colon, which expresses high levels of TGF-β1. Thus, it is plausible that, in normal cells, TGF-β1 results in a stable G_1 arrest without apoptosis, but should the cells acquire specific mutations or DNA damage this could lead to a TGF-β1-dependent apoptotic signal to remove damaged cells and reduce the risk of cancer development.

We have previously shown that γ-irradiation can induce apoptosis in colorectal tumour cells in vitro in a p53-independent pathway, although the induction of apoptosis is delayed[40]. We examined whether this p53-independent apoptotic response was delayed due to the treated cells differentiating prior to death; i.e. is p53-independent death induced by γ-irradiation a differentiation-dependent pathway to cell death? Although treatment with γ-irradiation induced significant apoptosis in adenoma and carcinoma cells, this did not result in an increase in either alkaline phosphatase activity or E-cadherin expression (A.J. Butt, A. Hague and C. Paraskeva, manuscript in preparation). We conclude that there are at least two pathways to apoptosis, a butyrate-mediated differentiation-dependent pathway, which may mimic apoptosis observed at the luminal surface in vivo, and a differentiation-independent pathway following TGF-β1-treatment or DNA damage.

Bcl-2 FAMILY MEMBERS AND APOPTOSIS

There has been considerable recent interest in the possible role of the Bcl-2 family proteins in cancer development. *Bcl-2* is a proto-oncogene which is activated by overexpression and protects cells from apoptosis induced by a wide variety of agents. The anti-apoptotic activity of Bcl-2 is antagonized by the homologous Bax protein, which is able to form heterodimers with Bcl-2[41]. It has been proposed that the ratio of Bax to Bcl-2 within the cell determines whether the cell undergoes apoptosis[41]. Their differential distributions within the colonic crypt suggest that these proteins are important in the control of cell survival and apoptosis in the colonic epithelium. Bcl-2 is expressed in the lower half of the crypt in the proliferation zone[5,6], whereas Bax has an opposing distribution, being expressed in the upper half of the crypt where cells have ceased proliferation[7]. Bcl-2 is expressed at high levels in many colonic adenoma and carcinoma cells[6,42–45] although there is evidence that the Bcl-2-positive carcinomas are less common than Bcl-2-positive adenomas[11,43,45]. A further Bcl-2 homologue which serves as a death promoter is Bak[46–48]. Bak expression has been reported in normal colonic epithelium[46,48] where there is a gradient of expression, with the strongest immunoreactivity in the cells at the top of the crypt[11]. Bak is expressed in the colonic adenocarcinoma cell line SW480[46]. However, colorectal tumours, both malignant and premalignant, have reduced Bak levels when compared with normal colonic epithelial cells[10].

Butyrate induces apoptosis in association with reduced levels of Bcl-2 or increased levels of Bak

Since butyrate, a natural component of the contents of the large bowel, is able to induce apoptosis in colonic tumour cells, we questioned whether members of the Bcl-2 family of proteins were involved in butyrate-induced apoptosis and, by investigating this, aimed to identify some of the components of the differentiation-dependent pathway to apoptosis. In spite of the potential importance of diet-gene interactions in the colonic epithelium, little research has been conducted in this area. One recent study has shown that butyrate treatment elevates levels of Bak protein in the HT29 colonic carcinoma cell line in conjunction with apoptosis[49]. However, these results were from only one cell line. Therefore, to gain further insight into the mechanisms by which butyrate induces apoptosis in colorectal tumour cells, we examined whether Bcl-2, Bax and Bak play a role in the induction of apoptosis by sodium butyrate in four cell lines: one carcinoma cell line (S/KS/FI) and three premalignant adenoma cell lines (PC/AA/C1,

S/RG/C2 and PC/BH/C1) (A. Hague and C. Paraskeva, manuscript in preparation). S/RG/C2 and PC/BH/C1 express Bcl-2 and in these two cell lines, butyrate treatment decreased Bcl-2 levels in association with apoptosis, whereas Bax and Bak levels remained constant. PC/AA/C1 and S/KS/FI contain no detectable Bcl-2 (examined using the monoclonal antibody Bcl-2/124[50]). In S/KS/FI, Bax or Bak levels did not change in response to butyrate. However, in AA/C1, butyrate-induced apoptosis was associated with increased Bak levels. Furthermore, butyrate also induced apoptosis and increased Bak levels in PC/AA/C1 cells transfected with a bcl-2 expression vector which expressed high levels of Bcl-2 protein under the control of an SV40 promoter (A. Hague and C. Paraskeva, manuscript in preparation). Therefore, in PC/AA/C1, butyrate-induced apoptosis appears to be mediated through Bak and the expression of Bcl-2 at high levels is unable to counter the effects of Bak. Different mechanisms appear to be involved in cell death signalling in different tumours since butyrate may induce apoptosis via elevated levels of Bak or reduced levels of Bcl-2. Understanding the cell death signalling pathways of an individual tumour may assist in the selection of relevant therapeutic strategies for some tumours. Butyrate may modulate the expression of Bcl-2 family members in colonic epithelial cells and therefore the diet may influence the balance between proliferation and apoptosis, suggesting a potential mechanism for the link between dietary fibre and reduced colorectal cancer risk.

Reduced Bcl-2 expression precedes TGF-β-induced apoptosis

Since TGF-β1 induces apoptosis in the adenoma cell lines PC/BH/C1 and S/RR/C1, we investigated whether TGF-β1 is able to reduce Bcl-2 levels in these colorectal adenoma cells. Both cell lines showed a decrease in Bcl-2 expression in response to TGF-β1. S/RR/C1 has low levels of Bcl-2 in control cultures[6], and in cells treated with TGF-β1 for 4 days the levels of Bcl-2 were undetectable by Western blotting (A. Hague and C. Paraskeva, unpublished observations). High levels of Bcl-2 were seen in the control cultures of PC/BH/C1, with reduced levels in the TGF-β1-treated cells. The level of Bcl-2 was reduced after 48 h of treatment: significant apoptosis was not detected at 48 h, but was detected after 72 h of treatment. The reduction in Bcl-2 levels prior to the appearance of apoptosis suggests that this change is part of the pathway by which TGF-β1 induces apoptosis and this is consistent with the reduction in levels of Bcl-2 in association with TGF-β1 apoptosis in myeloid leukaemia cells[51]. Therefore, although sodium butyrate induces apoptosis via differentiation and TGF-β1 induces apoptosis independent of differentiation in colonic adenoma cells, both of these agents reduce levels of Bcl-2 protein. These two agents must therefore share part of the biochemical pathways involved in the induction of apoptosis. Since TGF-β1 is present in the mature, differentiated cells at the top of the colonic crypt and absent from the proliferative compartment, whereas Bcl-2 is chiefly expressed at the base of the crypt in the proliferative compartment, it is possible that in vivo, TGF-β1 serves to down-regulate Bcl-2 expression, in addition to its other functions. However, TGF-β1 fails to down-regulate Bcl-2 in the adenoma cell line S/RG/C2, in which TGF-β1 induces growth inhibition, but not apoptosis. There is a clear requirement for further investigation into the role of TGF-β1 in the colonic epithelium and, in particular, into the question as to whether TGF-β1 induces differentiation and/or apoptosis in normal colonic epithelial cells.

CELL–CELL CONTACT AND SPECIFIC CYTOKINES, SUCH AS THE INSULIN-LIKE GROWTH FACTORS, INHIBIT APOPTOSIS OF COLONIC EPITHELIAL CELLS

It has been proposed that most mammalian cells are programmed to undergo apoptosis unless they are continuously signalled by other cells not to do so[33]. Cell death by apoptosis is thus considered a default pathway and withdrawal of specific factors that physiologically support the survival of the cell type can induce apoptosis. In addition, various cytokines may regulate cell survival and the survival factors required are specific to the tissue type.

Epithelial cells from normal adult human colon are notoriously difficult to culture. Buset et al.[52] have reported the short-term culture (2–4 days) of normal colonic epithelial cells. We have had similar experience with such primary cultures[53]. However, in our recent cultures large clumps of normal epithelial cells survived for many weeks. There are also few reports of successful establishment of premalignant colorectal adenoma cell lines. Nevertheless, the serial passage of adenoma-derived cells is possible if cell–cell contacts are maintained[54–56]. Adenoma cells can routinely be passaged using dispase, an enzyme which disrupts cell–substrate adhesion and retains cell–cell contacts, thus removing cells as clumps rather than single cells. We have previously shown that an important marker of tumour progression in colorectal carcinogenesis is the ability of cells to grow after single cell trypsinization (clonogenicity)[57,58]. Hence, normal colonocytes and early adenomas cannot be passaged using trypsin, whereas carcinomas and some later stage adenomas can be[57,58]. Bates et al.[59] showed that colonic epithelial cells undergo apoptosis in response to inhibition of intercellular contact by anti-integrin antibodies and we have recently shown that our non-clonogenic adenoma cell lines die by apoptosis if subjected to trypsinization[60]. This also occurs in adenomas derived from patients with familial adenomatous polyposis: *APC* mutations do not, therefore, confer resistance to cell death in response to loss of cell–cell contacts. In contrast, if cell–cell contacts are maintained non-clonogenic adenoma cells are capable of survival in suspension[60]. The ability to survive loss of cell–cell contacts and/or growth factor deprivation is a marker of tumour progression.

In addition to survival mediated by cell–cell contact, serum added to the medium to enable proliferation of the cells also provides factors for survival. Withdrawal of serum and growth factors from the medium is associated with an increase in the extent of apoptosis in some colorectal tumour cell cultures. This system was used to establish whether specific cytokines were able to act as survival factors for colonic epithelial cells, rescuing the cells from apoptosis induced by serum withdrawal[60]. After removal of serum and growth factors c-*myc* is down-regulated within 2 h. Therefore the induction of apoptosis is not an inappropriate response of the cells due to a deregulated *myc* gene. The apoptotic response is also p53-independent. Such cultures have been used to determine specific survival factors for colonic epithelial cells. Insulin, the insulin-like growth factors I and II, hydrocortisone and epidermal growth factor (EGF) each protect cells from the induction of apoptosis in the absence of serum over a short term period of 24 h[60]. This approach may give insight into the factors governing growth and survival of colonic epithelial cells *in vivo*.

THE EFFECT OF THE NON-STEROIDAL ANTI-INFLAMMATORY DRUGS ON THE GROWTH, DIFFERENTIATION AND APOPTOSIS OF COLORECTAL TUMOUR CELLS

Cyclooxygenase-2

A molecule that has recently been implicated in the regulation of apoptosis in intestinal epithelial cells is cyclooxygenase-2 (COX-2). This, the inducible isoform of cyclooxygenase, a key enzyme in the biosynthesis of prostaglandins, is induced by a variety of stimuli such as cytokines and growth factors and is an example of an immediate early gene product[61]. Nevertheless, stable transfection of COX-2 into rat intestinal epithelial (RIE) cells does not result in an increase in mito-genesis[62]. It does, however, decrease E-cadherin protein expression, elevate Bcl-2 protein expression and make the cells resistant to butyrate-induced apoptosis[62]. These acquired phenotypic characteristics are consistent with studies indicating that COX-2 is over-expressed in colorectal cancer. In normal colorectal mucosa COX-2 protein is either not detectable or detectable only at very low levels[63-65]. Of the colorectal tumour tissues analysed to date, COX-2 has been detected in 33% of adenomas and 85% of carcinomas[63-65]. The dramatic increase in COX-2 expression in carcinoma tissues appears to be localized largely to the tumour cells[65]. Over-expression of COX-2 may, in part, be responsible for deregulating the balance of cell proliferation and death in the colorectal epithelium and for the resistance of colorectal tumours to therapeutic agents which act by the induction of apoptosis.

NSAIDs are chemopreventive toward colorectal cancer

The importance of the role of COX-2 in colorectal carcinogenesis is perhaps indicated best (albeit indirectly) by the effect of the non-steroidal anti-inflam-matory drugs (NSAIDs) on this process. Currently used NSAIDs such as aspirin and sulindac, which inhibit the activity of COX-2 and that of the constitutively expressed COX isoform, COX-1, are effective chemopreventive agents for colorectal cancer[66]. This is indicated by a considerable body of evidence from epidemiological, clinical and animal studies. In epidemiological studies, the regular intake of aspirin has been shown to reduce the risk of developing colorectal adenomas or cancer by 40–50%[67]. The clinical trials are broadly supportive of the epidemiological studies in that they indicate the NSAID sulindac to cause the regression of colorectal adenomas in patients with FAP, a hereditary form of colorectal cancer[68].

NSAIDs induce apoptosis in colorectal tumour cells

Recent research, in addition to that on COX-2, has indicated possible mechanisms for the observed anti-neoplastic effects of NSAIDs. Our recent studies examined the effect of the aspirin metabolite salicylate on the growth of human colorectal tumour cell lines at varying stages of tumour progression[34]. Salicylate showed dose-dependent inhibitory effects on all of the cells lines (IC_{50} 1.65 ± 0.36 to 7.38 ± 1.08 mM, 4 day treatment), yet carcinoma and in vitro-transformed adenoma cell lines are more sensitive than adenoma cell lines. Salicylate caused all cell lines to accumulate in $G_0 - G_1$ and induced apoptosis in carcinoma and in vitro-transformed adenoma cell lines, but not in all adenoma cell lines. In those adenoma cell lines that did show significant levels of salicylate-induced apoptosis, the extent was considerably less than in the more transformed cell lines. The cell lines that were more sensitive to the growth inhibitory properties of salicylate did not necessarily exhibit an increased cell cycle arrest when compared with less sensitive cell lines. This suggests that the level of induction of apoptosis by salicylate was the major factor accounting for the differential sensitivities. Determining the molecular mechanism(s) underlying this differential will be important in understanding the biology of apoptosis and in the design of chemoprevention strategies. A candidate protein for the regulation of salicylate-induced apoptosis is the *p53* gene product. However, salicylate induced apoptosis by a *p53*-independent mechanism[34]. Is COX-2 potentially involved in determining sensitivity to salicylate-induced apoptosis? To test this we examined the expression of COX-2 protein in the tumour cell lines by Western blotting. COX-2 protein was readily detectable in two of three carcinoma cell lines yet was not detected in any of the four adenoma cell lines studied. Despite the in vitro-transformed and carcinoma cell lines being similarly sensitive to salicylate, the former failed to express detectable levels of COX-2 protein (D.J.E. Elder and C. Paraskeva, unpublished results). These data suggest that COX-2 expression alone does not determine the sensitivity of colorectal tumour cells to the aspirin metabolite salicylate. This is, perhaps, not surprising considering that salicylate potentially affects other cellular processes that are relevant to tumorigenesis, in addition to inhibiting COX activity. The inhibition of the activation of the transcription factor NFκB and the uncoupling of mitochondrial oxidative phosphorylation are two such examples[69,70]. There is also evidence to indicate that the chemopreventive effects of NSAIDs can be independent of the inhibition of COX activity[71]. Studies using a new class of NSAIDs[72] that are highly selective for COX-2 and do not uncouple oxidative phosphorylation will be invaluable in determining the extent of the role of COX-2 in regulating growth and apoptosis in colorectal tumour cells.

Our research indicates that the induction of apoptosis is a major anti-proliferative effect of the NSAIDs. This is consistent with other studies in which various NSAIDs have been shown to induce apoptosis in colorectal carcinoma cell lines[73,74], the rectal epithelium of FAP patients[75] and in small intestinal enterocytes of *Apc*[Min] mice[76]. There is also considerable in vitro evidence to indicate that NSAIDs cause colorectal tumour cells to arrest in the $G_0 - G_1$ phase of the cell cycle[34,74]. Both of these cellular responses are considered to be potentially chemopreventive, and almost certainly contribute to the observed chemopreventive effect of NSAIDs toward colorectal cancer. A further possible mechanism of chemoprevention is the induction of differentiation[77]. Using an increase in alkaline phosphatase (ALP) activity as an indicator of increased cell differentiation, Piazza et al.[73] showed that sulindac sulphide and sulindac sulphone do not cause differentiation of the colon carcinoma cell line HT29. However, Tsujii and DuBois demonstrated that the expression of COX-2 in rat intestinal epithelial cells decreased ALP activity, and sulindac sulphide, which inhibits COX-2 activity, reversed this effect[62]. Whether the HT29 cell line used in the study of Piazza et al.[73] expressed COX-2 protein is not stated. If it did not, then the ability of NSAIDs to increase colorectal cell differentiation may depend upon the expression of COX-2. Again, the effects of COX-2 selective inhibitors will be informative in this respect.

The current evidence suggests that NSAIDs may be effective in preventing colorectal cancer by restoring the balanced regulation of cell growth, differentiation and death. This is probably mediated, at least partly, through the inhibition of COX-2 activity, but other, as yet obscure, mechanisms cannot be ruled out. Elucidating the means by which NSAIDs exert their chemopreventive action has already contributed to the understanding of colorectal tumour cell biology and will continue to do so. Along with this understanding, the considerable potential of NSAIDs as chemopreventive agents for colorectal cancer is becoming increasingly apparent. Nonetheless, fundamental questions remain. Do COX-2 selective NSAIDs have the same anti-neoplastic effects in vitro and in vivo as currently available NSAIDs such as aspirin? If so, they are potentially ideal chemopreventives as they are considerably less toxic than current NSAIDs[72]. Might NSAIDs be effective as therapeutic agents for colorectal cancer, either alone or in combination with currently used therapeutics? Their ability to induce apoptosis, cause polyp regression and the apparent increased sensitivity to salicylate of cells at later stages of neoplastic progression, suggests that this may be so. Colorectal cancer remains one of the most common malignancies in the westernized world and current treatment strategies have little effect on survival. Consequently, novel strategies, such as the use of NSAIDs, for treatment and prevention are urgently required.

CONCLUDING REMARKS

Apoptosis may be induced in colonic epithelial cells by diverse signals. In the development of colon cancer, cells must develop resistance to death when encountering signals such as loss of cell–cell contacts, reduced survival factor availability and the presence of factors such as TGF-β1, which may induce apoptosis, if not in normal colonic epithelial cells, in cells with deregulated cell proliferation. As well as internal controls of proliferation, differentiation and cell death, the environment plays an important role in the regulation of tissue homeostasis. Butyrate, a luminal factor derived from bacterial fermentation of dietary fibre, can modulate apoptosis in colonic epithelial cells, a process involving decreased levels of Bcl-2 or increased levels of Bak. Some colonic carcinoma cells are resistant to butyrate-induced apoptosis (for example, the carcinoma cell line S/KS/FI). However, carcinoma cells are more sensitive to apoptosis induced by the aspirin metabolite salicylate than the premalignant adenoma cells. Furthermore, it is interesting that the S/KS/FI carcinoma cell line, which was relatively resistant to butyrate-induced apoptosis, is extremely sensitive to apoptosis induced by salicylate. Such observations offer promise of clinical therapies for colorectal cancer.

The kinetics of growth, differentiation and apoptosis in the colonic epithelium is tightly controlled to maintain the fine balance between cell proliferation, stable growth arrest and death that is required for the normal maintenance of a rapidly proliferating tissue. Colorectal tumorigenesis results from the progressive breakdown of this control. Determination of the factors that mediate this breakdown, has led to an increased understanding of tumorigenesis and, by extension, of the normal physiological mechanisms controlling the turnover of the colorectal epithelium.

References

1. Gavrieli Y, Sherman Y, Ben-Sasson SA. Identification of programmed cell death in situ via specific labelling of nuclear DNA fragmentation. J Cell Biol. 1992;119:493–501.
2. Hall PA, Coates PJ, Ansari B, Hopwood D. Regulation of cell number in the mammalian gastrointestinal tract: importance of apoptosis. J Cell Sci. 1994;107:3569–77.
3. Hague A, Manning AM, Hanlon KA, Huschtscha LI, Hart D, Paraskeva C. Sodium butyrate induces apoptosis in human colonic tumour cell lines in a p53-independent pathway: implications for the possible role of dietary fibre in the prevention of large bowel cancer. Int J Cancer. 1993;55:498–505.
4. Heerdt BG, Houston MA, Augenlicht LH. Potentiation by short chain fatty acids of differentiation and apoptosis in human colonic carcinoma cell lines. Cancer Res. 1994;54:3288–94.
5. Hockenbery DM, Zutter M, Hickey W, Nahm M, Korsmeyer SJ. Bcl-2 protein is topographically restricted in tissues characterized by apoptotic cell death. Proc Natl Acad Sci USA. 1991;88:6961–5.
6. Hague A, Moorghen M, Hicks D, Chapman M, Paraskeva C. Bcl-2 expression in human colorectal adenomas and carcinomas. Oncogene. 1994;9:3367–70.
7. Krajewski S, Krajewska M, Shabaik A, Miyashita T. Immunohistochemical determination of in vivo distribution of Bax, a dominant inhibitor of Bcl-2. Am J Pathol. 1994;145:1323–36.
8. Krajewski S, Krajewska M, Shabaik A et al. Immunohistochemical analysis of in vivo patterns of Bcl-X expression. Cancer Res. 1994;54:5501–7.
9. Krajewski S, Bodrug S, Krajewska M et al. Immunohistochemical analysis of mcl-1 protein in human tissues – differential regulation of mcl-1 and bcl-2 protein-production suggests a unique role for mcl-1 in control of programmed cell-death in vivo. Am J Pathol. 1995;146:1309–19.
10. Krajewska M, Moss SF, Krajewski S, Song K, Holt PR, Reed JC. Elevated expression of bcl-x and reduced bak in primary colorectal adenocarcinomas. Cancer Res. 1996;56:2422–7.
11. Krajewski S, Krajewska M, Reed JC. Immunohistochemical analysis of in vivo patterns of Bak expression, a proapoptotic member of the Bcl-2 family. Cancer Res. 1996;56:2849–55.
12. Clarke AR, Gledhill S, Hooper ML, Bird CC, Wyllie AH. p53 dependence of early apoptotic and proliferative responses within the mouse intestinal epithelium following gamma-irradiation. Oncogene. 1994;9:1767–73.
13. Merritt AJ, Potten CS, Kemp CJ et al. The role of p53 in spontaneous and radiation-induced apoptosis in the gastrointestinal tract of normal and p53-deficient mice. Cancer Res. 1994;54:614–17.
14. Donehower LA, Harvey M, Slagle BL et al. Mice deficient for p53 are developmentally normal but susceptible to spontaneous tumours. Nature. 1992;356:215–21.
15. Evan GI, Wyllie AH, Gilbert CS et al. Induction of apoptosis in fibroblasts by c-myc protein. Cell. 1992;69:119–28.
16. Avery A, Paraskeva C, Hall P, Flanders KC, Sporn M, Moorghen M. TGF-β expression in the human colon – differential immunostaining along crypt epithelium. Br J Cancer. 1993;68:137–9.

17. Barnard JA, Beauchamp RD, Coffey RJ, Moses HL. Regulation of intestinal epithelial cell growth by transforming growth factor β. Proc Natl Acad Sci USA. 1989;86:1578–82.
18. Hoosein HM, McKnight MK, Levine AE *et al*. Differential sensitivity of subclasses of human colon carcinoma cell lines to the growth inhibitory effects of transforming growth factor-β. Exp Cell Res. 1989;181:442–53.
19. Manning AM, Williams AC, Game SM, Paraskeva C. Differential sensitivity of human colonic adenoma and carcinoma cells to transforming growth factor β (TGF β): conversion of an adenoma cell line to a tumorigenic phenotype is accompanied by a reduced response to the inhibitory effects of TGF β. Oncogene. 1991;6:1471–6.
20. Geiser AG, Burmester JK, Werbink R, Roberts AB, Sporn MB. Inhibition of growth by transforming growth factor-β following fusion of two nonresponsive human carcinoma cell lines – implication of the type-II receptor in growth inhibitory responses. J Biol Chem. 1992;267:2588–93.
21. Wu SP, Theodorescu D, Kerbel RS *et al*. TGF-β1 is an autocrine-negative growth regulator of human colon carcinoma FET cells in vivo as revealed by transfection of an antisense expression vector. J Cell Biol. 1992;116:187–96.
22. Manning AM, Hague A, Paraskeva C. Role of transforming growth factor-β and the dietary factor sodium butyrate in the control of proliferation and apoptosis in colorectal carcinogenesis. In: Marks PA, Türler H, Weil R, eds. Pre-cancerous Lesions: A Multidisciplinary Approach. Ares–Serono symposia;1993;1:150.
23. Hsu S, Huang F, Hafez M, Winawer S, Friedman E. Colon carcinoma cells switch their response to transforming growth factor β1 with tumor progression. Cell Growth Diff. 1994;5:267–75.
24. Hague A, Manning AM, Van der Stappen JWJ, Paraskeva C. Escape from the negative regulation of growth by transforming growth factor β and from the induction of apoptosis by the dietary agent sodium butyrate may be important in colorectal carcinogenesis. Cancer Metastasis Rev. 1993; 12:227–37.
25. Burkitt DP. Epidemiology of cancer of the colon and rectum. Cancer. 1971;28:3–13.
26. Howe GR, Benito E, Castelleto R *et al*. Dietary intake of fiber and decreased risk of cancers of the colon and rectum – evidence from the combined analysis of 13 case–control studies. J Natl Cancer Inst. 1992;84:1887–96.
27. Sandler RS, Lyles CM, Peipins LA, McAuliffe CA, Woosley JT, Kupper LL. Diet and risk of colorectal adenomas: macronutrients, cholesterol, and fiber. J Natl Cancer Inst. 1993;85:884–91.
28. Cummings JH. Short chain fatty acids in the human colon. Gut. 1981;22:763–79.
29. Kim YS, Tsao D, Morita A, Bella A. Effect of sodium butyrate on three human colorectal adenocarcinoma cell lines in culture. In: Malt RA, editor, Colonic carcinogenesis. Lancaster: MTP Press Ltd, 1982:317–25.
30. Whitehead RH, Young GB, Bhathal PS. Effects of short chain fatty acids on a new human colon carcinoma cell line (LIM 1215). Gut. 1986;27:1457–63.
31. Barnard JA, Warwick G. Butyrate rapidly induces growth inhibition and differentiation in HT-29 cells. Cell Growth Diff. 1993;4:495–501.
32. Butt A. The role of sodium butyrate and transforming growth factor β1 in growth control in colorectal carcinogenesis. PhD Thesis, University of Bristol, 1996.
33. Raff MC. Social controls on cell survival and death: an extreme view. Nature. 1992;356:397–400.
34. Elder DJE, Hague A, Hicks DJ, Paraskeva C. Differential growth inhibition by the aspirin metabolite salicylate in human colorectal tumor cell lines: enhanced apoptosis in carcinoma and in vitro-transformed adenoma relative to adenoma cell lines. Cancer Res. 1996;56:2273–6.
35. Wang CY, Eshleman JR, Willson JKV, Markowitz S. Both transforming growth factor-β and substrate release are inducers of apoptosis in a human colon adenoma cell line. Cancer Res. 1995;55:5101–5.
36. Glick AB, Flanders KC, Danielpour D, Yuspa SH, Sporn MB. Retinoic acid induces transforming growth factor-β-2 in cultured keratinocytes and mouse epidermis. Cell Reg. 1989;1:87–97.
37. Schroy P, Rifkin J, Coffey RJ, Winawer S, Friedman E. Role of transforming growth factor β1 in induction of colon carcinoma differentiation by hexamethylene bisacetamide. Cancer Res. 1990;50:261–5.
38. Askew DS, Ashmun RA, Simmons BC, Cleveland JL. Constitutive c-*myc* expression in an IL-3-dependent myeloid cell line suppresses cell cycle arrest and accelerates apoptosis. Oncogene. 1991;6:1915–22.
39. Shi Y, Glynn JM, Guilbert LJ, Cotter TG, Bissonnette RP, Green DR. Role for c-*myc* in activation-induced apoptotic cell death in T cell hybridomas. Science. 1992;257:212–14.

40. Bracey TS, Miller JC, Preece A, Paraskeva C. γ-Radiation-induced apoptosis in human colorectal adenoma and carcinoma cell lines can occur in the absence of wild type p53. Oncogene. 1995;10:2391–6.
41. Oltvai ZN, Milliman CL, Korsmeyer SJ. Bcl-2 heterodimerizes in vivo with a conserved homolog, Bax, that accelerates programmed cell death. Cell. 1993;74:609–19.
42. Bronner MP, Culin C, Reed JC, Furth EE. The bcl-2 proto-oncogene and the gastrointestinal epithelial tumor progression model. Am J Pathol. 1995;146:20–6.
43. Sinicrope FA, Ruan SB, Cleary KR, Stephens LC, Lee JJ, Levin B. bcl-2 and p53 oncoprotein expression during colorectal tumorigenesis. Cancer Res. 1995;55:237–41.
44. Öfner D, Reihmann K, Maier H et al. Immunohistochemically detectable bcl-2 expression in colorectal carcinoma: correlation with tumour stage and patient survival. Br J Cancer. 1995;72:981–5.
45. Watson AJM, Merritt AJ, Jones LS et al. Evidence for reciprocity of bcl-2 and p53 expression in human colorectal adenomas and carcinomas. Br J Cancer. 1996;73:889–95.
46. Farrow SN, White JHM, Martinou I et al. Cloning of a bcl-2 homologue by interaction with adenovirus E1B 19K. Nature. 1995;374:731–3.
47. Chittenden T, Harrington EA, O'Connor R et al. Induction of apoptosis by the Bcl-2 homologue Bak. Nature. 1995;374:733–6.
48. Kiefer MC, Brauer MJ, Powers VC et al. Modulation of apoptosis by the widely distributed Bcl-2 homologue Bak. Nature. 1995;374:736–9.
49. Moss SF, Agarwal B, Arber N et al. Increased intestinal bak expression results in apoptosis. Biochem Biophys Res Commun. 1996;223:199–203.
50. Pezzella F, Tse AG, Cordell JL, Pulford KA, Gatter KC, Mason DY. Expression of the bcl-2 oncogene protein is not specific for the 14;18 chromosomal translocation. Am J Pathol. 1990;137:225–32.
51. Selvakumaran M, Lin HK, Miyashita T et al. Immediate early up-regulation of bax expression by p53 but not TGFβ1: a paradigm for distinct apoptotic pathways. Oncogene. 1994;9:1791–8.
52. Buset M, Winawer S, Friedmann E. Defining conditions to promote the attachment of adult human colonic epithelial cells. In Vitro. 1987;23:403–12.
53. Paraskeva C, Williams AC. The colon. In: Freshney RI, editor. Culture of epithelial cells. Chichester: John Wiley and Sons. 1992:81–105.
54. Paraskeva C, Buckle BG, Sheer D, Wigley CB. The isolation and characterization of colorectal epithelial cell lines at different stages in malignant transformation from familial polyposis coli patients. Int J Cancer. 1984;34:49–56.
55. Willson JKV, Bittner GN, Oberley TD, Meisner LF, Weese JL. Cell culture of human colon adenomas and carcinomas. Cancer Res. 1987;47:2704–13.
56. Whitehead RH, Vaneeden P, Lukeis RE. A cell line (LIM-2463) derived from a tubulovillous adenoma of the rectum. Int J Cancer. 1991;48:693–6.
57. Williams AC, Harper SJ, Paraskeva C. Neoplastic transformation of a human colonic epithelial cell line: in vitro evidence for the adenoma to carcinoma sequence. Cancer Res. 1990;50:4724–30.
58. Paraskeva C, Finerty S, Mountford RA, Powell SC. Specific cytogenetic abnormalities in two new human colorectal adenoma-derived epithelial cell lines. Cancer Res. 1989;49:1282–6.
59. Bates RC, Buret A, Van Helden DF, Horton MA, Burns GF. Apoptosis induced by inhibition of intercellular contact. J Cell Biol. 1994;125:403–15.
60. Hague A, Hicks DJ, Bracey TS, Paraskeva C. Cell-cell contact and specific cytokines inhibit apoptosis of colonic epithelial cells: growth factors protect against c-myc-independent apoptosis. Br J Cancer. 1997;75:960–8.
61. Williams CS, DuBois RN. Prostaglandin endoperoxide synthase: Why two isoforms? Am J Physiol. 1996;270:G393–400.
62. Tsujii M, DuBois RN. Alterations in cellular adhesion and apoptosis in epithelial cells over-expressing prostaglandin endoperoxide synthase 2. Cell. 1995;83:493–501.
63. Kargman SL, O'Neill GP, Vickers PJ, Evans JF, Mancini JA, Jothy S. Expression of prostaglandin G/H synthase-1 and -2 protein in human colon cancer. Cancer Res. 1995;55:2556–9.
64. Eberhart CE, Coffey RJ, Radhika A, Giardiello FM, Ferrenbach S, DuBois RN. Up-regulation of cyclooxygenase 2 gene expression in human colorectal adenomas and adenocarcinomas. Gastroenterology. 1995;107:1183–8.
65. Sano H, Kawahito Y, Wilder RL et al. Expression of cyclo-oxygenase -1 and -2 in human colorectal cancer. Cancer Res. 1995;55:3785–9.

66. Giardiello FM, Offerhaus GJA, Du Bois RN. The role of non-steroidal anti-inflammatory drugs in colorectal cancer prevention. Eur J Cancer. 1995;31A:1071–6.
67. Thun MJ. NSAID use and decreased risk of gastrointestinal cancers. Gastroenterol Clin N Am. 1996;25:333–48.
68. Giardiello FM. NSAID-induced polyp regression in familial adenomatous polyposis patients. Gastroenterol Clin N Am. 1996;25:349–61.
69. Koop E, Ghosh S. Inhibition of NFκB by sodium salicylate and aspirin. Science. 1994;265:956–9.
70. Hayllar J, Bjarnason I. NSAIDs, Cox-2 inhibitors, and the gut. Lancet. 1995;346:521–2.
71. Hanif R, Pittas A, Feng Y et al. Effects of non-steroidal anti-inflammatory drugs on proliferation and on induction of apoptosis in colon cancer cells by a prostaglandin-independent pathway. Biochem Pharmacol. 1996;52:237–45.
72. Masferrer JL, Isakson PC, Seibert K. Cyclooxygenase-2 inhibitors: A new class of anti-inflammatory agents that spare the gastrointestinal tract. Gastroenterol Clin N Am. 1996;25:363–72.
73. Piazza GA, Kulchak Rahm AL, Krutzsch M et al. Antineoplastic drugs sulindac sulfide and sulfone inhibit cell growth by inducing apoptosis. Cancer Res. 1995;55:3110–16.
74. Shiff SJ, Qiao L, Tsai L, Rigas B. Sulindac sulfide, an aspirin-like compound, inhibits proliferation, causes cell cycle quiescence, and induces apoptosis in HT-29 colon adenocarcinoma cells. J Clin Invest. 1995;96:491–503.
75. Pasricha PJ, Bedi A, O'Connor K et al. The effects of sulindac on colorectal proliferation and apoptosis in familial adenomatous polyposis. Gastroenterology. 1995;109:994–8.
76. Boolbol SK, Dannenberg AJ, Chadburn A et al. Cyclooxygenase-2 overexpression and tumor formation are blocked by sulindac in a murine model of familial adenomatous polyposis. Cancer Res. 1996;56:2556–60.
77. Kelloff GJ, Boone CW, Steele VE et al. Mechanistic considerations in chemopreventive drug development. J Cell Biochem. 1994;20(Suppl.)1–24.

25
A transgenic model for lactase down-regulation

J. T. TROELSEN, C. MITCHELMORE, N. SPODSBERG, A. MEHLUM, H. PRYDZ, O. NORÉN and H. SJÖSTRÖM

LACTASE-PHLORIZIN HYDROLASE

The total human LPH gene has been cloned and exon/intron organization determined[1]. The gene is about 55 kb and includes 17 exons ranging in size between 79 and 1551 bp. Southern blot analyses have revealed that only a single gene is present in humans[1], pigs[2] and rat[3]. In rabbits at least three different active genes exist[3]. The lactase gene has been localized to chromosome 2q21 in humans[4,5] and to chromosome 15q13 in pigs[2]. The localization to an autosomal chromosome also fits with the observation that adult-type hypolactasia is inherited in an autosomal recessive manner[6]. A 1 kb upstream fragment of the human gene was sequenced and was shown to contain two Alu sequences. A TATA-box is positioned 25 bp upstream of the transcription initiation site[1].

Computer analysis has identified several potential *cis* elements in the human LPH promoter: SP1 (−210), SRF (−250), AP-2 (−410), CTF/NF1 (−525), CREB (−635) and Oct1/Oct2 (−980)[1]. However, many of the elements are in the two Alu sequences of the human LPH promoter. As these Alu sequences are repetitive sequences specific for the human genome, the *cis* elements found within these regions are not likely to be transcriptionally important. No-one has yet demonstrated that any of the potential *cis* elements suggested by the computer search have a function in the transcriptional regulation of the human LPH gene.

The upstream LPH regions of the pig[7], rabbit[3] and rat[8,9] show a high degree of identity to the human promoter in the region close to the transcriptional initiation site (~150 bp), emphasizing the importance of this region. However, further upstream sequences show very little homology between the species.

LPH is expressed only in the enterocytes of the small intestine in adult mammals and it is regulated along the length of the small intestine, having the highest activities in the middle of the jejunum. In the proximal jejunum and distal ileum the LPH activity is low[10]. Along the crypt/villus axis the expression of LPH is initiated at the transition zone between the crypt and the villus. Two main phenotypes exist in the human population: lactase persistent and non-persistent (adult-type hypolactasia or lactose intolerant). Lactase-persistent individuals have high LPH expression throughout their lifetime, whereas the non-persistent individuals lose LPH activity in late childhood. The lack of LPH results in an inability to hydrolyse lactose and milk cannot be digested by those with the non-persistent phenotype[11]. Other mammals have a regulation of LPH that resembles the non-persistent phenotype in humans. Down-regulation of LPH is often referred to as the post-weaning decline of lactase.

TRANSGENIC MOUSE

In order to evaluate the importance of transcription in the regulation of LPH expression, a transgenic mouse line was established. The transgene contained 1 kb of pig LPH promoter in front of the rabbit β-globin gene as a reporter. Transgenic lines were generated by microinjection of oocytes and two mouse lines containing the transgenes were identified by Southern blot hybridization. One line contained a single transgene, while the other contained five copies positioned in a head to tail arrangement. However, Northern blot hybridization analysis revealed that only the transgenic mouse line with five copies of the transgene expressed the reporter gene. This mouse line was used for further studies[12].

Expression of the transgene was investigated in order to elucidate the importance of the 1 kb LPH promoter fragment in relation to post-weaning down-regulation, crypt/villus expression, longitudinal expression and enterocyte-specific expression of LPH. The level of transgene expression was measured by S1-nuclease protection assay using a ^{32}P-labelled 93-mer antisense β-globin oligonucleotide probe[13]. Using the S1-nuclease protection assay, only the correctly initiated reporter gene transcripts were measured, in contrast to many enzymatic reporter gene assays.

Transgenic mice 6–27 days of age were investigated for transgene expression. In this period the endogenous lactase expression is down-regulated in the mouse. The transgene mRNA declined in parallel with the LPH mRNA and lactase activity. This strongly emphasizes the importance of transcriptional regulation during the post-weaning decline. This result indicates that most (or all) of the regulatory sequences responsible for the lactase down-regulation in pigs are positioned in the 1 kb LPH promoter fragment, that the mouse expresses the transcription factors that are necessary for the down-regulation and that the mechanism behind the down-regulation is similar in pig and mouse.

The 1 kb LPH promoter region also controls the strict small intestinal expression of LPH. S1-nuclease protection assays of different tissues demonstrated that the transgene was expressed only in the small intestine. An in situ hybridization of the small intestine of an adult transgenic mouse using a digoxigenin-labelled anti-β-globin RNA probe revealed expression of the rabbit β-globin only in the enterocytes, with a maximum expression at the mid-villus. A weak labelling of β-globin mRNA in the crypt enterocytes was detected, whereas no LPH mRNA could be measured[14,15]. The longitudinal regulation of the transgene also resembles the expression of the endogenous LPH, except in the proximal jejunum where the expression of the transgene was high in contrast to the low level of endogenous LPH expression. The established transgene model for LPH regulation resembles the endogenous expression of LPH in aspects of post weaning down-regulation and small intestinal enterocyte-specific expression and longitudinal expression (except in the proximal jejunum).

CIS-ELEMENTS AND TRANSCRIPTION FACTORS INVOLVED IN LPH REGULATION

The transgenic mouse model has demonstrated that the 1 kb promoter region controls most facets of the LPH expression pattern. Thus, it is in this region we have to seek the mechanisms behind the transcriptional down-regulation of lactase. We have therefore started a functional characterization of the 1 kb LPH promoter region in order to find the *cis* elements and their corresponding transcription factors.

An initial deletion analysis of the 1 kb promoter in the lactase expressing cell line Caco-2[7] revealed two regions with transcriptional importance: a downstream region close to the transcriptional initiation site[7] and an upstream region located between − 143 and − 997. These two regions have now been studied in greater detail. The downstream region contains a typical TATA-box located 25 bp from the transcriptional initiation site. A region close to the TATA-box (− 40 to − 54) is protected in DNase I footprint experiments by a nuclear factor(s) from a small intestinal nuclear extract. No footprint was generated using a liver nuclear extract[7]. These results were confirmed by electrophoretic mobility shift assays (EMSAs). Thus, an intestinal specific nuclear factor binds to this *cis* element (named CE-LPH1a). Deletion of CE-LPH1a results in a 50% reduction of the transcriptional activity of the LPH promoter (Spodsberg et al., manuscript in preparation). In DNase I footprinting experiments using intestinal nuclear factors the protection of CE-LPH1a is bipartite[7]. A 2 bp mutation in the 5′ part of CE-LPH1a (named CEα-LPH1a) abolished protein binding in EMSA and the same mutation in the context of the 1 kb LPH promoter also caused a reduction of the transcriptional activity[32]. Supershift EMSAs demonstrated that the major CE-LPH1a binding protein in Caco-2 cells is Cdx-2, a homeodomain protein related to *caudal* from *Drosophila*. Cdx-2 is only expressed at detectable levels in the intestine. Co-transfection experiments with a Cdx-2 expression plasmid and wild-type or CE-LPH1a-mutated 1 kb LPH promoter/reporter constructs demonstrated that Cdx-2 activates transcription through the CEα-LPH1 site (Figure 1[32]). At least two other potential binding sites for Cdx-2 are located in the pig LPH promoter (CE-LPH1b and 1c; see Figure 1). We have also cloned another homeodomain protein HOXC11 from a differentiated Caco-2 cDNA library using a yeast genetic screening system (one hybrid system)[16]. HOXC11 binds to CEα-LPH1 with the same binding specificity as Cdx-2 (Mitchelmore et al., manuscript in preparation). However, future experiments have to be performed to examine whether HOXC11 activates LPH transcription.

Traber and co-workers identified a similar *cis* element (SIF1) in the promoter of the sucrase-isomaltase gene[17,18], to which Cdx-2 also binds. LPH and sucrase-isomaltase are regulated in the same way in many aspects, including small intestine/enterocyte-specific expression, initiation of transcription at the crypt/villus transition zone and longitudinal regulation. However, when LPH is down-regulated during weaning, sucrase-isomaltase is up-regulated. Detailed deletion analyses of the distal region (– 42 to – 997) of the pig LPH promoter have shown that this region contains *cis* elements that both activate and repress transcription (Spodsberg et al., manuscript in preparation). A region from – 894 to – 798 activates transcription. By supershift analysis it was shown that in this region two DNA elements (CE-LPH2a and CE-LPH2b) bind HNF1α or β. Furthermore a region at position – 85 to –73 in pig LPH promoter is a good HFN1 binding site (CE-LPH2c). HNF1 is a homeodomain transcription factor, which is expressed at high levels in liver, kidney and intestine[19]. Co-transfection experiments in HeLa and Caco-2 cells using the 1 kb LPH promoter region in front of a reporter gene (luciferase) and an HNF1α or β expression plasmid have shown that especially HNF1α is capable of activating the LPH promoter. HNF1 has also been shown to be involved in the expression of two other intestinal expressed genes: sucrase-isomaltase[20] and aminopeptidase[21,22]. When the region from – 894 to –798 is deleted the promoter activity is reduced to a low level. However, deleting a region from –299 to – 227 nearly restores the reporter gene transcription to the level of the 1 kb LPH promoter element. This indicates that a factor binds in this region and represses transcription. Analysis for potential *cis* elements in the region revealed that a perfect binding site for the FREAC factors is located at position – 278 to –264 (CE-LPH3). The FREAC factors are a family of fork head transcription factors showing homology to HNF3[23]. Recombinantly expressed FREAC 2 and 3 bind to CE-LPH3 in EMSAs and thus are potential factors repressing LPH transcription (Spodsberg et al., manuscript in preparation).

Our current view on how LPH transcription is regulated involves binding of four factors in the 1 kb region: Cdx-2 binds at CE-LPH1 (– 54 to – 46), HNF1 to CE-LPH2 (– 894 to – 881), FREAC (or related factors) to CE-LPH3 (– 275 to – 265) and an unknown factor in the region – 227 to – 142. The results of the promoter studies are summarized in Figure 1.

ADULT-TYPE HYPOLACTASIA

What is the implication of our results with the pig LPH promoter with respect to understanding the mechanism behind adult-type hypolactasia? We have demonstrated, using our transgenic mouse line, that the main mechanism behind the down-regulation of LPH is controlled by the 1 kb LPH promoter[12]. Our results have great relevance for the understanding of persistence/non-persistence, as the post-weaning decline of LPH is probably the event that leads to adult-type hypolactasia in humans. This is the normal situation for most humans in the world[24]. By resolving the mechanism behind the regulation of the pig LPH gene we describe a mechanism that is probably common for all mammals. This includes lactase non-persistent humans as in most cases of hypolactasia the low level of LPH is correlated to low LPH mRNA level[25–28], pointing to a transcriptional mechanism. However, examples of humans with low lactase activity and high mRNA level have been described[25,29]. As nobody has examined the lactase activities during childhood in these individuals, it is possible that they represent a phenotype that has a depressed lactase activity throughout their life. This could be caused by less severe mutations in an exon or altered processing of the LPH RNA or protein. Humans with high lactase activity throughout their life are a

Pig LPH promoter constructs

Results

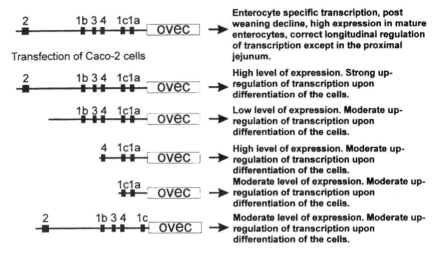

Transgenic mouse

Enterocyte specific transcription, post weaning decline, high expression in mature enterocytes, correct longitudinal regulation of transcription except in the proximal jejunum.

Transfection of Caco-2 cells

High level of expression. Strong up-regulation of transcription upon differentiation of the cells.

Low level of expression. Moderate up-regulation of transcription upon differentiation of the cells.

High level of expression. Moderate up-regulation of transcription upon differentiation of the cells.

Moderate level of expression. Moderate up-regulation of transcription upon differentiation of the cells.

Moderate level of expression. Moderate up-regulation of transcription upon differentiation of the cells.

Co- transfection of Caco-2 cells

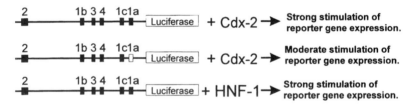

Strong stimulation of reporter gene expression.

Moderate stimulation of reporter gene expression.

Strong stimulation of reporter gene expression.

Figure 1 A summary of the results generated by the LPH promoter studies (Spodsberg et al., manuscript in preparation)[7,12,32]. The relative positions of the *cis* elements (filled squares) in the 1 kb LPH promoter region are shown. Our current opinion of candidate factors binding to the *cis* elements is: CE-LPH1a (1a) has been shown to bind Cdx-2 by supershift EMSAs. CE-LPH1b and c (1b and 1c) are sequences which are potential Cdx-2 binding sites. CE-LPH2 binds HNF-1. CE-LPH3 is a FREAC-binding site. We have no candidate for the factor binding to CE-LPH4. A mutation that abolishes Cdx-2 binding to CE-LPH1a is shown with an open square. The rabbit β-globin gene (OVEC) was used as reporter gene in the transgenic mouse line[7] and to generate stable Caco-2 cell lines[12]. The firefly luciferase gene was used as reporter in transient co-transfection experiments

minority among mammalians. The lactase-persistent phenotype probably arose late in evolution, as nobody drank animal milk before domestication around 4000 BC, but some human subpopulations have subsequently developed the ability to pro-duce lactase in adulthood. It has been estimated that if LPH-persistent individuals had 1% more children than lactose-intolerant individuals, then the present day differences in the distribution of the two phenotypes could develop in 400 generations (reviewed in Ref. 30). Our results imply that the change from a lactase non-persistence to a persistence phenotype probably comprises a mutation that destroys the normal transcriptional down-regulation of the LPH gene. The most likely explanation could be mutations either in some *cis* elements of the LPH promoter or changes in a transcription factor regulating LPH transcription. Nucleotide substitutions responsible for the lactase persistence/non-persistence polymorphism most likely are *cis* acting[31].

THE HUMAN LPH PROMOTER

Polymorphisms in the human LPH gene that correlate with low levels of lactase activity have been sought by other groups[1,25,28]. Four polymorphisms in the 1 kb upstream region of the human LPH gene have been described[1], but none correlates with low lactase activity[25]. However, the 1 kb region of the human promoter is not analogous to the 1 kb pig LPH promoter described here because of the two Alu sequences in the human LPH promoter. The CE-LPH2 element in the pig LPH promoter is not included in the 1 kb human LPH promoter sequence. In order to establish the human sequence of CE-LPH2 we have sequenced 600 bp further upstream (Spodsberg et al., manuscript in preparation). In this region the similarity between the human and pig sequence is low and no good conservation of CE-LPH2 can be found. However, two good HNF1 binding sites are present at position −1449 to −1421 in the human sequence, which might act like the CE-LPH2 site in the pig LPH promoter. Our future work will focus on the importance of the identified *cis* elements for the down-regulation of LPH transcription, focusing on the corresponding elements in the human LPH promoter and investigating whether sequence differences in the *cis* elements exist between persistent and non-persistent individuals.

Acknowledgements

We thank Anette Melchior Jensen and Annette Leerskov for the excellent technical assistance. This work was supported by grants from The Benzon Foundation, Denmark, The Danish Medical Research Council and The Danish Cancer Society. This project was part of a programme under The Biomembrane Research Center, Aarhus University.

References

1. Boll W, Wagner P, Mantei N. Structure of the chromosomal gene and cDNAs coding for lactase-phlorizin hydrolase in humans with adult-type hypolactasia or persistence of lactase. Am J Hum Genet. 1991;48:889–902.
2. Thomsen PD, Johansson M, Troelsen JT, Anderson L. The lactase phlorizin hydrolase (LCT) gene maps to pig chromosome 15q13. Anim Genet. 1995;26:49–52.
3. Villa M, Brunschwiler D, Gachter T, Boll W, Semenza G, Mantei N. Region-specific expression of multiple lactase-phlorizin hydrolase genes in intestine of rabbit. FEBS Lett. 1993;336:70–4.
4. Kruse TA, Bolund L, Grzeschik KH *et al*. The human lactase-phlorizin hydrolase gene is located on chromosome 2. FEBS Lett. 1988;240:123–6.

5. Harvey CB, Fox MF, Jeggo PA, Mantei N, Povey S, Swallow DM. Regional localization of the lactase-phlorizin hydrolase gene, LCT, to chromosome 2q21. Ann Hum Genet. 1993;57:179-85.
6. Sahi T, Isokoski M, Jussila J, Launiala K, Pyörälä K. Recessive inheritance of adult-type lactose malabsorption. Lancet. 1973;ii:823-8.
7. Troelsen JT, Olsen J, Norén O, Sjöström H. A novel intestinal trans-factor (NF-LPH1) interacts with the lactase-phlorizin hydrolase promoter and co-varies with the enzymatic activity. J Biol Chem. 1992;267:20407-11.
8. Boukamel R, Freund JN. The rat LPH gene 5' region: comparative structure with the human gene. DNA Sequence. 1992;3:119-21.
9. Verhave M, Krasinski SD, Maas SM et al. Further characterization of the 5'-flanking region of the rat lactase-phlorizin hydrolase gene. Biochem Biophys Res Commun. 1995;209:989-95.
10. Büller HA, Kothe MJC, Goldman DA et al. Coordinate expression of lactase-phlorizin hydrolase mRNA and enzyme levels in rat intestine during development. J Biol Chem. 1990;265:6978-83.
11. Auricchio S, Rubino A, Landolt M, Semenza G, Prader A. Isolated intestinal lactase deficiency in the adult. Lancet. 1963;ii:324-6.
12. Troelsen JT, Mehlum A, Olsen J et al. 1 kb of the lactase-phlorizin hydrolase promoter directs post-weaning decline and small intestinal-specific expression in transgenic mice. FEBS Lett. 1994; 342:291-6.
13. Westin G, Gester T, Møller MM, Schaffner G, Schaffner W. OVEC, a versatile system to study transcription in mammalian cells and cell-free extracts. Nucleic Acids Res. 1987;15:6787-98.
14. Maiuri L, Rossi M, Raia V et al. Mosaic regulation of lactase in human adult-type hypolactasia. Gastroenterology. 1994;107:54-60.
15. Rings EHHM, Büller HA, de Boer PA et al. Messenger RNA sorting in enterocytes. Co-localization with encoded proteins. FEBS Lett. 1992;300:183-7.
16. Wang MM, Reed RR. Molecular cloning of the olfactory neuronal transcription factor Olf-1 by genetic selection in yeast. Nature. 1993;364:121-6.
17. Wu GD, Wang W, Traber PG. Isolation and characterization of the human sucrase-isomaltase gene and demonstration of intestine-specific transcriptional elements. J Biol Chem. 1992;267:7863-70.
18. Traber PG, Wu GD, Wang W. Novel DNA-binding proteins regulate intestine-specific transcription of the sucrase-isomaltase gene. Mol Cell Biol. 1992;12:3614-27.
19. Xanthopoulus KG, Prezioso VR, Chen WS, Slakek FM, Cortese R, Darnell JE. The different tissue transcription patterns of genes for HNF-1, C/EBP, HNF-3 and HNF-4 protein factors that govern liver-specific transcription. Proc Natl Acad Sci USA. 1991;88:3807-11.
20. Wu GD, Chen L, Forslund K, Traber PG. Hepatocyte nuclear factor-1 alpha (HNF-1 alpha) and HNF-1 beta regulate transcription via two elements in an intestine-specific promoter. J Biol Chem. 1994;269:17080-5.
21. Olsen J, Laustsen L, Troelsen JT. HNF1α activates the aminopeptidase N promoter in intestinal (Caco-2) cells. FEBS Lett. 1994;342:325-8.
22. Olsen J, Laustsen L, Kärnström U, Sjöström H, Norén O. Tissue-specific interactions between nuclear proteins and the aminopeptidase N promoter. J Biol Chem. 1991;266:18089-96.
23. German MS, Wang J, Chadwick RB, Rutter WJ. Synergistic activation of the insulin gene by a LIM-homeo domain and a basic helix-loop-helix protein: building a functional insulin mini-enhancer complex. Genes Dev. 1992;6:2165-76.
24. Flatz G. The genetic polymorphism of intestinal lactase activity in adult humans. In: Scriver CR, Beaudet AL, Sly WS, Valle D, editors. The metabolic basis of inherited disease II. 6th edn. New York: McGraw-Hill, 1989:2999-3006.
25. Lloyd M, Mevissen G, Fischer M et al. Regulation of intestinal lactase in adult hypolactasia. J Clin Invest. 1992;89:524-9.
26. Escher JC, de Koning JD, van Engen CG et al. Molecular basis of lactase levels in adult humans. J Clin Invest. 1992;89:480-3.
27. Fajardo O, Naim HY, Lacey SW. The polymorphic expression of lactase in adults is regulated at the messenger RNA level. Gastroenterology. 1994;106:1233-41.
28. Harvey CB, Wang Y, Hughes LA et al. Studies on the expression of the intestinal lactase in different individuals. Gut. 1995;36:28-33.
29. Sebastio G, Villa M, Sartorio R et al. Control of lactase in human adult type hypolactasia and in weaning rabbits and rats. Am J Hum Genet. 189;45:489-97.
30. Simoons FJ. The geographic hypothesis and lactose malabsorption. A weighing of evidence. Am J Dig Dis. 1978;23:963-80.

31. Wang Y, Harvey CB, Pratt WS *et al.* The lactase persistence/non-persistence polymorphism is controlled by a *cis*-acting element. Hum Mol Genet. 1995;4:657–62.
32. Troelsen JT, Mitchelmore C, Spodsberg N, Jensen AM, Norén O, Sjöström H. Regulation of lactase phlorizin hydrolase gene expression by caudal-related homeodomain protein Cdx-2. Biochem J. 1997;322:833–8.

Index

Falk Symposium Series

43. Reutter W, Popper H, Arias IM, Heinrich PC, Keppler D, Landmann L, eds.: *Modulation of Liver Cell Expression*. Falk Symposium No. 43. 1987   ISBN: 0-85200-677-2*
44. Boyer JL, Bianchi L, eds.: *Liver Cirrhosis*. Falk Symposium No. 44. 1987
    ISBN: 0-85200-993-3*
45. Paumgartner G, Stiehl A, Gerok W, eds.: *Bile Acids and the Liver*. Falk Symposium No. 45. 1987   ISBN: 0-85200-675-6*
46. Goebell H, Peskar BM, Malchow H, eds.: *Inflammatory Bowel Diseases – Basic Research & Clinical Implications*. Falk Symposium No. 46. 1988   ISBN: 0-7462-0067-6*
47. Bianchi L, Holt P, James OFW, Butler RN, eds.: *Aging in Liver and Gastrointestinal Tract*. Falk Symposium No. 47. 1988   ISBN: 0-7462-0066-8*
48. Heilmann C, ed.: *Calcium-Dependent Processes in the Liver*. Falk Symposium No. 48. 1988   ISBN: 0-7462-0075-7*
50. Singer MV, Goebell H, eds.: *Nerves and the Gastrointestinal Tract*. Falk Symposium No. 50. 1989   ISBN: 0-7462-0114-1
51. Bannasch P, Keppler D, Weber G, eds.: *Liver Cell Carcinoma*. Falk Symposium No. 51. 1989   ISBN: 0-7462-0111-7
52. Paumgartner G, Stiehl A, Gerok W, eds.: *Trends in Bile Acid Research*. Falk Symposium No. 52. 1989   ISBN: 0-7462-0112-5
53. Paumgartner G, Stiehl A, Barbara L, Roda E, eds.: *Strategies for the Treatment of Hepatobiliary Diseases*. Falk Symposium No. 53. 1990   ISBN: 0-7923-8903-4
54. Bianchi L, Gerok W, Maier K-P, Deinhardt F, eds.: *Infectious Diseases of the Liver*. Falk Symposium No. 54. 1990   ISBN: 0-7923-8902-6
55. Falk Symposium No. 55 not published
55B. Hadziselimovic F, Herzog B, Bürgin-Wolff A, eds.: *Inflammatory Bowel Disease and Coeliac Disease in Children*. International Falk Symposium. 1990 ISBN 0-7462-0125-7
56. Williams CN, eds.: *Trends in Inflammatory Bowel Disease Therapy*. Falk Symposium No. 56. 1990   ISBN: 0-7923-8952-2
57. Bock KW, Gerok W, Matern S, Schmid R, eds.: *Hepatic Metabolism and Disposition of Endo- and Xenobiotics*. Falk Symposium No. 57. 1991   ISBN: 0-7923-8953-0
58. Paumgartner G, Stiehl A, Gerok W, eds.: *Bile Acids as Therapeutic Agents: From Basic Science to Clinical Practice*. Falk Symposium No. 58. 1991   ISBN: 0-7923-8954-9
59. Halter F, Garner A, Tytgat GNJ, eds.: *Mechanisms of Peptic Ulcer Healing*. Falk Symposium No. 59. 1991   ISBN: 0-7923-8955-7
60. Goebell H, Ewe K, Malchow H, Koelbel Ch, eds.: *Inflammatory Bowel Diseases – Progress in Basic Research and Clinical Implications*. Falk Symposium No. 60. 1991
    ISBN: 0-7923-8956-5
61. Falk Symposium No. 61 not published
62. Dowling RH, Folsch UR, Löser Ch, eds.: *Polyamines in the Gastrointestinal Tract*. Falk Symposium No. 62. 1992   ISBN: 0-7923-8976-X
63. Lentze MJ, Reichen J, eds.: *Paediatric Cholestasis: Novel Approaches to Treatment*. Falk Symposium No. 63. 1992   ISBN: 0-7923-8977-8
64. Demling L, Frühmorgen P, eds.: *Non-Neoplastic Diseases of the Anorectum*. Falk Symposium No. 64. 1992   ISBN: 0-7923-8979-4
64B. Gressner AM, Ramadori G, eds.: *Molecular and Cell Biology of Liver Fibrogenesis*. International Falk Symposium. 1992   ISBN: 0-7923-8980-8

*These titles were published under the MTP Press imprint.

Falk Symposium Series

65. Hadziselimovic F, Herzog B, eds.: *Inflammatory Bowel Diseases and Morbus Hirschprung.* Falk Symposium No. 65. 1992   ISBN: 0-7923-8995-6
66. Martin F, McLeod RS, Sutherland LR, Williams CN, eds.: *Trends in Inflammatory Bowel Disease Therapy.* Falk Symposium No. 66. 1993   ISBN: 0-7923-8827-5
67. Schölmerich J, Kruis W, Goebell H, Hohenberger W, Gross V, eds.: *Inflammatory Bowel Diseases – Pathophysiology as Basis of Treatment.* Falk Symposium No. 67. 1993   ISBN: 0-7923-8996-4
68. Paumgartner G, Stiehl A, Gerok W, eds.: *Bile Acids and The Hepatobiliary System: From Basic Science to Clinical Practice.* Falk Symposium No. 68. 1993   ISBN: 0-7923-8829-1
69. Schmid R, Bianchi L, Gerok W, Maier K-P, eds.: *Extrahepatic Manifestations in Liver Diseases.* Falk Symposium No. 69. 1993   ISBN: 0-7923-8821-6
70. Meyer zum Büschenfelde K-H, Hoofnagle J, Manns M, eds.: *Immunology and Liver.* Falk Symposium No. 70. 1993   ISBN: 0-7923-8830-5
71. Surrenti C, Casini A, Milani S, Pinzani M , eds.: *Fat-Storing Cells and Liver Fibrosis.* Falk Symposium No. 71. 1994   ISBN: 0-7923-8842-9
72. Rachmilewitz D, ed.: *Inflammatory Bowel Diseases – 1994.* Falk Symposium No. 72. 1994   ISBN: 0-7923-8845-3
73. Binder HJ, Cummings J, Soergel KH, eds.: *Short Chain Fatty Acids.* Falk Symposium No. 73. 1994   ISBN: 0-7923-8849-6
73B. Möllmann HW, May B, eds.: *Glucocorticoid Therapy in Chronic Inflammatory Bowel Disease: from basic principles to rational therapy.* International Falk Workshop. 1996   ISBN 0-7923-8708-2
74. Keppler D, Jungermann K, eds.: *Transport in the Liver.* Falk Symposium No. 74. 1994   ISBN: 0-7923-8858-5
74B. Stange EF, ed.: *Chronic Inflammatory Bowel Disease.* Falk Symposium. 1995   ISBN: 0-7923-8876-3
75. van Berge Henegouwen GP, van Hoek B, De Groote J, Matern S, Stockbrügger RW, eds.: *Cholestatic Liver Diseases: New Strategies for Prevention and Treatment of Hepatobiliary and Cholestatic Liver Diseases.* Falk Symposium 75. 1994.   ISBN: 0-7923-8867-4
76. Monteiro E, Tavarela Veloso F, eds.: *Inflammatory Bowel Diseases: New Insights into Mechanisms of Inflammation and Challenges in Diagnosis and Treatment.* Falk Symposium 76. 1995.   ISBN 0-7923-8884-4
77. Singer MV, Ziegler R, Rohr G, eds.: *Gastrointestinal Tract and Endocrine System.* Falk Symposium 77. 1995.   ISBN 0-7923-8877-1
78. Decker K, Gerok W, Andus T, Gross V, eds.: *Cytokines and the Liver.* Falk Symposium 78. 1995.   ISBN 0-7923-8878-X
79. Holstege A, Schölmerich J, Hahn EG, eds.: *Portal Hypertension.* Falk Symposium 79. 1995.   ISBN 0-7923-8879-8
80. Hofmann AF, Paumgartner G, Stiehl A, eds.: *Bile Acids in Gastroenterology: Basic and Clinical Aspects.* Falk Symposium 80. 1995   ISBN 0-7923-8880-1
81. Riecken EO, Stallmach A, Zeitz M, Heise W, eds.: *Malignancy and Chronic Inflammation in the Gastrointestinal Tract – New Concepts.* Falk Symposium 81. 1995   ISBN 0-7923-8889-5
82. Fleig WE, ed.: *Inflammatory Bowel Diseases: New Developments and Standards.* Falk Symposium 82. 1995   ISBN 0-7923-8890-6

Falk Symposium Series